CLINICAL BIOMECHANICS

CLINICAL BIOMECHANICS

ZEEVI DVIR, PhD, LLB

Department of Physical Therapy
Sackler Faculty of Medicine
Tel Aviv University
Ramat Aviv
Israel

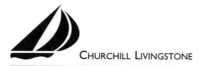

CHURCHILL LIVINGSTONE

A Harcourt Health Sciences Company
New York Edinburgh London Philadelphia

CHURCHILL LIVINGSTONE
A Harcourt Health Sciences Company

The Curtis Center
Independence Square West
Philadelphia, Pennsylvania 19106

Library of Congress Cataloging-in-Publication Data

Clinical biomechanics / [edited by] Zeevi Dvir.

p.   cm.

ISBN 0–443–07945–5

1. Orthopedics.   2. Human mechanics.   3. Musculoskeletal
   system—Mechanical properties.   I. Dvir, Zeevi.   [DNLM:
   1. Biomechanics.   WE 103 C6403 2000]

RD732. C575 2000   616.7—dc21

DNLM/DLC   99–37691

Acquisitions Editor: Andrew Allen
Manuscript Editor: Amy Norwitz
Production Manager: Natalie Ware
Illustration Specialist: Francis Moriarty

CLINICAL BIOMECHANICS   ISBN 0–443–07945–5

Printed in the United States of America.

Last digit is the print number: 9   8   7   6   5   4   3   2   1

In loving memory of my father.

CONTRIBUTORS

DAN L. BADER, PHD
Professor of Medical Engineering, Department of Engineering, Queen Mary and Westfield College, University of London, London, UK
Biomechanics of Soft Tissues

JOHN BEHIRI, PHD
Senior Lecturer, Department of Materials, Queen Mary and Westfield College, University of London, London, UK
Biomechanics of Bone

RICHARD W. BOHANNON, EDD, PT, NCS
Professor, Department of Physical Therapy, School of Allied Health, University of Connecticut, Storrs, Connecticut; Senior Scientist, Institute of Outcomes Research, Hartford Hospital, Hartford, Connecticut
Biomechanics of Neurologic Treatment

CARLIJN BOUTEN, PHD
University Lecturer, Department of Computational and Experimental Mechanics, Eindhoven University of Technology, Eindhoven, The Netherlands
Biomechanics of Soft Tissues

ELSIE CULHAM, PT, PHD
Associate Professor, School of Rehabilitation Therapy, Faculty of Health Science, Queen's University, Kingston, Ontario, Canada
Biomechanics of the Shoulder Complex

ZEEVI DVIR, PHD, LLB
Professor and Chairman, Department of Physical Therapy, Sackler Faculty of Medicine, Tel Aviv University, Ramat Aviv, Israel
Biomechanics of Muscle

JULIANNA GÁL, PHD
Senior Lecturer, School of Applied Sciences, University of Glamorgan, Pontypridd, Wales, UK
Biomechanics of Manual Therapy

WALTER HERZOG, PHD
Professor, Human Performance Laboratory, University of Calgary, Calgary, Alberta, Canada
Biomechanics of Manual Therapy

JUDITH LAPRADE, BSC(PT), MSC
Department of Anatomy and Cell Biology, Faculty of Health Science, Queen's University, Kingston, Ontario, Canada
Biomechanics of the Shoulder Complex

MICHAEL LEE, M BIOMED ENG
Lecturer, School of Exercise and Sport Science, and Department of Aeronautical Engineering, University of Sydney, Sydney, New South Wales, Australia
Biomechanics of Manual Therapy

STUART M. MCGILL, PHD
Professor of Spinal Biomechanics, Department of Kinesiology, Faculty of Applied Health Sciences, University of Waterloo, Waterloo, Ontario, Canada
Biomechanics of the Thoracolumbar Spine

JOSEPH MIZRAHI, DSC
Professor, Department of Biomedical Engineering, Julius Silver Institute of Biomedical Engineering Sciences, Technion–Israel Institute of Technology, Haifa, Israel
Biomechanics of Unperturbed Standing Balance

JOSEPH J. SARVER, BSME, MS BIOMED ENG
Teaching Assistant, School of Biomedical Engineering, Science and Health Systems, Drexel University, Philadelphia, Pennsylvania
Measurements in Biomechanics

RAMI SELIKTAR, PHD
Professor of Biomedical Engineering and Mechanical Engineering, Drexel University, Philadelphia, Pennsylvania
Measurements in Biomechanics

JOHN STALLARD, BTECH, CENG, FIMECH E, FIPEM

Technical Director, Orthotic Research and
 Locomotor Assessment Unit, Robert Jones &
 Agnes Hunt Hospital, Oswestry, Shropshire,
 UK

Lower Limb Orthotics

DEEPAK VASHISHTH, BE (HONS), MSME, PHD

Assistant Professor, Department of Biomedical
 Engineering, Rensselaer Polytechnic Institute,
 Troy, New York

Biomechanics of Bone

PREFACE

Back in 1975, as a first-year PhD student at the Bioengineering Unit, Strathclyde University in Glasgow, I was introduced to Biomechanics by one of the world leaders in this branch of science and engineering, Professor Robert M. Kenedi. It took "Bobby," as he was known in the professional and social circles, no less than five lecture sessions to encompass the vast domain of biomechanics. With the elegance of a great artist and the mastery of a distinguished conductor, he moved from components to systems, from tissue to organ and whole-body level, and from the most basic science concepts to the most applied. In so doing, he managed to instill in us the excitement as well as the humility with which one should view and approach this fascinating interdisciplinary subject. In years to come, we became very close, and in the course of many visits I paid to the Kenedis' home in beautiful Milngavie near Glasgow, his scientific curiosity, particularly with respect to several biomechanical aspects of the aging body, was as robust as ever. During my last meeting with him in February '98, I was so extremely pleased to learn that he would gladly write the preface to this book, but this plan was sadly frustrated by his untimely death a few months later. This book is a tribute to an absolutely outstanding teacher, scientist, and friend.

In formulating the guidelines to this book, I was advised that it should (1) be clinically oriented, particularly toward motor dysfunctions and rehabilitation; (2) aim at the postgraduate level; (3) serve more as a reference than as a textbook; and (4) be written by an international team of researchers who were involved with various aspects of musculoskeletal biomechanics. This joint authorship has inevitably led to a measure of heterogeneity, but I believe that it is a worthwhile price.

The opening chapter of the book introduces the reader to basic concepts and measurement methods; Chapters 2 through 4 relate to tissue biomechanics; Chapters 5 and 6 deal with two major joint-muscle systems, the spine and the shoulder; and Chapters 7 through 10 present the use of biomechanics in various clinical applications: treatment of patients with neurologic disorders, balance measurement and analysis, spinal manipulation, and orthotics. It was felt that these chapters presented an intellectual as well as practical challenge. On the other hand, it was decided not to include an independent chapter on gait analysis because this subject is well covered by other texts.

It is a great pleasure to offer my sincere appreciation and thank all contributors for a very fine piece of work. I am also indebted to Professor Otto Payton from the Medical College of Virginia, who paved the way for this book, as well as to the publishing team at WB Saunders for their persistent effort and kind help in bringing this project to a successful completion.

ZEEVI DVIR

NOTICE

Physical therapy is an ever-changing field. Standard safety precautions must be followed, but as new research and clinical experience broaden our knowledge, changes in treatment and drug therapy become necessary or appropriate. Readers are advised to check the product information currently provided by the manufacturer of each drug to be administered to verify the recommended dose, the method and duration of administration, and the contraindications. It is the responsibility of the treating physician, relying on experience and knowledge of the patient, to determine dosages and the best treatment for the patient. Neither the publisher nor the editor assumes any responsibility for any injury and/or damage to persons or property.

THE PUBLISHER

Contents

CHAPTER 1

MEASUREMENTS IN BIOMECHANICS

Rami Seliktar and Joseph J. Sarver

OVERVIEW

Measuring weight, length, speed, temperature, voltage, and other variables has become part of our modern lifestyle. We often question the *accuracy* of our measurement devices by asking such questions as, Is the $5 garden thermometer really showing the correct temperature? Isn't the bathroom scale reading a little high? Are we really going 65 miles per hour? Our doubts are perfectly legitimate because these devices are not *precision* instruments, and their readings involve a considerable margin of *error*. It is possible to increase the precision of the measuring instruments at some extra cost, but the measurement will never be absolute, and this is the first thing that we have to understand when we study the principles of measurement. Although it is important to perform a correct measurement, the price of greater accuracy may be high, whereas the benefit may be insignificant; therefore, the objective of the measurement should determine the desired margin of error. For example, for determining weather conditions, a thermometer that can read temperature with an accuracy of one thousandth of a degree Celsius is of no advantage to us over a thermometer that reads only up to one degree.

To this end, we need to have an appreciation of measurements and can begin by looking at our own sensory system and its measuring capabilities. The belief that "what you see is what the object actually is" is quite common and quite incorrect. People tend to believe that what they see, feel, or sense is absolute, that is, represents the actual size, shape, color, and weight of an object. Several aspects of measuring, however, affect how a person perceives a given object or a stimulus; this results in different perceptions among different people. For example, as the sun sets, the colors of objects appear to fade, until at some point they appear gray. Nothing physically changes in the object; rather, it is our perception that is *biased* by the lighting conditions at dusk. This example helps to clarify the measurement process, which typically involves at least two components, namely a sensor (transducer) and a conditioner. Our eyes (sensors or transducers) transform the light energy into neural signals, whereas our brain conditions these neural signals so that we perceive a color.

So far, we have used several terms, such as *accuracy, precision, error, bias,* and *sensor,* that have distinct definitions in the measurement jargon. Other terms commonly used to describe characteristics of measurement systems and measurands in general include *noise, sensitivity, discrimination, repeatability, reproducibility, hysteresis, resolution, linearity, drift, distortion, calibration, cross-talk, analog, discrete,* and *sampling.* At least some of these terms sound familiar because they are borrowed from expressions used daily. For example, the size of the setting sun appears larger than the midday sun, meaning there is obviously a perception (measurement) error. Lifting a heavy object biases our sense of force; consequently, a lighter object may feel much lighter. When we bake a cake, we weigh our ingredients to achieve good reproducibility. Formal definition of these terms is important because they describe the properties of the measuring system and the *measurands.*

A key to good measurement is understanding the process of measurement and the tools used to perform the measurement. More than anything else, however, it is important to know what to expect. Without this basic understanding, measurement errors may never be noticed and therefore may be assumed correct. For instance, most people can tell that if a speedometer in a car reads a speed of 250 miles per hour, it must have false calibration. Without prior information about the range of speeds to expect when driving a car, this measurement error would not have been noticed by the operator. On the other hand, if a person jumps from a chair and an acceleration gage shows that the acceleration of his head at landing is 50 m/s^2, few could tell whether that measurement is right or wrong.

The point of this chapter is to discuss the instrumentation commonly used when measuring biomechanical variables. Within this overview section, we provide a brief introduction to biomechanics and the variables of interest as well as a review of the different measurement terms mentioned earlier. A more detailed discussion of some biomechanical variables follows, and a more in-depth description of the instrumentation most commonly used to measure these variables is then presented, including a review of some clinical and research applications of such equipment.

WHAT IS BIOMECHANICS?

With the latest surge of interest in human motion and gait analysis, particularly on the part of nonengineering professionals, misconceptions about biomechanics have developed. For example, one can frequently find references to gait analysis as "biomechanics" in discussion forums as well as published works. Although gait analysis is a part of biomechanics, it is by no means representative of the spectrum of activities in biomechanics. A brief clarification of the definition, topics, and disciplines within biomechanics is therefore needed.

Because our existence and interaction with our environment is primarily mechanical, most of us develop an intuition with regard to "what happens if?" The following examples depict some aspects of the science of biomechanics:

- While swinging a tennis racquet, as in Figure 1–1, the tennis player's muscles need to exert *forces* that move his joints so that they reach the required *positions*.
- While swinging his racquet, synergistic muscles in the player's torso, shoulder, arm, and wrist act in concert to execute the motion, not only in terms of positioning but also in temporal precision and with the appropriate *velocity* and *acceleration* for impact with the ball (kinematics).
- Consequently, overexertion of the shoulder, arm, wrist, or lumbar spine can create excessive *stress* in the muscle, tendons, ligaments, joint cartilage, or even bone and can either cause acute failure or initiate a cumulative trauma disorder.

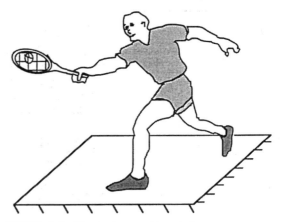

FIGURE 1–1   Tennis player striking a ball.

- If a ball hits the player's head, the impulse is transmitted through the skull to the brain, creating conditions that may result in brain injury. This may be caused by *shear* of the brain tissue, compression on the impact side, or cavitation on the opposite side. How do we determine what are the force and impulse thresholds that will cause injury?

Although there is no formal convention for classifying different biomechanical activities, the following broad categories encompass most of the research disciplines:

Mechanics of human performance, in which one of the objectives is to study the performance itself or, alternatively, to study the performance to determine the internal (musculoskeletal) forces

Mechanics of biologic tissues (including biofluid mechanics), in which the objective is to study the material behavior of the system's elements (e.g., bone, cartilage, tendons, body fluids).

BIOMECHANICAL VARIABLES OF INTEREST

The basic variables that need to be measured in any mechanical analysis and that therefore are of interest in a biomechanical analysis are *force, position* (and *displacement*), *mass,* and *time*. Other variables of interest, such as *moments, moments of inertia, velocity, acceleration,* and *stress,* can be derived from these basic variables. More compounded variables, such as work-energy, power, impulse, and internal muscle and joint forces, can subsequently be computed once these fundamental variables have been measured.

MEASUREMENT TERMS

As mentioned earlier, measurement is a process involving at least two components: a sensor/trans-

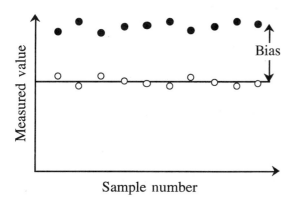

FIGURE 1–2 Depiction of accuracy and precision.

ducer and a conditioner. Either one of these components can be responsible for distortion of the measurement, which results in a production of errors.

An error, defined as the difference between the measured value and true value, can occur in either the sensor/transducer or the conditioner. The corresponding accuracy (A) of a measurement is defined by the ratio of the error to the true value, as follows:

$$A = 1 - \frac{(\text{Measured value} - \text{true value})}{\text{True value}}$$

Notice that both accuracy and error require knowledge of a measurand's true value. Unfortunately, it is impossible to know the true value of any given variable for several reasons, one of which is noise. Noise is defined as a random variation of a given value that is of no interest to the measurement itself. For example, when one is listening to music (i.e., sound at specific frequencies and amplitudes), a jackhammer being used outside would add noise, altering the perceived (measured) sound. Noise is unavoidable and is present in every measurement, making the true value of a given measurand intangible.

To minimize the effects of errors resulting from various sources such as noise, it is advisable to first calibrate the measuring instrumentation by performing repeated measurements of the variable while in a controlled system. Upon doing so, we encounter a distinction between accuracy and precision (repeatability).

In Figure 1–2, for example, we see 10 random measurements from instruments A and B (filled and hollow circles, respectively) of the same variable, whose true value is seen as a line. Clearly, both instruments have repeatable (reproducible) measurements and therefore have a low precision

error; however, instrument A is obviously less accurate than instrument B.

It is interesting to apply some basic principles of statistics and probability to the example in Figure 1–2 that can help us to understand the nature of measurements. If we were to compare the mean measurements from instruments A and B, we would see that indeed instrument A's mean measurement is significantly larger than that of B as well as the true value. The bias of instrument A could then be defined as the difference between its mean measurement and the true measurement. Furthermore, the *standard deviations* of either instrument give an indication of the precision error, that is, the larger the standard deviation, the larger the precision error. In fact, the equation that defines precision error is as follows:

$$\%E_R = \frac{2\sigma}{R} \times 100\%$$

where σ is the standard deviation and R is the range (maximum minus minimum) of the measuring device.

The sensitivity, defined as the ratio between the change in output (Y) for the given change in input (X), or $S = \Delta Y/\Delta X$ (the slope of the line in Fig. 1–3), can sometimes be too low or too high. A sensitivity that is too low results in minimal output for a significant change in input, whereas a sensitivity that is too high results in a large change in output for an insignificant change in input. Notice in Figure 1–3 that the data (hollow circles) follow a nearly straight line. In such a case, the instrument is said to have a relatively low linearity error, defined by the following equation:

$$\%(e_L)_{max} = \frac{(e_L)_{max}}{R} \times 100\%$$

where $(e_L)_{max}$ is the maximum expected error between the measurement and a linear approxima-

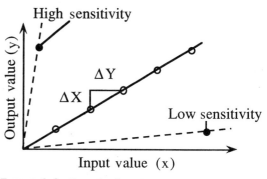

FIGURE 1–3 Example of sensitivity.

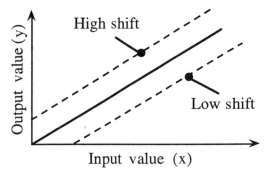

FIGURE 1–4 Example of drift.

tion of the measurement system's behavior (in Fig. 1–3 the difference between the circle values and the solid line approximation).

A particular error commonly encountered is drift. Drift, particularly zero drift, can occur to instrumentation for a variety of reasons, one of which is temperature. In the example shown in Figure 1–4, we see that a high shift results in zero output at nonzero input. Drift, then, is described by the shifting of the linear model of the measuring system. Other common errors, such as cross-talk, are discussed in a later section of this chapter.

Because a "true" measurement is realistically nonexistent, it is common practice to measure a given variable repeatedly in hope of reducing errors associated with either noise or the measuring device itself. The measurement (X) is then typically reported as a mean with a certain confidence interval, or $X = \mu \pm c$. A variable's confidence interval can be increased by increasing the number of measurements according to the central limit theorem. One way to increase the number of sam-

ples is to use multiple instruments to measure the same variable simultaneously. Some disadvantages to this method are the cost and the impracticality, given the nature of the measuring device. Another way to increase the number of samples is to measure the same variable repeatedly given approximately the same conditions. The problem with this method is that the variable being measured must be independent of time (unfortunately, most biomechanical variables are time dependent). Indeed, recording sample measurements from a nonstationary (i.e., time-dependent) system leads to another measurement issue, namely sampling frequency.

The *sampling frequency* (time between samples) one uses must be small enough so that no relevant portions of the signal are lost. The simplest way to understand this is to examine a nonstationary signal such as the one seen in Figure 1–5. This signal has only one frequency of 1 Hz. If we were to take sample measurements of this signal at the same frequency (square sample points), plot our measurements, and attempt to reconstruct our original signal (dashed line), we would obviously have an inaccurate reconstruction. If we sampled at twice the system's frequency (2 Hz), our reconstructed signal might be better than before, and at four times the system's frequency (4 Hz), our reconstructed signal is even better. According to the Nyquist theorem, the minimum frequency at which one can sample is at least two times the system's frequency. However, the Nyquist frequency is not always the best choice. For example, in Figure 1–5, if we began our sampling at t = 0.25 s instead of t = 0 s, the reconstructed signal would have been fairly inaccurate.

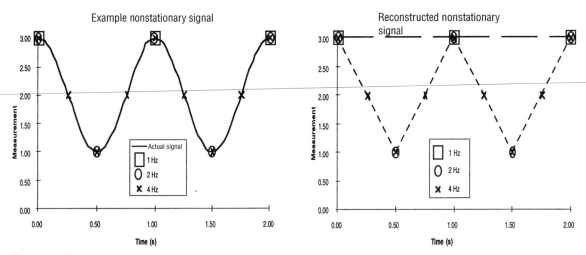

FIGURE 1–5 Example of a nonstationary signal and sampling frequencies.

In reality, a measured signal is unlikely to have only one frequency component, and therefore determining a system's frequency and the corresponding sampling frequency is not as simple as in the previous example. In fact, there is an entire science dedicated to measuring and analyzing non-stationary signals (digital signal processing), and although many of the details involved in signal processing, such as filtering or analog-to-digital conversion, are beyond the scope of this chapter, one concept useful to mention here is a signal's distribution.

A signal's, or in more general terms, a variable's distribution allows for determination of the minimum number of samples, or sampling frequency. Most commonly, variables are assigned a normal (gaussian) distribution, but this is not necessarily the case for all variables. Other common distributions are even (white), log-normal, Poisson, Weibull, and student-t. The student-t distribution is commonly used when dealing with relatively few samples (10 < number of samples < 50). Unfortunately, it is not always possible to know the distribution of a given variable; in such cases, nonparametric statistics can be used to estimate the number of samples needed.

The review of the measurement jargon presented here is simplified and is meant to provide a familiarity with the terminology, not a detailed description. For a more detailed description of measurements, the reader is urged to examine some of the measurement literature provided at the end of this chapter.

MECHANICS OVERVIEW

It is generally appropriate to assume that, in biomechanical analyses, we use mechanical tools and methods to model and analyze biologic systems. Our subsequent discussion, therefore, focuses on the mechanical modeling of the human body, its response to the application of forces, and its performance as an active force-generating system. A brief discussion of applicable mechanical variables and methods follows.

The first step in analyzing any mechanical system is to create a model that describes the physical system's behavior with a set of simplified elements. These elements can in turn be subjected to the corresponding laws of physics and formulated in a mathematical way to derive conclusions about the system's behavior.

In mechanical modeling, we describe physical objects that have specific geometries, masses, and material properties. The type of mechanical model we choose is primarily a function of the information we hope to extract from the physical system.

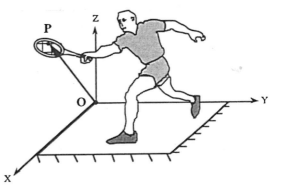

FIGURE 1–6   Position of the tennis ball (point P) relative to the origin point (point O) located in the floor.

If, for example, we are interested in the *ballistic motion* of an athlete performing a long jump, we can model the athlete's body as if the entire mass of the person were concentrated at a single point (the center of mass). Such a model is referred to as a *particle model,* in which all forces act at the center of mass and the motion trajectory is the motion of the center of mass. Determining the location of the center of mass of an athlete, however, is by no means simple because as the jumper changes his or her segmental orientation, the location of the athlete's center of mass also changes. Therefore, one cannot assume that the center of mass is fixed at the level of the navel, regardless of the configuration of the body segments.

A simpler example of a particle model is given in Figure 1–6, in which the tennis ball is approximated by a particle with its center of mass at point P. Although it might seem that modeling the ball as a particle is obviously appropriate, intrinsic to the particle model is the assumption that the orientation of the object being modeled is unimportant or unrelated to the objectives. In other words, the particle model does not account for rotational motion of the ball during its flight, which may prove very important when considering aerodynamic effects! To account for such rotations, it is necessary to model the object as a *body.*

In general, a body has a specific mass, geometry, and material properties. As is commonly the case when studying human performance, however, we often simplify our analysis by ignoring the compliance of the body and assume that it is *rigid.* Furthermore, it is possible to combine several rigid bodies into a multilink or segment model, such as the model of the tennis player's various body segments and racquet as depicted in Figure 1–7.

The implication of the rigid body assumption in the case of human performance analysis would be that the various body segments are assumed to

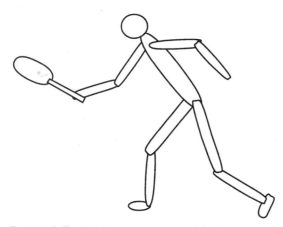

FIGURE 1–7   Multilink and segment model of tennis player.

maintain a constant shape and mass distribution throughout the task studied. However, our body segments change shape and mass distribution significantly as a result of muscle contraction and forces applied to the soft tissue. Even acceleration alone can cause substantial deformation to body parts and shift the positions of internal organs. The compromise involved in assuming rigidity of the body segments while dynamic performance is studied is relatively insignificant. On the other hand, if the objective were to study the compliance of the tissue, such as in the case of the stump–socket interface in limb prostheses or in the study of bed sores, no rigidity assumption would be legitimate. Instead, we would need to apply methods employed in analyzing mechanics of biologic tissues.

After formulating a satisfactory mechanical model, we can construct a *free body diagram* of our modeled system. Next, we can apply the condition of equilibrium, if the system is static, to determine unknown forces. For example, as a person stands (neglecting postural sway or adjustments), we can consider the person static. We can therefore apply the static equilibrium condition and determine such forces as the ground reaction force. If the system is dynamic, we formulate the dynamic equations of motion to analyze the interactive forces (kinetics), to determine the nature of motion, (kinematics), or both (dynamics). For example, knowing its mass, we can use the acceleration and velocity of the tennis ball to determine the force exerted by the racquet. With the multisegment model of the tennis player, on the other hand, knowing the ground reaction force, we can determine the moment exerted at the different anatomic joints.

In the subsequent section, we will discuss the variables of interest in a human performance analysis assuming either particles or rigid bodies. We then briefly present the variables representing the material behavior factors relevant to this text.

THE VARIABLES

CLASSIC MECHANICS VARIABLES

As an introduction to our discussion of biomechanical variables, we review the fundamentals of classic mechanics and its variables, including *mass, position, force,* and *time.* Most of us are familiar with the concepts of these variables; however, a more strict "mechanical" definition is needed before we can proceed. It is important to note at this point that units of measurement have to be specified when dealing with quantitative values of variables. The most common system of units in mechanics is the SI system, by which force is measured in Newtons (N), position in meters, mass in kilograms, and time in seconds.

Mass

An object has mass, which is defined as some impedance (resistance) to motion. For example, in Figure 1–8, the tennis ball has a mass and therefore resists any change to its motion, meaning that the player must exert a force to alter the motion of the ball. Mass is a *scalar quantity;* that is, it can be described by a single number. For example, we would say that the tennis ball has a mass of 0.1 kg. Mass can also be viewed as a material

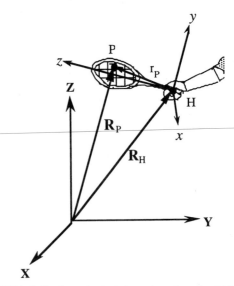

FIGURE 1–8   Example depicting orientation of a rigid body (tennis racquet).

property, which is usually measured indirectly through its weight. The weight of the mass, however, may change in accordance with the geographic position where the weighing takes place owing to changes in the gravitational field.

Position (and Its Time Derivatives)

The following section may sound complicated to readers who do not have the appropriate mathematical background. However, understanding the concept of describing position and viewing the same position from different frames of reference is extremely important when dealing with motion measurement and analysis and with musculoskeletal forces. A somewhat detailed discussion is therefore necessary, but this is in no way sufficient to provide the necessary skills to perform such analyses; our intention is merely to make the reader aware of some of the issues involved.

Position describes the location and orientation of an object relative to some reference frame. For example, in Figure 1–6, we describe the position of the ball (modeled as a *particle* with its center of mass at point P) relative to the reference frame located in the floor at point O. Notice that to describe the position of point P, we need to have an array of three measurements in the X, Y, and Z directions; position is a vector quantity, and by convention, we describe the position vector of a point (P) as $\vec{R}_p$. The dimensionality of the position variable, however, is dependent on the modeling tools used (particle versus rigid body).

The position of a particle is indeed a three-dimensional (X, Y, Z) quantity; however, when modeling the racquet as a rigid body, we need six dimensions (coordinates) to describe its position—three to describe the location of some reference point on the body and three to describe its orientation, such as seen in Figure 1–8. We may choose to use a set of coordinates describing the position of a point at the location of the palm of the hand ($\vec{R}_H$) (X, Y, Z) and a set of angles to describe the orientation of the racquet relative to the XYZ global coordinates. Such angles describe the orientation of the tennis racquet's (local) coordinate system (lowercase x, y, and z in Fig. 1–8) relative to the global coordinate system (X, Y, Z). Keep in mind that the local coordinate system is fixed to the racquet and is hence fully representative of the position of the racquet as a rigid body.

Coordinate systems of the kind discussed here are usually represented by a set of three orthogonal vectors whose dimensions are one unit (unit vectors). Considering that each unit vector representing the axes of the local coordinates x, y, and z can be specified by three angles with respect to

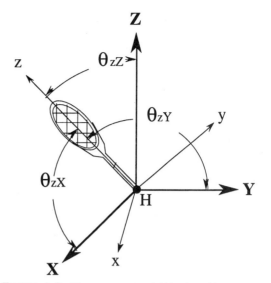

FIGURE 1–9   The racquet as a rigid body and its orientation defined relative to the global coordinates.

the three global coordinates (e.g., the racquet's z unit vector has three angles relative to the global [θzX, θzY, θzZ], as in Fig. 1–9), then it seems like *nine* values are needed to define an orientation of one coordinate system relative to another. These nine values, however, contain a substantial redundancy of information, and it can be shown that only three angles are necessary for such description. In other words, only three independent coordinates (*degrees of freedom*) are sufficient to define the orientation of a body (or for that matter, a coordinate system) in space.

In fact, these nine values (of which only three are independent) are used to define the 3 × 3 directional cosines (DC) matrix [C], which is used to describe mathematically the orientation of a rigid body (or local coordinate system) relative to a global coordinate system (see Fig. 1–9). Transforming from one coordinate system to another is accomplished by multiplying the position of a point by the DC matrix [C]. It is important to note, however, that such transformations can be performed between any two coordinate systems, regardless of whether one of the systems is fixed in space (global) or both coordinate systems are moving.

Typical to the subject of this discussion is, for example, the case of viewing a body with one camera and trying to determine how the body would appear to a second camera that is displaced and rotated relative to the first. This process of either description of an object relative to a coordinate system or transformation of position information from one frame of reference to another is

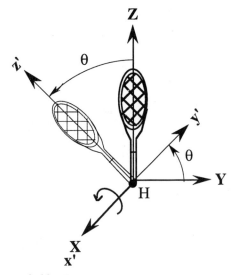

$$\vec{R}_P \begin{Bmatrix} R_{P_x} \\ R_{P_y} \\ R_{P_z} \end{Bmatrix}$$

We can calculate the position of the ball in terms of the tennis racquet's reference frame according to the following equation:

$$\vec{R}_{P(x,y,z)} = \begin{Bmatrix} R_{P_x} \\ R_{P_y} \\ R_{P_z} \end{Bmatrix} = [C]\vec{R}_{P(XYZ)}$$

$$= \begin{bmatrix} 1 & 0 & 0 \\ 0 & \cos\theta & \sin\theta \\ 0 & -\sin\theta & \cos\theta \end{bmatrix} \begin{Bmatrix} R_{P_x} \\ R_{P_y} \\ R_{P_z} \end{Bmatrix}$$

$$= \begin{bmatrix} R_{P_x} \\ R_{P_y}\cos\theta + R_{P_z}\sin\theta \\ -R_{P_y}\sin\theta + R_{P_z}\cos\theta \end{bmatrix}$$

This, however, is an extremely simple example in which the rotation occurred around only one axis; in general, rotations occur around all three axes, making the transformation matrix [C] much more complicated. Regardless of the complexity of the directional cosine [C], the method is the same as that described previously.

We have concluded, therefore, that it takes six coordinates to define the position of a rigid body in space: three regular cartesian coordinates to define translation and three angular coordinates to define orientation (rotation). Unfortunately, unlike cartesian position coordinates, *angular coordinates are not vectors.* Angular displacements do not obey the law of commutativity, nor can they be added or subtracted by using a parallelogram law. To state this severe restriction in a simpler language: we cannot sequentially add angular displacements that occur in a three-dimentional space to obtain a unique resulting orientation. Changing the sequential order changes the result obtained. Conversely, we cannot resolve angular motion into cartesian components as we do with linear position vectors. An exception to this rule is planar motion, in which case only one axis of rotation is possible, or an isolated motion around a single axis, such as the spinning motion of a propeller of a fan. When the angular displacements are very small, however, they do obey the commutativity law and can therefore be added as if they were vectors. The main relief resulting from this exception is that *angular velocities are vectors* because they are derived from infinitely small angular displacements.

To summarize, the position of an object can be treated as a three-dimensional or six-dimensional

bidirectional and is mathematically done by inversion of the DC matrix. The inversion of a matrix may be a somewhat tedious process, but in the case of the direction cosines, the matrix belongs to a class of orthonormal matrices in which the inverse equals the transpose: $[C]^{-1} = [C]^T$. What that means is that inversion of the matrix can be obtained by exchanging rows with columns.

For example, if we want to transform the position of the ball, whose motion is originally given in terms of the global coordinates (X, Y, Z), into the racquet's local coordinate system (x, y, z), we take the product of the position vector and the transformation matrix [C], as follows:

$$\vec{R}_{P(xyz)} = [C]\,\vec{R}_{P(XYZ)}$$

The advantage of such representation may be in viewing the approach of the ball from the perspective of the racquet. The matrix [C] contains the angles associated with the orientation of the racquet's local coordinate system relative to the global system. For the purpose of simplicity of illustration, let us assume that the racquet was rotated only around the X-axis by angle θ, as in Figure 1–10.

In this case, the matrix [C] would be calculated as follows:

$$[C] = \begin{bmatrix} 1 & 0 & 0 \\ 0 & \cos\theta & \sin\theta \\ 0 & -\sin\theta & \cos\theta \end{bmatrix}$$

The global position of the ball is calculated as follows:

variable, depending on the modeling tools selected. When using a particle model, in which an object is represented as a point-concentrated mass, such as the tennis ball, the orientation of the particle is meaningless and the location (X, Y, Z) of a single point on the body is sufficient to describe its position. Otherwise, if the rigid body model is used, then both the location (X, Y, Z) and orientation need to be specified, and hence six coordinates are necessary per rigid body (segment).

Displacement and Velocity

If we imagine that the tennis ball continues to travel after the player strikes it and we then track the motion of the ball, we will see a trajectory as in Figure 1–11, where the ball moves from point P to point A and finally to point B. The *displacement* vector that describes the motion from point P to point A is given by $\Delta \vec{r}_{A/P}$ and is equal to the difference between the position vectors at points A and P, or $\Delta \vec{r}_{A/P} = \vec{r}_A - \vec{r}_P$. Furthermore, a displacement serves to define *velocity*, which is the rate of change of the position vector:

$$\vec{V}_A = \frac{d\vec{r}}{dt} = \lim_{\Delta t \to 0} \left(\frac{\Delta \vec{r}_{A/P}}{\Delta t} \right)$$

The displacement and velocity vectors, therefore, lie in the same direction because, like mass, time is a scalar value and the direction of a vector that is divided by a scalar remains unchanged.

Considering the restrictions imposed on the angular coordinate as discussed earlier, one cannot simply differentiate angles to obtain angular velocity ($\vec{\omega}$) or, conversely, integrate angular velocity to obtain position. Such simple differentiation can be performed only if the angular position (orientation) is represented by a set of three independent angular coordinates, such as *Euler's angles*. For dynamic analysis purpose, however, we are often able to define the angular velocity

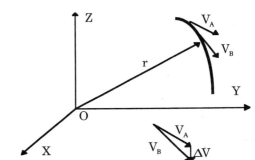

FIGURE 1–12   Change in velocity from A to B.

vector without the need to derive it from the orientation coordinates.

Acceleration

Finally, as the ball follows the trajectory seen in Figure 1–12, the velocity of the ball changes as it moves from point A to point B. Note that the velocity, being a vector, can change in magnitude as well as in orientation. The change in velocity from point A to point B is defined as the difference between the velocity vectors at points B and A, or $\Delta \vec{V}_{B/A} = \vec{V}_B - \vec{V}_A$, and can be seen in Figure 1–12. We refer to the change in velocity versus time as *acceleration*, which is defined as follows:

$$\vec{a}_B = \frac{d\vec{V}}{dt} = \lim_{\Delta t \to 0} \left(\frac{\Delta \vec{V}_{B/A}}{\Delta t} \right)$$

The acceleration of the tennis ball at point B ($\vec{a}_B$) will have the same direction as the change in velocity vector $\Delta \vec{V}_{B/A}$. Thus, position and its corresponding time derivatives (velocity and acceleration) are vector variables. Note, however, that unlike displacement and velocity, which are always in the direction of motion, acceleration is not! An object can move in a curved path at a constant speed (absolute value of the velocity), and yet its acceleration is not zero. This is because the change of direction of the velocity vector by itself, even without change of magnitude, constitutes a change in the velocity vector. In this example, if the speed does not change, the acceleration is perpendicular to the direction of motion.

In analogy to linear acceleration, *angular acceleration* is defined as the rate of change of the angular velocity vector:

$$\vec{\alpha} = \frac{d\vec{\omega}}{dt}$$

Force

Force is defined as the ability to accelerate a mass or according to Newton's second law: $\vec{F} =$

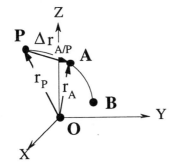

FIGURE 1–11   Displacement of the tennis ball.

$\vec{ma}$, where F is force, m is mass, and $\vec{a}$ is acceleration. More specifically, Newton's second law states that the sum of all forces ($\Sigma\vec{F}$) acting on a body of a given mass (m) equals the mass times acceleration (a) of that body, or $\Sigma\vec{F} = \vec{ma}$. Thus, the fact that the ball is accelerating as depicted in Figure 1–12 implies that all external forces acting on the ball sum to provide a vector in the same direction as the ball's acceleration ($\vec{a}_B$). For example, consider the forces exerted on the ball by the racquet ($\vec{F}_{raq}$) and by gravity ($\vec{W}_{ball}$) as depicted in Figure 1–13. The force vector resulting from summation of these two forces ($\Sigma\vec{F}_{ball}$) has the same direction as the acceleration of the ball.

In fact, the summation of forces seen in Figure 1–13 is an example of one of the most fundamental aspect of mechanical modeling, a *free body diagram* (FBD).

DERIVED VARIABLES

The basic mechanical variables described previously are used to develop further relations that lead to other variables of interest in a biomechanical analysis. The following discussion is concerned with the most commonly used (in biomechanics) class of derived variables.

Moment

Moment is the product of position and force. Because both force and position are vectors, we have to define the nature of the product, which in this case is a cross-product, yielding a vector, or $\vec{M} = \vec{r} \times \vec{F}$. It is important to note that $\vec{r}$ is a position vector originating at a reference point (O) and leads to any point on the line of action of the force $\vec{F}$ as depicted in Figure 1–14.

Consider, for example, the ground reaction

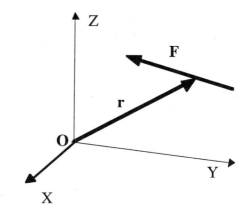

FIGURE 1–14   Depiction of moment.

force ($\vec{R}$) acting on the foot in Figure 1–15. If we want to calculate the moment of this force around the knee joint, we have to determine the $\vec{M} = \vec{r} \times \vec{F}$ product, which could be expressed as the following determinant:

$$\vec{M}_k = \vec{r} \times \vec{R} = \begin{vmatrix} \hat{i} & \hat{j} & \hat{k} \\ r_x & r_y & r_z \\ R_x & R_y & R_z \end{vmatrix}$$

where $\hat{i}$, $\hat{j}$, and $\hat{k}$ are the unit vectors of the coordinate system where $\vec{r}$ and $\vec{R}$ are described.

Momentum

Momentum is defined as the product of mass and velocity ($\vec{G} = m\vec{v}$) and is representative of the persistence (inertia) of the object in its motion.

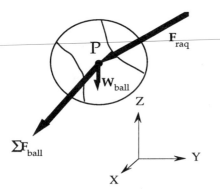

FIGURE 1–13   Sum of external forces acting on the tennis ball.

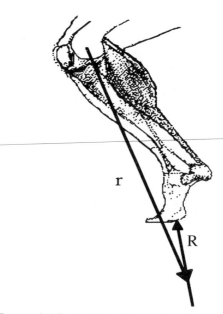

FIGURE 1–15   Depiction of ground reaction moment.

Impulse

Impulse is defined as the time integral of the force and equals the difference of momenta,

$$\vec{I} = \int \vec{F} dt = \Delta(m\vec{v})$$

Angular Momentum

Angular momentum is defined as $\vec{H} = \Sigma \vec{r} \times m\vec{v}$, where the summation sign Σ represents an overall contribution of all elements (particles) toward such momentum, $\vec{r}$ is a position vector of any such element of the system, and mv is the linear momentum of such element. An actual detailed discussion of the specific formulation of the angular momentum is beyond the scope of the present discussion but can be found in any advanced textbook of engineering dynamics.[1]

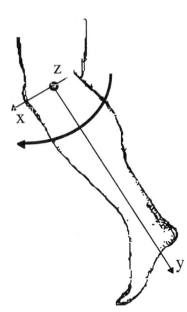

<u>FIGURE 1-16</u>   Demonstration of the leg inertia properties.

Moment and Product of Inertia

The *moment of inertia* is a rotational inertia property that is somewhat equivalent to mass in translational motion. Unlike mass, however, which is a scalar variable, the moment of inertia is a much more complex variable, called a *tensor,* which is made up of nine components. The inertia tensor is described by the following matrix:

$$[I] = \begin{bmatrix} I_{xx} & -I_{xy} & -I_{xz} \\ -I_{yx} & I_{yy} & -I_{yz} \\ -I_{zx} & -I_{zy} & I_{zz} \end{bmatrix}$$

The definition of the different terms of the matrix is mathematical and depends on the coordinate system selected. The terms designated by equal suffices are called moments of inertia, and the ones with the mixed suffices are called *products of inertia.*

Moments of inertia and products of inertia are defined mathematically as follows:

$$I_{xx} = \int (x^2 + y^2) dm$$

and

$$I_{xy} = \int xy dm$$

The products of inertia are more difficult to measure or assess and are often ignored in biomechan-

ical analyses, although not always with sufficient justification.

To illustrate the meaning of these inertial properties, let us consider the leg described in Figure 1–16. Without getting involved with the intricacies of the dynamic equations of motion, a moment exerted at the knee joint about the z axis causes the shank to swing forward. The greater the moment of inertia of the shank around the knee I_{zz}, the greater the moment required to accelerate the shank. Considering now the possible existence of products of inertia, such as I_{xz} or I_{yz}, such inertia components cause the shank to swing (rotate) around the x axis and the y axis, merely as a byproduct of its rotation around the z axis. Such a cross-effect is often referred to as *dynamic imbalance.*

The elimination of such cross-effects by eliminating the products of inertia is referred to as *diagonalizing* of the inertia matrix, so that it obtains the following form:

$$[I] = \begin{bmatrix} I_{xx} & 0 & 0 \\ 0 & I_{yy} & 0 \\ 0 & 0 & I_{zz} \end{bmatrix}$$

Work

Work is defined analytically as $W = \int \vec{F} \cdot \vec{dr}$, where W designates work, $\vec{F}$ is the force under consideration, and dr is the displacement that the force has undergone. Note that the force has to move to produce work. It is also important to understand that work is a scalar and therefore that there is no directionality attached to it.

Energy

Energy is a rather complicated variable, and only some basic features are discussed here. In mechanics, we distinguish between two types of energy: *kinetic energy* and *potential energy*. Both kinetic and potential energy are usually assessed on a differential basis, namely, the change in kinetic or potential energy is the actual variable being assessed and not the energy level as such.

Kinetic Energy. The kinetic energy is derived directly from the definition of work and the application of Newton's second law. The change in kinetic energy of a particle can be expressed in the following form:

$$W = \int \vec{F} \cdot \vec{dr} = \int_1^2 m\vec{a} \cdot \vec{dr} = \frac{m\vec{v}_2^2 - m\vec{v}_1^2}{2}$$

$$= \Delta\left(\frac{m\vec{v}^2}{2}\right) = \Delta(KE)$$

Kinetic energy of a rigid body is based on the same principle but constitutes a summation process over all the particles that make up the rigid body. This summation yields an expression of the form (note that for simplicity, only moments of inertia have been included; i.e., the inertia matrix is diagonalized):

$$\Delta(KE) = \Delta\left(\frac{m\vec{v}_G^2}{2}\right) + \Delta\left(\frac{I\vec{\omega}^2}{2}\right)$$

Potential Energy. Potential energy is the negative of the work done exclusively by "conservative" forces. The principle of *conservation* is again a complicated one, and the objective of this discussion is to prevent mistaken assumptions about conservation of energy. To minimize complication of the discussion, we use certain terms or definitions without getting too analytical.

A simple definition of the characteristics of a conservative force is that its work does not depend on the path, or *the work done by such force when performing a closed path equals zero*. Analytically, a conservative force is defined as one that can be derived as a *gradient* of a *potential* function (V):

$$\vec{F}_{consv} = -\frac{\delta V}{\delta x}\vec{i} - \frac{\delta V}{\delta y}\vec{j} - \frac{\delta V}{\delta z}\vec{k}$$

$$= F_x\vec{i} + F_y\vec{j} + F_z\vec{k}$$

hence:

$$W = \int \vec{F} \cdot \vec{dr} = -\Delta V$$

Since we have shown above that

$$W = \int \vec{F} \cdot \vec{dr} = -\Delta(KE)$$

and for a conservative force system that

$$W = \Delta V$$

we can write

$$W = \Delta(KE) = -\Delta V$$

or

$$\Delta(KE) + \Delta V = 0$$

which is the principle of conservation of mechanical energy.

To verify that a system is conservative and that the principle of conservation of energy can be used, one has to examine the force system and ensure that the *nonconservative forces are not doing work*. For example, applying force to stretch a spring stores potential energy in the spring. When the force is released, the work done to stretch the spring is recovered almost completely, through utilization of the stored energy, if the spring is elastic. On the other hand, when sliding a box on the ground against friction (a nonconservative force), the entire work is dissipated and cannot be recovered.

In a biomechanical context, consider a person jumping from some height and hitting the ground with taught gastrocnemius and quadriceps muscles. As the person approaches the ground, he or she loses potential energy of gravitation and acquires kinetic energy. When the person comes in contact with the ground, knees slightly flexed and ankle plantar-flexed, the muscles and connective tissues act as a combined spring and damper. The spring elements store some of the energy, but most of it is dissipated by the damping components, and therefore the jumper's rebound is minimal. If the muscles acted as fully conservative springs, the person would probably rebound to the same height that he or she jumped from. It is to our benefit, however, to dissipate such impact energy.

Power

Power is defined as the work done per unit of time. Power is also a scalar and is useful in assessing the instantaneous energy consumption during performance activities.

MECHANICS OF MATERIALS (STRESS AND STRAIN)

Overview

It is important to consider the mechanical behavior of materials when subjected to forces for the purpose of understanding both the behavior of biologic tissues and some operational principles of force-measuring instruments. Mechanics of materials can be studied on different levels, depending on the complexity of the material properties and the complexity of the loading conditions as well as on the geometry of the object under consideration. Our discussion focuses on the most simple relation between stresses acting on materials and the corresponding deformation that results from the application of such stresses.

Stress

Imagine the underside of the tennis player's right shoe as seen in Figure 1–17. The ground reaction force acting on the bottom of the shoe produces a *stress* on the surface area of the shoe in contact with the ground, labeled A_f. Stresses are forces applied on an area; therefore, unlike force, which is a vector, and time, which is a scalar, stress is specified through another quantity, called a *tensor.* Unlike scalars and vectors, tensors are represented by a combination of two vectors, and in the case of the stress tensor, one vector is the force and the other is normal to the area on which such force is acting.

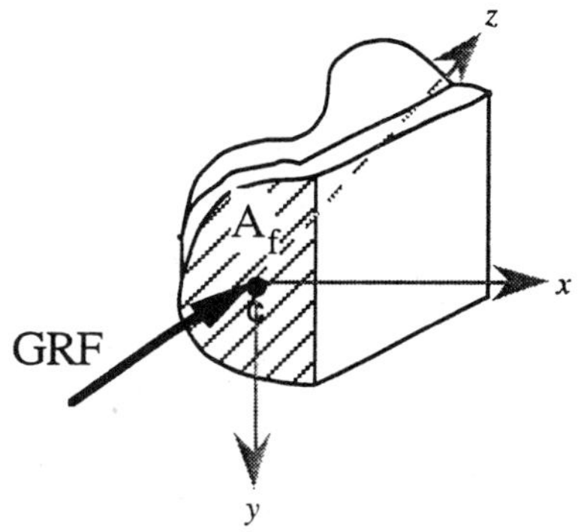

FIGURE 1–17 Depiction of the stresses acting on the tennis player's shoe.

In the example depicted in Figure 1–17, the ground reaction force (GRF) and the vector normal to the surface area A_f (in this case, a vector pointing in the negative z direction) combine to produce a stress tensor acting on the surface of the shoe:

$$(\tau_{ij}] = \begin{bmatrix} \sigma_{xx} & \tau_{xy} & \tau_{xz} \\ \tau_{xy} & \sigma_{yy} & \tau_{yz} \\ \tau_{xz} & \tau_{yz} & \sigma_{zz} \end{bmatrix}$$

Looking at this stress tensor, we see that it has nine components; however, owing to the direction of A_f and the symmetric nature of the stress tensor, only three are of interest: the axial stress (σ_{zz}) and two shearing stresses (τ_{zx} and τ_{zy}). The axial stress is given by the z component of the GRF according to the following equation:

$$\sigma_{zz} = \frac{GRFz}{A_f}$$

On the other hand, the shearing stresses (τ_{zx} and τ_{zy} are given by the x and y components of the GRF respectively, as follows:

$$\tau_{zx} = \frac{GRFx}{A_f} \text{ and } \tau_{zy} = \frac{GRFy}{A_f}$$

The situation described in Figure 1–17 is a simple case in which only one load was applied at the center of the surface area A_f. If, however, an object is subjected to bending in a typical three-point situation such as depicted in Figure 1–18, compressive (negative) stresses develop in the upper layers of the object shown, and tensile (positive) stresses develop in the bottom layers. As a result, we anticipate a deformation of the kind depicted on the right of the figure.

Strain

Because in real loading conditions the stresses vary throughout the material, deformations are considered on a local basis. Furthermore, deformations are usually expressed as nondimensional local changes in the size of small elements. Typically, if we mark a very short line on the surface of the material under consideration and subject the material to its loading, the line will change its dimensions. The relative deformation, namely *strain,* is defined as the ratio of the change in length and the original length:

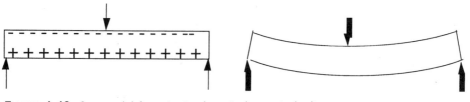

<u>FIGURE 1-18</u>   Stress and deformation in a beam in three-point loading.

$$\epsilon = \frac{\Delta l}{l}$$

Linear Elasticity

Often, material properties are expressed in terms of the relation between stress and strain. In solid materials such as metals, wood, and bone, one simple characterization of the material can be made by the stress–strain relation by assuming linear (elastic) behavior. Under such an assumption, we can refer to a material's modulus of elasticity (E), which is the ratio of stress to strain:

$$E = \frac{\sigma}{\epsilon}$$

This relation is the most simple manner in which mechanical behavior of materials can be represented. Otherwise, like stress, strain is also represented by a 3×3 tensor, and the general relation between stress and strain can be described by the relation between each component of the stress tensor and corresponding components of the strain tensor. Such relations, however, are beyond the scope of the present discussion. Because the objective of this chapter is to describe the application of mechanics in biomechanical measurements and not to teach applied mechanics, it is confined to simple examples.

MEASUREMENT INSTRUMENTATION

OVERVIEW

As concluded earlier, the basic variables of biomechanical measurement are position, mass, force, and time. Theoretically, once these basic variables have been defined or measured, we can proceed to derive other kinematic and dynamic variables, such as velocity, acceleration, jerk, moments, momentum, impulse, work, and energy. In practice, however, such derivation may not be simple; hence, the primary variables and measuring tools that we select depend on the designated use of the information. For example, the kinematics of the knee joint can be studied by using an optical motion-analysis system. However, if we were interested in only the flexion and extension of the knee, we might be better off using a goniometric linkage that directly measures the joint angle and its variation. On the other hand, to study the accelerations acting on a person riding an agricultural tractor, no motion-analysis system is sensitive enough to produce a differentiable motion data representing the higher frequencies of vibrations that may be particularly harmful to the spine. In such an event, the choice would clearly be to use accelerometers.

To study repetitive exposure to musculoskeletal stresses of a postal worker sorting mail and depositing it into boxes, clearly an optoelectronic motion system would be preferred. Supplemental force information can be acquired from GRF transducers, and effects of muscle fatigue can be detected by an appropriate electromyogram (EMG) system. Moreover, an EMG may be required to facilitate modeling of the musculoskeletal system by reducing the computational redundancy, namely identifying the active muscles.

Clearly, the measuring tools employed depend on the application, and there is definitely no duplication or redundancy in the existence of the different kinematic and dynamic measuring tools.

MEASURING FORCE

Force can be measured through the effects that it creates. According to Newton's law, force causes acceleration. If we know the mass of the object that is subjected to such force, and if we could measure the acceleration of the object, we could compute the force from the equation $\vec{F} = m\vec{a}$. Unfortunately, single forces seldom appear in isolation and therefore may not necessarily cause motion because other forces are concurrently opposing them. For example, an object resting on the ground is subjected to its own gravitational force (weight). At the same time, the ground applies a reactive force to the object (according to Newton's third law) that is equal in magnitude and opposite in direction, and the object remains in static equilibrium, as illustrated in Figure 1–19.

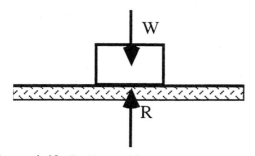

FIGURE 1-19   Equilibrium of forces.

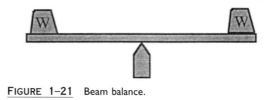

FIGURE 1-21   Beam balance.

example of such electronic force transducers that are commonly used is based on *strain gage* technology.

Strain Gages

The basic principles behind strain gage technology are discussed first, and the applications of strain gages in measuring force, acceleration, and other related variables are reviewed subsequently. A variety of sensors referred to as strain gages exist, and for simplicity, we discuss the most common type of resistance strain gage while keeping in mind that other types exist and use similar concepts of measurement.

The classic strain gage is an electrically conductive material that, when deformed, undergoes a change in its resistance that is directly proportional to the change in its length (strain). For example, pulling on either end of a wire causes a positive strain and increases the resistance of the wire. By passing an electrical current through the wire, the change in resistance can be measured as a change in voltage. Furthermore, by choosing appropriate materials, we can develop a linear relationship between the pulling force and the corresponding change in voltage.

Specific materials are chosen to serve as gages based on several material properties, one of which is the linearity between strain and resistance. In addition, the strain values that allow this linearity are typically rather small, meaning that the force (or other loading condition) that can be applied to such strain gages is also relatively small. As a result, strain gages are typically mounted to metal bases so that forces (or loading conditions), which are the magnitude of interest, can be evaluated. In such a system, the strain on the surface of the base is passed on to the gage, and the material of the base is chosen so as not to exceed strains outside the linear range of the gage under the expected loading conditions.

The resistor and semiconductor (or piezoresistive) strain gages are the most commonly used in biomechanical measurements. The resistor strain gage is more linear, is less sensitive to temperature changes, and can measure higher values of strain, but it is by far less sensitive than the semiconduc-

As a result, a more convenient effect that can be used is the deformation caused to the object by the force. For example, when we apply a force to a spring, the spring compresses, and the amount of its compression is measurable. Likewise, many solid engineering materials exhibit elastic properties similar to the spring. If the spring or the solid material has linear force displacement characteristics, its deflection is directly proportional to the force applied. Technically, the relative change in length is referred to as strain, and therefore many force transducers act as strain sensors.

The most common form of force measuring is weighing. Traditionally, weighing was performed by using some type of a spring mechanism (Fig. 1-20) or by comparing between the moments of the weights of masses by balancing a beam on a fulcrum, as illustrated in Figure 1-21. Although such force-measuring equipment has lasted through the centuries, the spring and beam balances have limitations when it comes to measuring dynamic forces. As a result, alternative technologies for measuring force have evolved and are based on force transducers that can be electronically monitored, thereby allowing the measured information to be stored and further processed. An

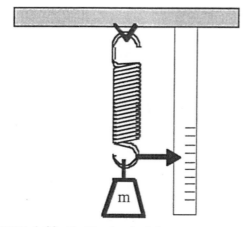

FIGURE 1-20   Traditional spring balance.

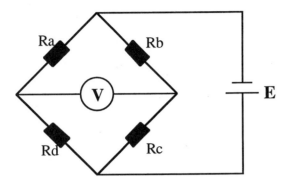

FIGURE 1-22 Schematic description of the wheatstone bridge.

$$V = E \frac{R_c R_a + R_c R_d - R_d R_b - R_c R_d}{(R_b + R_c)(R_a + R_d)} \qquad \text{Equation 1}$$

If all resistors were identical, V would be zero and the bridge would be said to be *balanced*. This, however, is unlikely to happen in practice because of small manufacturing differences in resistance and the high sensitivity of the bridge. A variable resistor is typically added in a calibration circuit to counteract such effects and facilitate balancing of the bridge. Of importance when measuring force, acceleration, or other variables while using strain gages is the linearity of both the gage and the material to which the gage is mounted. With appropriate materials, it is possible to develop a linear relation between the applied force, acceleration, and so forth and the change in resistance of the conductive strain gage and corresponding output voltage of the Wheatstone bridge. For example, the case presented in detail in the following subsection describes the use of strain gages attached to a base used to measure force, which is conventionally known as a *load cell*.

tor strain gage. Typically the *gage factor,* representing the relation between strain and change in resistance, is about 2 for a resistor gage and 125 for a semiconductor strain gage.

Strain is usually measured in nondimensional units of microstrain, which describes the relative change of dimensions in the underlying material (or strain gage). In most applications, the strain is kept well below the yield value of the metals serving as the structural component of the load cell. For example, mild steel begins to yield at about 1400 microstrains, whereas some other materials can obtain up to 40,000 microstrains. Therefore, the more common useful range of strain gages designed to be mounted on metal is within 10^{-5} to 10^{-2} of relative resistance change.

Because of this small change in relative resistance, strain gages are typically placed into an electrical circuit called a *Wheatstone bridge*. Strain gages are connected in either one or several of the positions described by the resistors Ra, Rb, Rc, and Rd in Figure 1–22. A bridge containing only two strain gages as active resistors is referred to as a *half-bridge* configuration, whereas a bridge containing four active resistors is referred to as a *full bridge*.

The Wheatstone Bridge Equations

Assuming that the bridge's input voltage E is constant, the output voltage V can be described as follows:

Showing the Relation Between Resistance and Force

The intent of the load cell depicted in Figure 1–23 is to measure the axial force P. Strain gages are mounted on the top and bottom surfaces of the metal base so as to increase sensitivity while reducing measurement errors, such as those resulting from temperature changes, as will be shown within the following analysis. Furthermore, these strain gages are placed into a Wheatstone bridge in the positions of resistors Ra and Rd. As described in the variables section of this chapter, the loading of the metal base, as seen in the figure, results in compressive stresses on the top and tensile stresses on the bottom surfaces, as follows:

$$\sigma_{top} = -\sigma_a - \sigma_b \qquad \text{Equation 2}$$

$$\sigma_{bot} = -\sigma_a + \sigma_b \qquad \text{Equation 3}$$

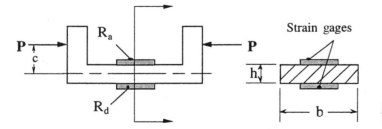

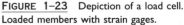

FIGURE 1-23 Depiction of a load cell. Loaded members with strain gages.

Thus, common to both strain gages is the compressive axial stress (σ_a), whereas the bending stresses (σ_b) have opposite signs. Furthermore, recall from our discussion of stress and strain that for a linearly elastic element such as the metal base in our example load cell, stress is linearly related to strain as follows:

$$\sigma = E \cdot \epsilon$$

Substituting this relation into equations 2 and 3, we have the relation between the strains on the top (Ra) and bottom (Rd) strain gages:

$$\epsilon_{top} = \frac{1}{E}(-\epsilon_a - \epsilon_b) \qquad \text{Equation 4}$$

$$\epsilon_{bot} = \frac{1}{E}(+\epsilon_a + \epsilon_b) \qquad \text{Equation 5}$$

Finally, we link our mechanical analysis with the Wheatstone bridge by chosing a linear gage that has the resistance-strain properties described as follows:

$$\frac{\delta R}{R} = G_f\epsilon \qquad \text{Equation 6}$$

where G_f is the manufacturer's gage factor, δR is the change in gage resistance associated with an applied strain, and R is the resistance of the gage with zero strain.

We now revisit the original bridge circuit equation with the basic assumption that before any strain is applied, the bridge is balanced, or Ra ≈ Rb ≈ Rc ≈ Rd = R (recall that Ra and Rd are the strain gages). We can then simplify as follows:

$$V = E \cdot \frac{\delta R_d - \delta R_a}{2(2R + \delta R_d + \delta R_a)} \qquad \text{Equation 7}$$

However, we know that the change in the gage's resistance associated with the applied strain (δR) will be much smaller than the original resistance in both Ra and Rd, or mathematically, δR_a, δR_d << R. We can therefore simplify equation 7 as follows:

$$V = \frac{E}{4} \cdot \frac{\delta R_d - \delta R_a}{R} \qquad \text{Equation 8}$$

Recalling that Ra was the strain gage on the top surface and Rd on the bottom, and combining equation 6 with equation 8, we have the following:

$$V = \frac{E}{4}G_f[(-\epsilon_a - \epsilon_b) - (-\epsilon_a + \epsilon_b)] \qquad \text{Equation 9}$$

In equation 9, we see that the axial strains (i.e., the common strains) cancel each other, while the bending strains sum together, such that we get the following:

$$V = -\frac{E}{2}G_f\epsilon_b \qquad \text{Equation 10}$$

Thus, any strain that is common to both surfaces, such as the axial stresses, or the effects of temperature are canceled with the Wheatstone bridge in this configuration. Finally, it can be shown that the bending strain (ϵ_b) is linearly dependent on the applied load P, as follows:

$$V = -E\frac{G_f}{2}\frac{6c}{bh^2}P \qquad \text{Equation 11}$$

where c, b, and h are constants associated with the load cell's geometry (see Fig. 1–23), G_f is a constant associated with the gage, and E is the constant input voltage to the Wheatstone bridge. Thus, the output voltage of the bridge, V, is linearly dependent on the applied force, P.

Measuring Force in General

The previous example of the load cell is only a generic description of such a device. Specific load cells are designed to measure forces in unidimensional, two-dimensional, and three-dimensional configurations, as discussed in the following section. Although most force transducers are made from either resistive strain gages or piezoelectric crystals, it is possible to use other elements, such as conductors or fiberoptics. Regardless of the nature of the transducer used within the load cell, one major problem is how to design the cell so that force measured in one direction is not affected by forces acting in other directions, a phenomenon referred to as *cross-talk*. To facilitate automation of the collection, processing, and storage of data, as well as to compensate for known transducer errors, it is customary to place the cell into a data acquisition system, as seen in the block diagram of Figure 1–24.

The Dynamic Forceplate

The *dynamic forceplate* is a force transducer designed to measure forces applied to the ground by an individual while walking or while performing other athletic, occupational, or leisurely activities. Traditionally, forceplates consist of a rectangular plate mounted on four pillar transducers, one at each corner of the plate. Each transducer measures

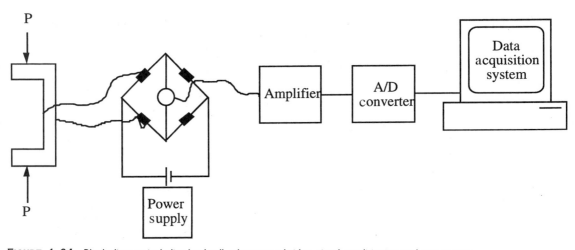

FIGURE 1–24 Block diagram including load cell, wheatstone bridge, signal conditioning, and appropriate data acquisition equipment.

three force components, one vertical and two shear, as depicted in Figure 1–25. For simplicity, only one such set of forces is illustrated.

A variety of forceplate models were built over the years using either strain gage or piezoelectric technology. Generally, the piezoelectric transducers were treated with skepticism because of the relatively poor response and stability at the low frequency range. However, good charge amplifiers can provide excellent stability and reliability of the signal and a very good response to low frequency signals up to a full directional cosine response (constant force). The major advantage of the piezoelectric forceplates is their high sensitivity and compact load cells, whereas their major drawback is the cost of the electronics.

Considering the forces measured by the four load cells, if all four vertical components are summed, the total vertical force is obtained: $F_{vertical} = \Sigma F_z = F_{z1} + F_{z2} + F_{z3} + F_{z4}$. The same summation procedure applies to F_y and F_x. Typically, the person walks in the y direction, and therefore F_y represents the anteroposterior ground force, and F_x represents the transverse or mediolateral force. These three components (F_x, F_y, and F_z) can be reassembled into a single vector, representing the total foot-to-ground force.

In addition to the force itself, the foot applies a moment around the z axis, which can be computed from the 12 force components described. The z moment, however, is also influenced by the eccentricity of the total ground force with respect to the center of the forceplate; therefore, the location of the insertion point of the resultant ground force must be identified. Once again, these x and y coordinates of the insertion point (or center of pressure) can be computed from the 12 measured force components. The actual formulas for the determination of the position coordinate and the z moment are not given here, but the general concept can be stated as follows: the forceplate measures a total of six components: three forces and three moments. The three force components are the actual forces exerted by the foot to the ground (or by the ground to the foot). The z moment (after processing) is an actual moment exerted by the foot on the ground; however, the moments around the x and y axes are not actual moments applied to the ground but rather are merely moments of the resultant force owing to its offset from the sensitive axes located (theoretically) at

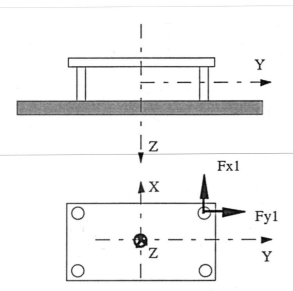

FIGURE 1–25 Schematic description of forceplate illustrating the sensitivity axes and the shear force components acting on one corner transducer.

the geometric center of the forceplate. These moments are therefore used to determine the coordinates of the center of pressure. In summary, each forceplate provides information on F_x, F_y, and F_z and on M_z, X, and Y of the center of pressure of the foot.

It is important to be aware of the following:

- When the objective is to study the dynamics of the human body, the forces to be considered are the GRFs, namely the forces exerted on the person and not those exerted by the person on the ground.
- For any computational purpose involving the ground forces, one should be aware of the location of the sensitive axes of the forceplate.
- Because the forceplate is a highly constrained transducer, there is a high probability for cross-talk. Usually, cross-talk values are provided by the manufacturers, but it is highly recommended to perform calibration tests.
- Cross-talk is particularly detrimental when accuracy of the position coordinates of the center of pressure is sought.
- At least two forceplates are needed to monitor the ground forces during gait. Measuring forces on one foot at a time is not a good practice because gait can be significantly biased owing to "aiming" and environmental disturbances; therefore, data gathered from different walk cycles may be inconsistent.
- The forceplates can be placed either one beside the other or one in front of the other with 50% overlap. We prefer the latter.
- For the forces to be measured, the walker needs to "hit" the forceplate. This is often found to be biasing and distorting to the gait patterns. The question of whether to mark the location of the forceplates and ask the walker to aim at them, or to completely conceal the forceplates, has been a controversial issue. Discussion of the advantages and limitation of the aiming approach can be found elsewhere.[2–4]

MEASURING POSITION

In biomechanics, we are concerned with several classes of position measurements:

1. Small displacements, such as those measured when subjecting a biologic tissue to stresses to study its mechanical properties. Such small displacement measurements are considered irrelevant to the present text and are not discussed here.
2. Relative movement between body segments, typically angular displacements.
3. General purpose motion documentation and

analysis, such as in human locomotion, athletics, and ergonomics.

In all of these classes, we are usually interested in more than just position measurements, and we often compute or measure velocities and accelerations. For example, we may want to study the behavior of a given biologic tissue, such as tendon, while it is subjected to different rates of stretching; the variation of angular velocity at a given joint; or the speed at which a tennis player swings his racquet. Moreover, derivation of the dynamic equations of motion require that we know the acceleration and velocities. Thus, the higher derivatives of the position variable are essential and can be calculated based on the recorded position measurements or can be measured independently.

When data processing, such as differentiation, integration, or transformation into frequency domain, is being considered, it is almost impractical to perform such operations manually. Particularly when considering measurement of fast movements such as those occurring in most human performance tasks, including normal locomotion, there is an obvious advantage to automating the collection and storage of position data. It is therefore desirable to convert position measurements into electric signals, which in turn can be recorded on a computer and made available for further processing.

The following section discusses the fundamental principles behind different position measuring systems as they apply to measuring the different classes of biomechanical position measurements.

Intersegmental Motion

Goniometers

A goniometer is a device that typically converts the angles between two rigid bodies connected by some joint into an electrical signal. The most common form of a goniometer is a rotary potentiometer (a variable resistor), which is attached to two arms (calipers). One arm is attached to its base and the other to its shaft. When the arms rotate one relative to the other, the potentiometer changes its resistance in a manner that is proportional to the angular displacement and in this way provides a measure of the angle between the calipers. In biomechanics, goniometers are placed over an anatomic joint (such as the knee), and the calipers are fastened to the adjacent body segments (e.g., the thigh and shank). A simple electric circuit can be wired to generate voltages proportional to the potentiometer's resistance, which is then calibrated to read the angle between these two segments. The output voltage can be readily recorded by a data acquisition system.

A variety of methods exist for the transduction of angular position into an electrical signal. Perhaps the most common in biomechanics is the potentiometer described previously. There are different types of potentiometers; the two most common are the wound wire and the conductive plastic. The wound wire type is a goniometer in which the conductive element is made of a thin long wire that is wound around a circular core and a slider that slides on the coil transversely and contacts the coils sequentially. The disadvantage of such a potentiometer is that its resolution is limited to the resistance of a single coil (there are jumps in readings between the coils). However, the precision and linearity of such measurement are much better than those of the conductive plastic. Conductive plastic, on the other hand, gives a smooth and continuous measurement (usually classified as *infinite resolution*), but its accuracy and linearity depend on the manufacturing process and hence its cost. Good-quality precision potentiometers can be very expensive.

Another popular transducer uses the Hall effect, whereby a magnet within the goniometer is oriented in such a way that as the joint moves, the magnet moves. Hall effect sensors within the goniometer produce a voltage directly proportional to the angle of the magnet; thus, a change in joint angle is seen as a change in voltage. In fact, Hall sensors have been developed that use the earth's magnetic field rather than a magnet within the goniometer. In such a system, the change in the orientation in the wires relative to the fixed magnetic field produces voltage signals that are readily recordable. Although such a system can be configured to detect angular displacements, it is beyond what is considered the traditional goniometer.

Goniometers are intended primarily to measure single joint motion and not to serve as a whole-body kinematic system. A major difficulty associated with the design and mounting of a goniometric system is in the fact that all skeletal joints are either multiaxial or polycentric. As a result, one needs to develop fairly complicated linkages that allow precise measurement of the desired motion while minimizing the constraining effects of the linkage. In other words, consider a knee joint and a pair of calipers mounted on top of it, so as to measure exclusive flexion and extension (see Fig. 1–26). If the center of articulation of the knee does not coincide with the hinge of the calipers, there will be resistance to the knee flexion, which will force the calipers to slide on the thigh and the shank. Moreover, the rotation of the anatomic

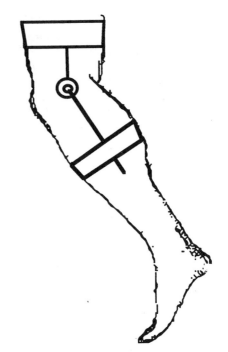

FIGURE 1–26   Schematic illustration of a knee goniometer.

knee joint around the other two axes causes further inconvenience and interference.

Goniometric linkages range in complexity from measuring one angular rotation to measuring all three angles. Multiaxial goniometric systems are mechanically complicated and are seldom used because of their high cost and inconvenience. At 3 degrees of freedom, linkage that fully separates the rotations and aligns itself with the anatomic axes is not only complicated but also cumbersome and interferes with the naturality of the human performance. Such complexity is detrimental to its viability as a clinical or even a research tool.

Although most applications of potentiometers are in measuring intersegmental motion, there are other forms of applications. In one such application, an open chain of links is formed from rods interconnected by multiaxial joints equipped with potentiometers. Knowing the relative positions of the links relative to each other can facilitate the determination of the position of the end point of the device. Such equipment is not suitable for monitoring free motion of a point in space but is useful for any quasistatic motion, or in particularly for describing trajectories and anatomic configurations. One typical application is to describe the curvature of a scholiotic spine.

General Purpose Motion Documentation

Optical Imaging Systems

Historically, the use of optical images to measure position and subsequently motion dates back to the mid 1880s and the work of Muybridge,[5] who captured a series of photographic images of humans performing various locomotive tasks. Although advances in both the film and digital imaging technologies have progressed rapidly in the past century, the basic traditional principles regarding machine and image calibration are still valid. To begin, the image capturing device, usually a camera, needs to be calibrated.

Camera Accuracy. Regardless of the image medium (film, video, or digital), several aspects of camera operation have an effect on the accuracy of any position measurements that might later be extracted from recorded images. For example, with some systems, the cameras first need to be focused on the subject being studied. Although this might seem trivial, consider capturing frontal plane images of a subject walking. It is necessary that the cameras stay focused on the subject as he or she walks away or toward the cameras. By decreasing the aperture of the camera, one can extend the camera's depth of field, thus allowing the subject to remain in focus for most of the recorded motion, at the cost of reducing the amount of light reaching the recording medium as well as measurement accuracy.

The time between recorded images and length of exposure (e.g., shutter speed, frames per second, sampling frequency) onto any of the media (film, video, or digital) must be appropriately adjusted so that no significant motion is lost between images. As discussed earlier, choosing the appropriate sampling frequency for a specific task depends on a detailed analysis of the frequency components of the given motion. For example, the frequency components of a hand tremor (8 to 12 Hz) are significantly different from those in a gait cycle, and therefore the sampling frequency (for tremor at least 24 Hz, but typically 50 Hz) depends on the recorded motion. Imperfections in the curvature of the lens lead to distortion of the image and must therefore be taken into account when extracting measurements. Careful examination of both the motion to be recorded and the proposed camera equipment is needed.

Recording Media. Intrinsic to the choice of a camera system is the image medium. Cinematographic medium has been used for many years, and cinematographic analysis has the advantage of high image resolution and shutter speed. However, extracting information from cine images is complicated and time-consuming, and the costs of developing and storing film can be high. High-quality video cassettes can also be used to record human motion, although with relatively poor image resolution and significantly lower shutter speeds. Again, extracting information from video tape is not a simple matter, but software that can perform such image processing is available (in some cases on the Internet). Finally, video and digital cameras that use a variety of optoelectronic principles can also be used to capture motion. Such cameras can produce either analog or digital output signals, which can be readily recorded by a computer.

A digital camera's resolution is described by several features, including the number of pixels that capture the light, the type of photoelectric equipment being used (e.g., charged couple device [CCD]), and the bit resolution of each pixel. For example, a common resolution is a 256×256 8-bit CCD camera, which is to say that there are 65526 CCD pixels, each with an 8-bit resolution.

The clearest advantage of digital cameras is the ease in image storage and processing. One disadvantage of the system is that most digital cameras require a separate computer for storing the images, although some cameras have been designed with small internal computers. Although relatively inexpensive digital cameras have a modest resolution (8-bit 256×256) and sampling rates as high as 500 frames per second, the rapid progress of computer technology is likely to improve, making the storage, resolution, and sampling rate deficiencies of current systems a thing of the past.

Image Calibration. One aspect of using images to measure position that is not likely to change in the near future is the need for image calibration. Several different techniques for calibrating images are available, but each method essentially establishes the distance between camera and subject. Without this calibration, the positions of the various body segments extracted from the image have no units and therefore cannot be compared with results of other studies, even those with the same camera system.

The most rudimentary form of calibration is to have the subject move in front of some background of known dimension. By combining the background's height, anthropometric measurements of the subject, and camera focal length, the images can be calibrated. More recently developed digital tracking systems are supplied with a calibration frame of known dimension. By placing the calibration frame in view of the camera, the system's software performs a self-calibration. When the distance between camera and subject has been determined, it is possible to extract features, such as the position of the knee throughout a gait cycle, from the recorded images. When analyzing human motion, the features being extracted are the positions of specific points on the various body segments.

Conversion From Two to Three Dimensions. Image media are currently limited to two dimensions; therefore, extracting the three-dimensional position of any given point on a body segment requires at least two cameras. Thus, when using multiple cameras, each camera, as well as the combination of all cameras, must be calibrated. This calibration is by no means simple and relies heavily on statistical averaging to estimate the three-dimensional position of any point. As a result, using more than two cameras has the benefit of reducing these estimation errors owing to the increased number of samples. Although it is true that "the more cameras, the more accurate," the decrease in error associated with the addition of another camera becomes less significant with each additional camera, making configurations with more than six cameras impractical. Furthermore, having multiple cameras allows for occlusion of a given marker from any one camera's point of view—meaning that throughout a recorded motion, at least two (typically more) cameras can view all body segments.

Reconstruction of the three-dimensional position of a point based on the combination of images from several cameras has several sources of errors that affect the accuracy of the position's measurement. For example, by increasing the volume of space from which we want to record a given motion, we significantly reduce the accuracy of the position calculation. The sources of these errors are far too numerous and complex to discuss here, but it is important to note that the larger the recording volume (i.e., depth of field), the greater the error. According to system specifications on certain equipment, it is possible to achieve accuracies to the nearest 0.5 mm for a 1.5-m cubic volume, or less than 0.05%! Such accuracy, however, is highly dependent on several site-specific issues, including the position of the various cameras, the lighting of the room, and objects in the field of view. Such issues have been investigated thoroughly by numerous investigators; however, there appears to be no decisive conclusion about which aspect of capturing human motion is more correct for every situation, and the photogrammetry literature should be reviewed before deciding what camera configuration is best for a particular task.

Feature Extraction. To be able to extract positions of body segments from images, one must be able to define a body segment by some features of an image. In the early cinematography work, feature extraction, or *digitizing*, was done by identifying bony landmarks on the body segments of interest from each exposure. The positions of these various bony landmarks, in combination with the calibration information, were used to extract the positions of the various body segments. This is a tedious and inaccurate means of measuring position. By adding markers on the bony landmarks, the accuracy of film digitizing is increased, but the feature extraction process is still time-consuming.

With the advent of computers and of video and digital cameras, image storage and manipulation (such as feature extraction) became readily available. Systems typically in use today have taken several different approaches to both feature extraction and storage. For example, some systems store all the digital images captured by each camera. Later, during analysis, the user places "virtual" markers on the various body segments and can then track the position of these markers (and therefore the body segments) through time. These systems have the advantage of not requiring any markers to be placed on a subject. Because the digital cameras typically capture light from the visible spectrum, they can be used in almost any environment. However, because these systems store entire images, the demands on computer memory for data storage are high, especially if one considers a multiple camera system with a high sampling rate. For example, if one were to record with a *single* 256 × 256 8-bit camera for 10 seconds at a sampling rate of 50 Hz, the entire recording session would produce more than 32 megabytes of data!

Other systems (known as tracking systems) rely on markers placed on the body at specific locations. The system then records (tracks) the positions of the markers through time. Typically, these systems use multiple cameras (four or five) to capture the same image simultaneously. Through some image processing done through either hardware or software in real time, it is possible to extract the three-dimensional coordinates of each marker. The information of interest is usually not the position of a particular point on a body segment, but rather the position and orientation of the entire segment (recall the discussion of the position variable). For this reason, when capturing the three-dimensional motion of body segments, it is necessary to place at least three markers on any given segment. Although many image-capturing systems designed for analyzing human motion have software packages that, when provided sufficient information, can calculate the orientation of body segments, it is beneficial to describe the

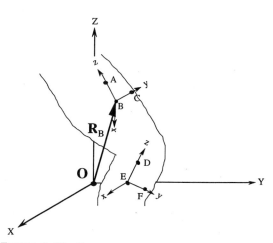

FIGURE 1–27 Determining the six-dimensional coordinates of a segment using kinematic data where A, B, and C are located on the thigh and D, E, and F are on the shank.

founding principles behind such analyses. Imagine the situation as depicted in Figure 1–27.

Example of Extracting the Six-Dimensional Position of Body Segments. The vector describing the position of C relative to B, that is $R_{C/B}$, describes the x direction of the thigh's local coordinate system and can be calculated using simple vector arithmetic:

$$\vec{R}_{C/B} = \vec{R}_C - \vec{R}_B = \begin{Bmatrix} (R_{Cx} - R_{Bx}) \\ (R_{Cy} - R_{By}) \\ (R_{Cz} - R_{Bz}) \end{Bmatrix}$$

In addition, the vector $\vec{R}_{C/B}$, which describes the z direction of the thigh's local coordinate system, can also be calculated. Finally the y direction of the thigh's coordinate system can be calculated by taking the cross-product of the z ($\vec{R}_{A/B}$) and x ($\vec{R}_{C/B}$) directions, or y direction = $\vec{R}_{A/B} \times \vec{R}_{C/B}$. With these three vectors, it is possible to determine the orientation of the thigh's local coordinate system relative to the global coordinates. This can be done by first remembering the discussion of multiaxis position from the variables section, where it was shown that it is possible to transform a vector in the global space into a vector in the local space using the matrix $[C_T]$.

The matrix $[C_T]$ contains the angles with which the local coordinate system has been rotated relative to the global coordinate system. Although several transformations are acceptable (e.g., Cardan-Euler or helical), the joint coordinate system is most readily understandable to the clinical audi-

ence in that the transformation results in angles like flexion and extension, varsus-valgus, and internal and external rotation of the shank. The matrix $[C_T]$ can be calculated using linear algebra if, for example, we use the position of point B relative to point A in both the global ($\vec{R}_{A/B}$) and local ($\vec{r}_{A/B}$) coordinates:

$$\vec{r}_{A/B} = [C_T] \cdot \vec{R}_{A/B} \Rightarrow \vec{r}_{A/B} \cdot \vec{R}_{A/B}^{-1} = [C_T]$$

The solution from $[C_T]$ will be the angles of rotation of the thigh relative to the global coordinate system; however, of more interest to us is the angular rotation of the shank relative to the thigh. We can determine this by first transforming the global positions of points D, E, and F into the thigh's coordinate system, or $\vec{r}_{D, E, F} = [C_T] \cdot \vec{R}_{D, E, F}$. Next, we determine the transformation matrix of the shank relative to the thigh, $[C_{S/T}]$, in the same way we calculated the thigh's transformation matrix. Within the matrix $[C_{S/T}]$ will be the flexion and extension, varus-valgus, and internal and external rotation angles of the shank relative to the thigh, which is typically how clinicians refer to joint rotations.

Markers. Several different techniques have been developed based solely on the type of markers used in any given tracking system. Reflective, or passive, markers are not likely to interfere with the motion being measured; however, because each marker is the same, it is not possible to distinguish between markers based solely on one image. Instead, image processing must track the position of the marker for identification purposes. Light-emitting, or active, markers, on the other hand, are labeled by a central module and can be readily identified by, for instance, sequencing their ignition. This sequencing or labeling control requires some form of wiring, which renders the method cumbersome, especially for use in monitoring athletic performance. Because tracking systems automatically determine the position of the markers, efforts have been made to minimize the error associated with extracting the three-dimensional coordinates of a marker's position. Some researchers have used the infrared light spectrum to detect markers, thereby reducing problems associated with reflections within the visible-light spectrum. Furthermore, software and hardware exist that use pattern recognition, whereby the pattern of interest is the image of a marker. The camera is then automatically adjusted so that only the marker's positions are recognized, significantly reducing the amount of information stored for each image.

Nonoptical Imaging Systems

Another way of measuring body motion from a global reference frame that uses magnetic fields has been developed. These systems use electrically conductive coil markers placed on the subject. The flux from the magnetic field (either generated or natural) induces a current in the marker's coils, which is proportional to the angle between each coil's sensitive axis and the magnetic flux lines. By placing three coils with sensitive axes in orthogonal directions within a given marker, it is possible for such systems to record the six-dimensional positions of various markers. These magnetic systems have the advantage that the human body is "invisible" to the detector, meaning that no marker occlusion occurs. Systems of this type have the problem that large ferrous objects in the room interfere with the detection of marker position as a result of the metal's interaction with the magnetic flux, and thus the operating environment is limited.

Marker Systems in General

In any of the marker-based motion-analysis systems, the placement of the markers is crucial to the accuracy of the measurements recorded. Most complete motion analysis systems provide detailed instructions for placing the markers on a subject. One particular problem with all such marker-based measurement systems is the fact that all positions being measured are truly positions on the skin, not necessarily of the bones underneath the skin. Particular applications that require a more precise measure of bone position might use x-ray or magnetic resonance imaging technology; however, as of yet these imaging systems are not designed for obtaining rapid motion images, and needless to say the costs of acquiring multiple images from these systems is prohibitively high.

Various Applications

As one can well imagine, the applications of the previously described measuring devices to the field of biomechanics in the evaluation of human performance are nearly endless. Various researchers have used systems to monitor athletic activities, examine workplace tasks, perform gait analyses, and evaluate pretreatment and posttreatment of various musculoskeletal conditions.

POSITION TIME DERIVATIVES

The kinematic variables of velocity, acceleration, and jerk (if needed) can be derived through differ-

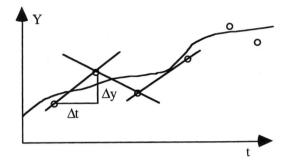

FIGURE 1–28   Differentiating the y-component dimension of a position vector.

entiation. Differentiation of experimental data, however, may be a "noisy" process and is not always as simple as it sounds; therefore, alternative methods that measure velocity and acceleration directly are sometimes considered. For example, in Figure 1–28, the derivative of y with respect to time is described as follows:

$$\frac{dy}{dt} = \lim_{\Delta t \to 0} \left(\frac{\Delta y}{\Delta t} \right)$$

If the curve in Figure 1–28 represents the best fit to the experimental data points (circles) and hence the actual process monitored, then obviously, as seen from the figure, the slope described by two adjacent points is in no way representative of the actual derivative of the curve at the same point. Moreover, if we take the second and third points and draw the connecting line to determine the slope (derivative), we can see that there is a substantial difference between the slopes of the two lines. A graph representing such derivatives based on computation of tangents of adjacent data points would therefore appear to be a very dispersed one. Hence, performing a second process of differentiation to estimate acceleration would yield results that are totally useless. A rather complicated smoothing process has to be applied to obtain a close determination of the actual derivatives of Y.

VELOCITY

Direct measurements of velocity have not been popular in biomechanics because velocity transducers are relatively complicated when multivariable human performance is being considered. Velocity can be measured directly by moving a permanent magnet in the vicinity of a fixed conductive coil. The motion of the flux lines of the permanent magnetic field through the coil generate electric current that can be measured. The voltage generated is proportional to the velocity, but to obtain meaningful readings, the geometry of the system has to be predetermined and the motion must be highly constrained.

Alternatively, with ultrasound, the Doppler effect can be used to measure velocity. The Doppler effect is based on the change of frequency of a beam generated by a stationary ultrasonic emitter and reflected from a moving object. Such measurements are therefore practical with respect to a translating object when only a single motion variable is being measured. Alternatively, when multidimensionality is required, emitters can be mounted on the moving object and can be picked up by stationary receivers. Here again, reconstruction of a three-dimensional motion data can be a complicated process.

Of course, both the electromagnetic and the ultrasonic Doppler concept can be adapted to measure multidimensional movement, but the cost can then become prohibitive, accuracy may be compromised, and the technical arrangement may become constraining to the moving object. Both methods have their advantages and disadvantages, but neither has been very popular in human motion analysis.

One rather crude but useful method of velocity measurement is based on conversion of linear motion into angular velocity. For example, a string wound on a spool when unwound will cause the spool to spin. The angular motion is easier to sense because it can be measured with an electromagnetic tachometer. Moreover, unlike linear motion, angular motion generates centripetal acceleration, which in turn can be sensed by a force transducer. A speed transducer of this kind had been in use at the gait laboratory of Moss Rehabilitation Hospital in Philadelphia and was used to document walking speed of test subjects. The string was tied to the waist of the subject and its other end was wrapped around a spring biased spool attached to the tachometer. Of course, such a system measures a scalar value velocity at the point of attachment of the string, and special attention should be paid to the concurrence between the direction of the string and the direction of the velocity.

ACCELERATION

The fact that acceleration is related to force through the second law of Newton is of major advantage to its measurement. Acceleration measurements are usually performed by measuring the strain that is exerted on a cantilever beam to

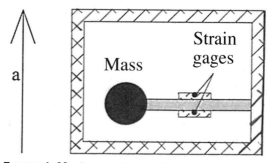

FIGURE 1–29 Example of an accelerometer.

accelerate a mass. Figure 1–29 depicts a typical configuration of an accelerometer.

The mass is mounted on a cantilever beam, and strain gages are mounted on both sides of the beam. As the accelerometer accelerates in the direction of the sensitive axis (indicated by the arrow), the mass lags behind owing to its inertia and causes the beam to bend. This bending causes strain in the cantilever beam, which is detected by the gages. This strain is related to the force exerted by the mass on the beam and is therefore proportional to the acceleration of the accelerometer.

As in many other types of dynamic equipment, such excitation of the beam causes it to oscillate around the nominal deflection caused by accelerating force, and to obtain a correct and stationary reading, these oscillations need to be damped. Efficient damping, under such conditions, may be achieved by filling the box with viscous fluid.

One feature of the accelerometer that is important to understand is the fact that its effective measurement is the force applied on the mass by the beam, and vice versa. As a result, when the accelerometer is placed in the gravitational field, the beam deflects, even if the box remains stationary owing to the weight of the mass, as seen in Figure 1–30.

The effect of gravity is an advantage as well as a disadvantage. The disadvantage is that the accelerometer will always sense a false acceleration value equal to 1 g, as illustrated in Figure 1–30. If the sensitive axis is aligned with the direction of gravity, then it will produce a signal equivalent to 1 g (about 9.81 m/s²). If the sensitive axis is rotated at an angle with respect to gravity line, then the accelerometer will read 1 g multiplied by the cosine of such an angle. If the sensitive axis is once again aligned with gravity but pointing in the opposite direction, then the accelerometer will read $(-)1$ g.

The advantage, however, is that this effect can be used for a relatively simple static calibration of the accelerometer by flipping it from positive to

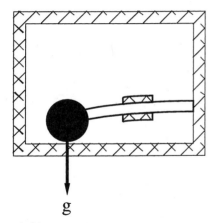

g

FIGURE 1–30 Effect of gravity.

negative around the horizontal axis. Doing so should produce a difference of 2 g provided that the sensitive axis is kept vertical.

Although accelerometers in general are highly accurate, placing an accelerometer on the skin to measure the acceleration of the bone can lead to rather large errors, depending on the motion. Imagine placing an accelerometer on the skin over the triceps and asking the subject to wave his or hand frantically. Obviously, the muscle and skin are compliant and move differently than the underlying bone, and therefore extracting the acceleration of the humerus is rather circumspect. In addition, because most accelerometers have cabled power supply and signal transmission, too many accelerometers on a subject can become cumbersome. Furthermore, although it is possible to integrate the acceleration signal to determine velocity and then position, this is rarely done because of the rather large errors resulting from the summation process of integration, which tends to accumulate errors resulting from drifts or constant offsets of the signal.

How Are Accelerometers Used to Monitor Biomechanical Phenomena?

Most of the applications of accelerometers in biomechanics are in the measurement of *impulsive* or *oscillatory* motion, in which either the axes of the body's fixed coordinates are easily identifiable or directionality is not of major importance. Often, accelerometers are used as expensive *event markers* to identify the onset of an event, such as heel-strike during locomotion.

Monitoring Human Motion With Accelerometers

The idea of using accelerometers for the measurement of human motion was inspired by the con-

cept of inertial navigation in air and space applications. However, inertial navigation equipment is by far less restricted than motion-analysis systems in terms of weight, volume, and cost. To define the motion of one segment of the human body in space, at least six uniaxial accelerometers need to be placed on the segment such that the accelerometers' sensitive axes are aligned with the segments' local coordinate system. The solution of the resulting six kinematic equations, to obtain the translation and orientation position variables, is complicated and computation intensive and is not presented here. In navigation systems, gyroscopes are often used to maintain constant attitude of the accelerometric platform (axes); thus, the integration of the accelerations remains uncoupled at all times. Inertial platforms of the kind used for navigation are extremely costly, heavy, and generally impractical for application to human motion. Moreover, one complete inertial set is needed per body segment, thus rendering this concept virtually useless for three-dimensional motion monitoring.

Oscillatory Motion (Vibrational Effects)

The purpose of measuring oscillatory motion of the human body is varied. In diagnostics, vibrational properties of bone have been studied for the purpose of monitoring the healing process of long bones and loosening of prosthetic implants. In pathogenesis, vibrations are believed to bear some responsibility for the development of degenerative changes in bone and cartilage (osteoarthritis). In any of the applications, the understanding of the oscillatory properties, that is, the natural frequency of the musculoskeletal elements and their transmissibility, were of primary concern.

Natural frequency is the frequency of oscillation of an object, such as in the case of a swing or a pendulum of a clock or the oscillation of a spring mass system, as shown in Figure 1–31.

The importance of knowing the natural frequency or of generally understanding the oscillatory behavior of a system is for the determination of the harm that can be sustained by the musculoskeletal system when subjected to such an environment. Mechanical systems have a tendency to resonate when subjected to vibrations whose frequency is close to their natural frequency. The mechanical energy that enters the system during such excitation gets trapped there, at least in part, and the disturbance to the mechanical equilibrium of the system continues to grow and may ultimately produce stresses that are damaging to its constituents.

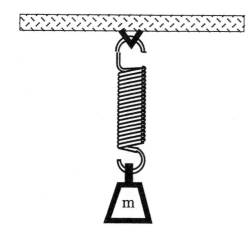

FIGURE 1-31 Illustration of an oscillatory system.

It has been determined with a reasonable degree of confidence that most humans can be adversely affected when chronically exposed to vibrations ranging from 0 to 16 Hz. Although the low frequency range, 0 to 1 Hz, primarily affects the vestibular organs (causing seasickness) without much known cumulative damage, portions of the human spine have a natural frequency that ranges between 4 and 16 Hz and can sustain permanent damage if subjected to vibrations on that level. The International Standardization Organization (ISO) has developed some guidelines with regard to such exposure. For example, a driver operating a truck is chronically exposed to vibrations generated by the machine (motor plus components). If the vibrations transmitted to the driver are within the frequency range of 4 to 16 Hz, cumulative trauma disorder to the spine may result. In this situation, the critical values pertaining to injury susceptibility are the frequency and amplitude of the accelerations. Although the frequency of oscillation of the environment can be obtained through either displacement or velocity measurement, the variable that most closely represents force is the acceleration.

Bone Fracture Healing

An accelerometer is mounted at one end of the bone, while the other end is subjected to a mechanical impulse such as by a hammer strike (Fig. 1–32). The impulse causes the bone to oscillate at its natural frequency, which is picked up by the accelerometer. As the union between the fractured bone pieces progresses, it is expected that a shift in both the natural frequency of the bone and the transmissibility of the oscillation through the bone will occur. Some problems associated with this method include the following:

- Because the method is noninvasive, both the excitation and the measurement of the acceleration are conveyed through soft tissue, which impedes and filters the signal.
- If the excitation is produced by a vibration generator, one has to watch carefully that the resonant frequencies of the generator are not perceived as those of the bone.
- Despite the natural appeal of the method, because of its noninvasiveness, it never reached a clinical level of applicability.

Vehicle Vibration

Vehicles are complex multibody dynamic systems whose different components are connected by constraining elements, such as bearings, springs, and shock absorbers. Because of this composition, the vehicle has a whole spectrum of natural frequencies that are excited either by the motor or by the humps of the terrain. From the biomechanical standpoint, of major importance are the vibrational components transmitted to the driver. One should keep in mind that vibrations can be filtered even if they are generated. One type of filter is the suspension of the vehicle. Another type of filtering that is more localized is the seat cushion or the seat suspension. To study the exposure of a vehicle operator to vibrations, accelerometers should be placed on the seat surface, and measurements

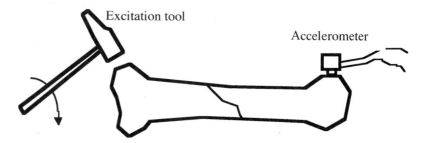

Excitation tool

Accelerometer

FIGURE 1-32 Schematic illustration of an accelerometer used to monitor healing.

should be performed while the operator sits in his or her normal position and posture.

Human Response to Vibrations

Various researchers attempted to study or simulate the response of the human system to vibrational excitation. In such an event, a seated or standing person is subjected to oscillations produced by a base on which he or she sits or stands. Accelerometers are mounted at different levels on the body, in the proximity of the spinal column. Ideally, one wants to determine what is the transmissibility at the different levels of the spine because the intervertebral disks are the most vulnerable elements. In vivo invasive measurements on humans, in which accelerometers are physically affixed to the bone, are prohibited, and thus the data must be obtained from gages mounted on the surface of the body. Such surface measurements are obviously influenced by soft tissue compliance and have to be treated with great caution.

On the other hand, to obtain information on transmissibility through the higher levels of the spinal column up to the head, one can mount an accelerometer to a "biting block" (Fig. 1–33). Such an attachment presents a reliable measurement of the vibrations reaching the head, and one can compare the ratio of the head acceleration amplitude with that of the excitation. This, however, does not solve the problem of studying the lumbar spine, which is most likely to sustain such injuries.

Impulsive Motion

One of the most common uses of accelerometers is in impulsive motion, often referred to as high acceleration environment. In the automotive industry, human surrogates (dummies) are used to assess the biomechanical consequences of collisions. The dummies are equipped with load cells and accelerometers that measure the force and acceleration patterns at different anatomic sites. Concurrently, studies are performed by research-

ers, on human cadavers, to relate as well as possible the measured accelerations and injury patterns. A vast amount of relevant literature can be found primarily in publications issued by the Society for Automotive Engineering (SAE).

Selection of Equipment

Because the accelerations differ substantially between the different body locations, one has to be careful with the choice of the mounting site and mounting method. For example, when the head impacts the windshield, accelerations at the front end of the skull reach hundreds of g's. Placement of an accelerometer at the rear or top of the cranium produces much lower acceleration values. Moreover, which portion of this acceleration is transmitted to the frontal lobes of the brain can only be estimated or measured indirectly using pressure transducers.

Acceleration values as high as 200 g are common in traumatic incidents, such as body impact against the vehicle interior during automobile accidents. The duration of such acceleration peaks is short, however, and is measured in milliseconds. If the peak value occurs for a very short period of time, it may have no injurious consequences. For example, in cases of head trauma, peak values of acceleration of 200 g extending over a period of 2 ms or less are often considered harmless.

Of course, for such measurements one needs to select the appropriate characteristics of the accelerometric equipment. The accelerometer must be capable of measuring values of the order of hundreds of g's and respond to frequencies of the order of 1000 Hz without much distortion. On the other hand, one should ensure that the natural frequency of the accelerometer remains outside the frequency range of the event being measured.

JERK

Jerk is the time derivative of acceleration or, alternatively, can be defined as the third time derivative of the position vector. Of course, the position vector can be differentiated any number of times, but such derivatives may totally lack physical significance. Jerk is a borderline variable in biomechanics and is seldom discussed. To try to visualize the physical meaning of jerk, one can imagine riding a vehicle that negotiates a turn and concurrently bounces from side to side (such as roller coaster). Although in a steady turn, the person senses a constant centripetal acceleration and therefore is made to lean away from the center of curvature. The added lateral bounces affect his or her acceleration (increasing and decreasing it) and in turn causes added discomfort. One way of de-

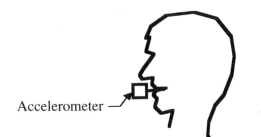

FIGURE 1–33 Measurement of vibration transmissibility by an accelerometer mounted on a biting block.

scribing such jerky motion is as the degree of the riding discomfort. Because jerk is not directly measurable, one has to measure acceleration and differentiate it.

Another example of the consideration of jerk in biomechanics is from the area of control of human motion. In the determination of the strategies employed by the human nervous system for the synthesis of motion trajectories, it has been hypothesized that one of the control objectives is to minimize jerk. This may sound like a somewhat far-reaching interpretation, but if we consider that jerk, or its absence, reflects a degree of smoothness of the path, it does make sense. Moreover, jerk is also representative of the derivative of the force characteristic; hence, such minimization of jerk is consistent with maintenance of an unperturbed muscle tone.

ANGULAR VELOCITY AND ANGULAR ACCELERATION MEASUREMENT

Unlike linear (translational) velocity and acceleration, angular velocity is not usually derived by differentiation of the position coordinates, owing to the restrictions imposed by the noncommutativity of the angular displacement coordinates. An exception to this concept is planar motion. The angular acceleration, however, can be derived by direct differentiation of the angular velocity vector. In general, dealing with angular motion in a three-dimensional space is a complicated subject that may require the use of representation of the vectors in terms of rotating coordinate systems. Such representation complicates the relevant differentiation criteria and is not discussed here. The basic concept of measuring angular velocity and angular acceleration is important, however, and is discussed in an implicit way.

As discussed earlier, six coordinates are needed to describe the state of a rigid body in space. The angular velocity and angular acceleration, therefore, require the identification of six such independent coordinates (degrees of freedom). The motion of three points on the rigid body have to be measured to facilitate determination of all the degrees of freedom. After such measurement has been performed, two equations describing the relative motion between the points are written and solved simultaneously to obtain a solution for the corresponding angular velocity coordinates. The form of these equations is as follows:

$$\vec{V}_B = \vec{V}_A + \vec{\omega} \times \vec{R}_{B/A}$$

$$\vec{V}_C = \vec{V}_A + \vec{\omega} \times \vec{R}_{C/A}$$

where $\vec{V}_B$ is the velocity of point B, $\vec{V}_A$ is the velocity of point A, $\vec{V}_C$ is the velocity of point C, $\vec{\omega}$ is the angular velocity vector of the rigid body, and $\vec{V}_{B/A}$ and $\vec{V}_{C/A}$ are the corresponding relative velocities between the points.

Resolution of these vector equations into scalar equations produces six such scalar equations, but because of redundancy, only three of the equations are independent, and their solutions renders three values for ω_x, ω_y, and ω_z.

After the angular velocity vector has been defined, the angular acceleration can be determined either in a similar procedure by relating linear accelerations of three points or by direct differentiation of the angular velocity.

MEASUREMENT OF MOMENTS AND PRODUCTS OF INERTIA

Moments and products of inertia can be computed, assessed, or measured. For geometrically defined shapes of rigid bodies, the integration as defined earlier can be performed. If the body has a complicated geometry, its volume can be divided into a finite number of geometric elements by forming a mesh, the simplest being a parallel piped, and then summing the contribution of these mass elements toward the total moment or product of inertia.

Actual measurement of the inertia matrix components can be performed by performing a dynamic test, such as mounting the rigid body on a pendulum and measuring the forces and moments generated by this motion with the aid of load cells. The measured forces and moments can then be substituted into the dynamic equations of motion, with the moments of inertia as the unknown variables. The solution of these equations will produce the inertia values. The actual equations are complicated and are not discussed here.

Because our primary interest is the biomechanical application of the moments of inertia and our limb segments are not detachable, the above method is hardly practical for in vivo testing. However, a number of cadaver tests have been performed for such definition of the inertia properties of the human body segments.

A compromised alternative to cadaver testing is the experimental swinging of a distal limb segment, such as the shank of the lower limb, and monitoring its motion. Substituting the kinematic variables into the corresponding dynamic equations of motion and solving these equations can produce some values for the moments of inertia. Unfortunately, this method can be applied only to distal segments.

PRESSURE MEASUREMENTS

Pressure is used extensively in engineering primarily to describe phenomena related to fluid (and gas) mechanics. It is a less popular term in solids, where our preference is to talk about stress rather than pressure. Biomechanical application of pressure sensors is primarily for the purpose of monitoring stresses applied on the interface of soft tissue. Because of its nature of describing force distribution over contact area, pressure is often used to describe the way the GRF is distributed throughout the contact area of the foot or the shoe. Qualitatively speaking, we can appreciate the amount of pressure we exert as we walk by examining the imprints left by our feet in the sand as we stroll along the beach. Clearly, the sand's displacement is proportional to the pressure applied by one's feet. Although the materials used in modern pressure transducers are somewhat more complicated, reliable, and expensive than sand, the basic concept of measuring the displacement of various points on a surface is still valid.

Industrial pressure transducers are typically load cells that use the strain gage or piezoelectric transduction technology, and the electrical output is used for direct monitoring or further processing and control. Such sensors, however, are seldom suitable to measure biomechanical pressure distribution. In biomechanics, usually an array of force transducers is arranged in a specific geometry to conform to the surface area on which pressure is to be measured. Conventional (strain gage or piezoelectric) pressure transducers are by far too bulky and complicated to form such arrays. Moreover, their power supply and signal conditioning systems use conducting cable connections, which renders such systems impractical. For example, using ordinary strain gage pressure transducers to measure pressure on the surface of the residual limb of an amputee while using a prosthesis can be done only at several sample locations rather than at the entire interface. Using more than 10 such points makes the system heavy and cumbersome as a result of cabling. Furthermore, the procedure is invasive, transducers have to be installed into the material, and the prosthesis can be used only experimentally.

More biomechanically suitable methods of measuring distributed force or pressure have been explored extensively with some degree of success. *Conductive polymers* constitute one group of materials studied in connection with such applications, but their suitability is still questionable. Several problems are associated with conductive polymers: usually only measurement that is relative to a calibrated value can be made, and the measurement has poor repeatability, considerable hysteresis, and drift of the signal; also, the polymers are sensitive to high temperatures.

Another concept has been explored that is based on optical monitoring of interference fringes created by *polarized light* reflection from an appropriate polymer due to impression of rigid cylinders. Although no cables are needed to acquire the data, quantification of this technique involves optical imaging and a considerable processing of the image information (per single frame), which renders it computation intensive and cost prohibitive in dynamic applications.

A method that gained considerable popularity is based on *capacitance sensing* technology. A conductive mesh is imprinted between layers of dielectric compressible polymer in such a way that the pattern of one conductor is perpendicular to the other. Basically, a matrix of rows and columns is created, forming $N \times M$ sensing points. The information is acquired by only $N + M$ wires, however, which is a substantial saving over $N \times M$, which would be necessary under ordinary wiring conditions. Some systems of this type have reached a full commercial application and are used primarily in foot pressure monitoring. Several problems associated with this technology are similar to those listed for conductive plastics. The considerable advantage of this technology is in the multiplexed nature of the output signals, which economizes considerably on the number of output channels. The materials are not sufficiently developed at this point to comply with complicated surfaces, such as the interior of a prosthesis or the shape of the body in contact with a seat. Foot pressure is measured adequately, however, provided that proper calibration is performed.

Another concept of pressure distribution measurement involves pressure sheets whereby *microcapsules of dye* enclosed between translucent sheets burst and form stain patterns corresponding to the pressure intensity. A similar method of staining loose microcapsules was popular in assessing excessive pressure on residual limb-socket interfaces. Of course, this method is quantitative and most likely highly nonlinear in the calibration of transparency versus pressure of the film.

A variety of other attempts to measure pressure have been made.[8]

The major deficiency of the methods of pressure distribution measurement described here is that they are genuine "bearing stress" measuring systems and do not provide information on shearing stresses at the interface. Such shearing stresses may be crucial to certain applications.

SUMMARY

This chapter has presented several concepts ranging in complexity from mass (a scalar measurement) to the six-dimensional position of a rigid body in space and finally to the stress tensor. Note, however, that the discussion in the variables section was not intended to provide absolute definitions. Rather, the point of this section was to illustrate to the reader that such variables are complex and require a detailed analysis. Several appropriate references can be found at the end of this chapter that will aid the reader in obtaining a more fundamental understanding of the biomechanical variables presented in this text.

We then examined some of the instrumentation used to measure variables of interest in many biomechanical analyses. Again, a detailed analysis into the acquisition and underlying theory of many of the presented transducers was beyond the scope of this text. Instead, we examined in detail some simplified examples of different instrumentation to illustrate the transduction nature of measurement systems.

Throughout this chapter, we have repeatedly seen that the choice of measuring equipment is primarily dependent on the type of biomechanical analysis of interest. Thus, as has been stated, determining the appropriate measuring equipment requires a detailed analysis of the variables of interest as well as an understanding of the measuring devices themselves. Although manufacturer and product analysis literature exists, when purchasing equipment for any biomechanical study, it is beneficial to contact informed authorities about the appropriateness of certain equipment in measuring specific tasks. With the advances of the Internet, worldwide web, and so forth, such resources are readily available to clinicians worldwide.

References

1. Greenwood DT: Principles of Dynamics, 2nd ed. Englewood, NJ, Prentice Hall, 1988, p 552.
2. Seliktar R, Mizrahi J, Vachranukunkeit T, et al: Human performance with prosthetic devices and surgically modified skeletal elements. Automedica 11:145, 1989.
3. Seliktar R, Susak Z, Najenson T, Solsi P: Dynamic features of standing and their correlation with neurological disorders. Scand J Rehabil Med 10:59, 1978.
4. Seliktar R: Integrated information approach to clinical analysis of gait. *In* Johnson CP (ed): Proceedings of the Third ASCE/Engineering Mechanical Division Speciality Conference, Austin, TX, 1979, p 586.
5. Muybridge E: The male and female figure in motion. Mineola, NY, Dover Publications Inc., 1984.
6. Backaitis SH (ed): Biomechanics of impact injury and injury tolerance of the head and neck complex. Warandale, PA, SAE Publications (SAE PT-43), 1993, p 1200.
7. Backaitis SH (ed): Biomechanics of impact injury and injury tolerance of the thorax-shoulder complex. Warandale, PA, SAE Publications (SAE PT-45), 1994, p 1306.
8. Doebelin EO: Measurement Systems, Applications and Design, 4th ed. New York, McGraw-Hill Inc., 1990.

Suggested Reading

Allard P, Stokes IAF, Blanchi JP: Three-Dimensional Analysis of Human Movement. Champaign, IL, Human Kinetics, 1995.

Amirouche FML: Modeling of human reactions to whole-body vibration. Trans AMSE 109:210, 1987.

Andriacchi TP, Ogle JA, Glanate JO: Walking speed as a basis for normal and abnormal gait measurements. J Biomechanics 10:261, 1977.

Asada H, Slotine J-JE: Robot Analysis and Control. New York, John Wiley Interscience, 1985, p 266.

Brash JI, Skorecki J: Determination of the modulus of elasticity of bone by a vibration method. Med Biol Engineering 8:389, 1970.

Braune CW, Fisher O: Der gang des menschen. i teil versuche unbelasten und belasten menschen. Abhandl J Math-Phys Cldk Sachs Gesellsch 21:153, 1985.

Bur AJ: Measurements of the dynamic piezoelectric properties of bone as a function of temperature and humidity. J Biomech 9:495, 1976.

Butler DL, Stouffer DC: Tension-torque characteristics of the canine anterior cruciate ligament. II. Experimental observations. Trans ASME 105:160, 1983.

Campbell JN, Jurist JM: Mechanical impedance of the femur: A preliminary report. J Biomechanics 4:319, 1971.

Chesnin KJ, Besser MP, Selby-Silverstein L, et al: A fourteen segment geometric-based multiple linear regression model for calculating segment masses. Proceedings of the ASB Conference, Atlanta, 1996.

Corradini ML, Gentilucci M, Leo T, Rizzolatti G: Motor control of voluntary arm movements: Kinematic and modelling study. Biol Cybern 67:347, 1992.

Czerniecki JM, Gitter A, Munro C: Joint moment and muscle power output characteristics of below knee amputees during running: The influence of energy storing prosthetic feet. J Biomech 24:1, 1991.

Doebelin EO: Measurement Systems Application and Design, 4th ed. New York, McGraw-Hill, 1990, p 960.

Dorlot JM, Ait Ba Sidi M, Tremblay GM, Drouin G: Load elongation behavior of the canine anterior cruciate ligament. Trans ASME 102:190, 1980.

Doud JR, Walsh JM: Muscle fatigue and muscle length interaction: Effect on the EMG frequency components. Electromyogr Clin Neurophysiol 35:331, 1995.

Elftman H: A cinematic study of the distribution of pressure in the human foot. Anat Rec 59:481, 1934.

Elftman H: Experimental studies on the dynamics of human walking. N Y Acad Sci Ser 26:1, 1943.

Elftman H: Scientific apparatus and laboratory methods: The measurement of external force in walking. Science 88:2276, 1938.

Esquenazi A, Talaty M, Silktar R, Hirai B: Dynamic EMG during walking as an objective measurement of lower limb orthotic alignment. Basic Applied Myology 7(2):103, 1997.

Evaluation of human exposure to whole-body vibration. 1. General requirements. International Organization for Standardization. ISO 2631/1–1095 (E).

Figiola RS, Beasley DE: Theory and Design for Mechanical Measurements. New York, John Wiley & Sons, 1991.

Foux A, Seliktar R, Valeiro A: Effects of lower body negative pressure on the distribution of the body fluid. J Appl Physiol 41:5, 1976.

Gage JR: The clinical use of kinetics for evaluation of pathological gait in cerebral palsy. J Bone Joint Surg 76-A:4, 1994.

Galante J: Human Motion Research. Proceedings of the 48th Annual Meeting of the American Academy of Orthopaedic Surgeons, Las Vegas, 1981.

Grassino AE, Clanton T: Mechanisms of muscle fatigue. Monaldi Arch Chest Dis 48:1, 1993.

Griffin MJ: Handbook of Human Vibrations. New York, Academic Press, 1990, p 988.

Guzelsu N, Saha S: Diagnostic capacity of flexural waves in wet bones. ASME Biomechanics Symposium, 1983, p 197.

Guzelsu N, Saha S: Electro-mechanical wave propigation in long bones. J Biomechanics 14:19, 1981.

Holman JP: Experimental Methods for Engineers, 6th ed. New York, McGraw-Hill, 1994, p 616.

Isacson J, Brostrom LA: Gait in rheumatoid arthritis: An electrogoniometric investigation. J Biomech 21:6, 1988.

Judge G: Measurement of knee torque during the swing phase of gait. Engineering in Medicine 4:3, 1976.

Katz K, Susak Z, Seliktar R, Najenson T: End bearing characteristics of patellar-tendon bearing prosthesis. Bulletin on Prosthetic Research 10–32:55, 1979.

Kettelkamp DB, Chao EY: A method for quantitative analysis of medial and lateral compression forces at the knee during standing. Clin Orthop 83:202, 1972.

King AI, Mital NK: Computation of rigid-body rotation in three-dimensional space from body-fixed linear acceleration measurements. J Appl Mech 46:4, 1979.

Kirsch RF, Rymer WZ: Neural compensation for muscular fatigue: Evidence for significant force regulation in man. J Neurophysiol 57:6, 1987.

Krebs DE, Wong D, Jevsevar D, et al: Trunk kinematics during locomotor activities. Phys Ther 72:7, 1992.

Lewis JL: A dynamic model of healing fractured long bone. J Biomech 8:17, 1975.

Lindinger MI, Heigenhauser GJF: The role of ion fluxes in skeletal muscle fatigue. Can J Physiol Pharmacol 69:246, 1991.

Loeb GE, Gans C: Electromyography for experimentalists. Chicago, University of Chicago Press, 1986.

Mansour JM, Lesh MD, Nowak MD, Simon SR: A three dimensional multi-segmental analysis of the energetics of normal and pathological human gait. J Biomech 15:1, 1982.

Marey EJ, Demeny: Etudes experimentales de la locomotion humain. Compt Rendu Acad d Sc 105:544, 1873.

Mederios J: Automated measurement systems for clinical motion analysis. Phys Ther 64:12, 1984.

Meijer GA, Westerterp KR, Verhoeven FM, et al: Methods to assess physical activity with special references to motion sensors and accelerometers. IEEE Trans Biomed Eng 38:3, 1991.

Morris JRW: Accelerometery: A technique for the measurement of human body movements. J Biomech 6:729, 1973.

Morrison JB: Bioengineering analysis of force actions transmitted by the knee joint. Biomed Eng 3:164, 1968.

Nigg BE, Herzog W: Biomechanics of the Musculo-Skeletal System. New York, John Wiley & Sons, 1995.

Noyes DH, Clark JW, Watson CE: Mechanical input impedance of human teeth in vivo. Med Biol Eng 6:487, 1968.

Ozgirgin N, Bolukbasi N, Beyazova M, Orkun S: Kinematic gait analysis in hemiplegic patients. Scand J Rehabil Med 25:51, 1993.

Padgaonkar AJ, Krieger KW, King AI: Measurement of angular acceleration of a rigid body using linear accelerometers. J Appl Mech 42:3, 1975.

Patriarco AG, Mann RW, Simon SR, Mansour JM: An evaluation of the approaches of optimization models in the prediction of muscle forces during human gait. J Biomech 14:8, 1981.

Pope MH, Wilder DG, Jorneus L: The response of the seated human to sinusoidal vibration and impact. J Biomech Eng 109:279, 1987.

Rosenstein AD, McLardy-Smith PD, Cunningham JL, Turner-Smith AR: The differentiation of loose and secure femoral implants in total hip replacement using a vibrational technique: An anatomical and pilot clinical study. Proc Inst Mech Eng 203:77, 1989.

Roy SH, DeLuca CJ, Casavant DA: Lumbar muscle fatigue and chronic lower back pain. Spine 14:9, 1989.

Ryker NJ, Bartholomew SH: Determination of acceleration by use of accelerometers. Advisory Committee on Artificial Limbs National Research Council II:7, 1951.

Saha S, Lakes RS: The effect of soft tissue on wave-propagation and vibration tests for determining the in vivo properties of bone. J Biomech 10:393, 1977.

Sarver JJ, Smith BT, Seliktar R: A quantitative analysis of shoulder motion used for controlling FES systems in adolescents with C4 level SCI.

Proceedings of the RESNA Conference, Pittsburgh, 1997.

Seliktar R, Mizrahi J: Gait characteristics of below-knee amputees and their reflection in the ground reaction forces. Eng Med 15:1, 1986.

Seliktar R, Mizrahi J: Partial immobilization of the ankle and talar joints complex and its effects on the ground-foot force characteristics. Eng Med (UK) 13:1, 1984.

Seliktar R, Susak Z, Najenson T, Solsi P: Dynamic features of standing and their correlation with neurological disorders. Scand J Rehabil Med 10:59, 1978.

Seliktar R, Susak Z: Limits of applicability of force plates in clinical examination of human movement. Agressology 24:2, 1983.

Seliktar R: Biomechanics of prosthetic gait. *In* Esquenazi A (ed): Physical Medicine and Rehabilitation: State of the Art Review. Philadelphia, Hanley & Belfus, 1994, p 89.

Seliktar R: The use of impulse momentum for quantification of gait disorders. *In* DeLuc C (ed): Proceedings of the 4th International Congress of the International Society for Electrophysiological Kinesiology, Boston, 1979, p 224.

Sonstegard DA, Mathews LS: Sonic diagnosis of bone fracture healing: A preliminary study. J Biomech 9:689, 1976.

Stokes IAF, Medlicott PA, Wilder PA: Measurement of movement in painful intervertebral joints. Med Biol Eng Comput 18:694, 1980.

Stouffer DC, Butler DJ, Kim H: Tension-torque characteristics of the canine anterior cruciate ligament. 1. Theoretical framework. Trans ASME 105:154, 1983.

Susak Z, Katz K, Seliktar R: Persistence of waddling gait after total hip replacement for congenital dislocation of the hip. Scand J Rehabil Med 12:113, 1980.

Sutherland DH, Hagy JL: Measurement of gait movements from motion picture film. J Bone Joint Surg 54-A:4, 1972.

Threshold Limit Values for Chemical Substances and Physical Agents Biological Exposure Indices. ACGIH Worldwide, second printing, 1996, p. 138.

Vaughan CL, Davis BL, O'Connor JC: Dynamics of Human Gait. Champaign, IL, Human Kinetics Publishers, 1992.

Webster G: Medical Instrumentation: Application and Design. Princeton, NJ, Houghton Mifflin, 1991.

Wiker SF, Chaffin DB, Langolf GD: Shoulder posture and localized muscle fatigue and discomfort. Ergonomics 32:211, 1989.

Winter DA: Biomechanics and Motor Control of Human Movement, 2nd ed. New York, John Wiley & Sons, 1990.

Winter DA: Biomechanics of normal and pathological gait: Implications for understanding human locomotor control. J Motor Behav 21:4, 1989.

Yang L, Condie DN, Granat MH, et al: Effects of joint motion constraints on the gait of normal subjects and their implications on the further development of hybrid FES orthosis for paraplegic persons. J Biomech 29:2, 1996.

CHAPTER 2

BIOMECHANICS OF SOFT TISSUES

Dan L. Bader and Carlijn Bouten

Many noncalcified skeletal connective tissues, such as articular cartilage, intervertebral disk, ligaments, and tendons, have a biomechanical function in response to the dynamic mechanical loads applied in a repetitive manner during normal physiologic activity. Each of these tissue structures constitutes a biologic composite, which contains the ubiquitous biologic macromolecule collagen in fibrous form. The building block of collagen fibers is the tropocollagen molecule, 300 nm long and 1.5 nm wide, with a molecular weight of about 300,000 daltons. Its molecular form is ideally designed to support tensile loads, to which the structural composites are subjected. Its precise role in a biologic composite depends, however, on the nature of loading present when the individual soft tissues perform their various functions. This role is illustrated in this chapter in relation to a series of soft tissues.

The vascularity of most soft tissues is generally poor and in some cases is nonexistent. Thus, the natural self-healing response of soft tissues is limited. Impairment of these soft tissue structures as a result of mechanical overload, such as repetitive strain injury, and of low back pain or disease, such as osteoarthritis, often seriously affects body posture and movement and hence normal daily functioning. These conditions, which affect people of all ages, are commonly presented in hospital clinics. Indeed, it has recently been estimated that soft tissue replacements constitute about 35% of the world market for all medical devices.[1]

ARTICULAR CARTILAGE

GENERAL FEATURES

Three types of cartilaginous soft tissue are found in the body: elastic cartilage, fibrocartilage, and hyaline cartilage. Hyaline cartilage located in sy-

novial joints is generally termed *articular cartilage*. Articular cartilage is the soft tissue that covers the articulating ends of the bones that terminate at a synovial joint (Fig. 2–1). In this position, cartilage is subjected to the forces that pass through the joint. Thus, the main functions of articular cartilage are to reduce the contact stresses to safe values, protect the subchondral bone, and provide the joint with low-friction, low-wear surfaces. Indeed, articular cartilage in conjunction with its lubricant, synovial fluid, produces a coefficient of friction in healthy joints that is lower than can be achieved for any manmade engineering system.

The thickness of cartilage varies from joint to joint and by location on a joint surface. Cartilage thickness in major load-bearing joints is generally between 1.5 and 3.5 mm, although cartilage located on the lateral facet of the patella can be 5 mm thick. Young tissue is usually white or bluish white and translucent, but with increasing age, articular cartilage tends to become yellowish and opaque.

Normal human articular cartilage does not contain blood vessels. Thus, pathways must exist to supply its cells with the vital nutrients to maintain viability and remove waste products. In addition, articular cartilage is devoid of nerve endings. Therefore, any perceived pain from its location within the joint is probably a direct result of abnormal bone contact or other structural damage from within the joints.

STRUCTURE AND COMPOSITION

Articular cartilage consists of cells known as *chondrocytes* and an abundant extracellular matrix that contains three major constituents, water, collagen fibers, and proteoglycans, in the approximate proportions given in Table 2–1. The properties of

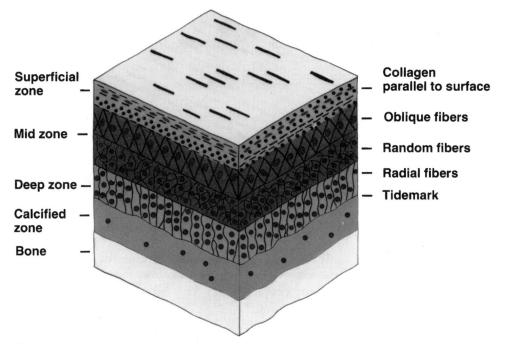

Superficial zone —

Mid zone —

Deep zone —

Calcified zone —

Bone —

— **Collagen parallel to surface**

— **Oblique fibers**

— **Random fibers**

— **Radial fibers**

— **Tidemark**

FIGURE 2–1   Structural variation through the thickness of articular cartilage showing zonal arrangement of collagen fibers and chondrocytes.

these extracellular components and their interactions determine the physical and mechanical properties of the tissue.

Chondrocytes

The chondrocytes are responsible for the synthesis and maintenance of the extracellular constituents of cartilage. The chondrocytes are on average between 10 and 30 μm in diameter and are contained within spaces called *lacunae*. The ratio of cell volume to tissue volume is lower in chondrocytes than in most tissues, accounting for between 1% and 10% of the tissue volume, with a reported mean chondrocyte density of 14,000 cells/mm³.[2] The chondrocytes are most numerous near the articular surface.

The characteristics of chondrocytes change with depth from the articular surface. In normal adult articular cartilage, four cellular zones can be identified under the light microscope:

- A *superficial zone* beneath the articular surface in which the cells are flattened and orientated parallel to the surface
- A *transition zone* in which the cells are more ellipsoidal, with their axes oblique to the articular surface
- A *deep zone,* sometimes called the *proliferative zone,* which contains ellipsoidal or spherical cells in groups of four to eight arranged in columns perpendicular to the articular surface
- A *calcified zone* beneath the uneven basophilic line, known as the *tidemark,* marking the transition to calcified cartilage

It is the cells in the transition zone and deep zone, with relatively large cytoplasmic volumes containing well-developed endoplasmic reticulum and Golgi complexes that produce the main synthetic activity in cartilage.

The chondocytes in articular cartilage are supplied by nutrients in the synovial fluid, which are transported across the cartilage surfaces. Clearly, the permeability of cartilage affects nutrition by means of fluid transport; thus, structural changes that occur with age and disease certainly affect these pathways.

The extracellular matrix (ECM) surrounding

TABLE 2–1   Relative Proportion of Noncellular Components in Adult Human Articular Cartilage

COMPONENT	WET WEIGHT (%)
Collagen	15–20
Ground substance	3–15
Water	65–80
Noncollagenous proteins and lipids	1
Cartilage oligomeric matrix protein (COMP)	

each chondrocyte can also be divided into three regions, known as the *pericellular, territorial,* and *interterritorial* regions. These regions differ in both their proximity to the chondrocytes and their structure and organization. The interterritorial region is the largest and thus the main contributor to the mechanical properties of the matrix.

Collagen

A large proportion of the nonaqueous ECM of cartilage is composed of a network of collagen fibrils. The building blocks of collagen, the *tropocollagen molecules,* consist of three polypeptide chains, designated α *chains,* coiled together in a right-handed helical structure. Each α chain contains about 1000 amino acid residues. With the exception of the short nonhelical sequences at the end of each chain, one third of the amino acid residues are composed of the small molecule glycine. The remainder are composed of large quantities of proline and hydroxyproline, both of which have inherent rigidity in their ring structure and hence confer stability to the triple helix. The precise sequence of amino acids determines the type of collagen present.

Collagens are conventionally classified according to the structures of the three α chains. Articular cartilage contains type II collagen, in which each of three identical polypeptide chains contains a specific content of hydroxylysine residues and linked prosthetic groups. In the past few years, other types of collagen have been reported within cartilage, namely types VI, IX, X, XI, and XIV. These may have important roles in the overall structure of the tissue.[3]

Collagen fibrils undergo a slow maturation process during which intermolecular and intramolecular cross-links are formed. The formation of these cross-links requires a degree of overlap between adjacent molecules, which is consistent with the 64-nm periodicity observed in the fibrils (Fig. 2–2). Intermolecular cross-links may also be formed between residues located in the helical regions of the adjacent molecules. The reducible cross-links formed in immature cartilage are intermediate processes in the formation of more stable, nonreducible cross-links. There is also an increase in the intermolecular covalent cross-links with age in human tissues. Such observations are consistent with the marked increase in chemical stability of the collagen fibers in mature adult cartilage.

Collagen Microstructure

Both the diameter and orientation of collagen fibers in articular cartilage vary with depth below the articular surface. Zones were referred to earlier when describing chondrocyte variation according to depth. The superficial zone, including the articular surface, extends to a depth of about 200 μm below the surface and contains fibrils about 300 nm in diameter. The fibrils are arranged in sheets that lie parallel to the articular surface, and in each sheet, the direction of the fibrils is approximately constant. The fiber orientation varies, however, in subjacent sheets. Fibrils and fiber bundles are closely packed with little intervening proteoglycans when compared with the deeper zones.[4] At the surface of the superficial zone, there is a thin layer composed of fine fibrils, about 5 nm in diameter, associated with abundant proteoglycans.[4, 5]

Immediately subjacent to the superficial zone is the transition zone, occupying up to 45% of the matrix volume, in which the collagen fibrils vary in diameter between 30 and 60 nm. There are fewer fiber bundles, and the interfibrillar spacing is increased with larger amounts of proteoglycans. The fibrils in this zone, which is about 50 μm thick, are more randomly disposed, although there is evidence to suggest a principally radial array.[6]

The deep zone of cartilage occupies the remainder of the uncalcified tissue thickness. The collagen fibers surround the columns of cells and thus also tend to be orientated perpendicularly to the interface between the cartilage and the subchondral bone.[7, 8] In the calcified region, there are increasing deposits of calcium salts in the matrix surrounding the few cells. The collagen fibrils are radially aligned in this region, which occupies between 5% and 10% of the matrix volume.

Proteoglycans

The high-molecular-weight macromolecules of connective tissue are complexes of carbohydrates and proteins in which the carbohydrate consists of repeating disaccharide units. The disaccharide unit is composed of an amino sugar and a uronic acid or galactose. Three main glycosaminoglycans exist in cartilage: chondroitin sulfate (CS), keratan sulphate (KS), and hyaluronan, in proportions that vary with the type of cartilage and with age.

The term *proteoglycan* describes macromolecules of connective tissues composed of a protein core to which a large number of glycosaminoglycan chains are attached laterally. A unique feature of cartilage proteoglycans is their ability to form large multimolecular aggregates, named *aggrecans,* with molecular weights on the order of 50 million daltons. The aggrecan consists of a core protein to which both CS and KS chains and O-linked and N-linked oligosaccharides are attached

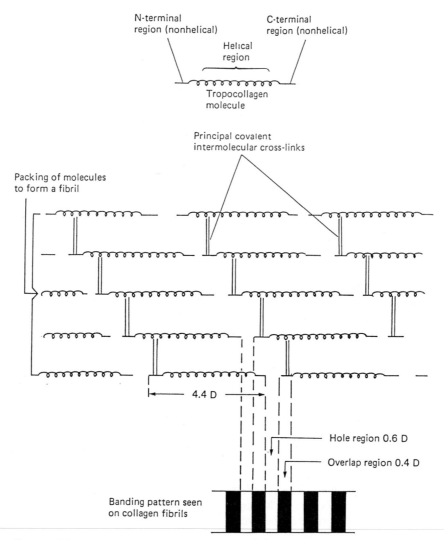

N-terminal
region (nonhelical)

C-terminal
region (nonhelical)

Helical
region

Tropocollagen
molecule

Principal covalent
intermolecular cross-links

Packing of molecules
to form a fibril

4.4 D

Hole region 0.6 D

Overlap region 0.4 D

Banding pattern seen
on collagen fibrils

FIGURE 2–2   Diagram of tropocollagen molecules and their packing arrangement in a collagen fibril (D is the periodicity seen in the native fibril).

(Fig. 2–3).[9] The core protein has three different globular domains: the G1, G2, and G3 domains. The G1 domain is situated at the amino-terminal end of the core protein and binds the aggrecan to hyaluronan (see Fig. 2–3). This interaction is stabilized by a link protein that binds to hyaluronan as well as to the G1 region of the aggrecan. The aggrecan–hyaluronan interaction retains the aggrecan within the matrix. When there is a large excess of proteoglycan over hyaluronan, as in cartilage, a large number of proteoglycan molecules interact with a single chain of hyaluronan, as shown in Fig. 2–4.[9]

Other smaller proteoglycans exist in articular cartilage, including biglycan, decorin, and fibromodulin. Their functions are largely unknown, but the latter two small proteoglycans are thought to be involved in collagen fibrillogenesis.

Proteoglycans are polyanions as a result of the negatively charged groups associated with KS and CS along their molecular chains. These properties control the ability of proteoglycans to bind water osmotically, and the polyelectrolyte gels may be considered osmotic systems. The gel behaves like a solution in that it tends to dilute itself with solvent. In cartilage, this process is limited by the extensibility of the collagen fibers with which the proteoglycans are enmeshed.

The proteoglycan content is inhomogeneously distributed throughout the depth of cartilage. In the superficial zone, there is little hyaluronan and, as a consequence, only small amounts of aggrecan. Instead, the proteoglycans present in this zone are strongly associated with the densely packed collagen fibers. The content of proteoglycans increases significantly with distance from the articu-

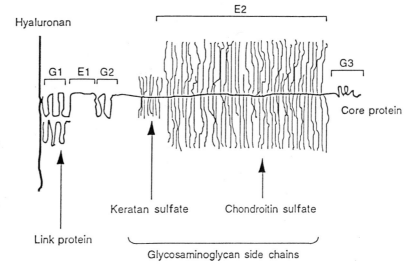

FIGURE 2–3 Schematic representation of an aggrecan molecule bonded to hyaluronan by means of a link protein. (From Knight MM: Deformation of Isolated Articular Chondrocytes Cultured in Agarose Constructs. PhD Thesis. London, University of London, 1997.)

lar surface, attaining a maximum value in the middle and deep zones.

Interstitial Water

Water readily enters articular cartilage because of the hydrophilic nature of the proteoglycans. The highest water content is found near the articular surface, and the amount of water decreases toward the subchondral bone, attaining a value of about 65% in the deep zone.[10]

Only a small proportion of the total water in cartilage is intracellular. It is now well established that the interstitial water can exist in two distinct compartments. About 30% of the interstitial water is strongly associated with the collagenous network. The remaining water is associated with the proteoglycan domains and is freely exchangeable during joint loading and unloading. It is this movement that is important in joint lubrication and in maintenance of chondrocyte viability. Furthermore, the tissue fluid–containing mobile-

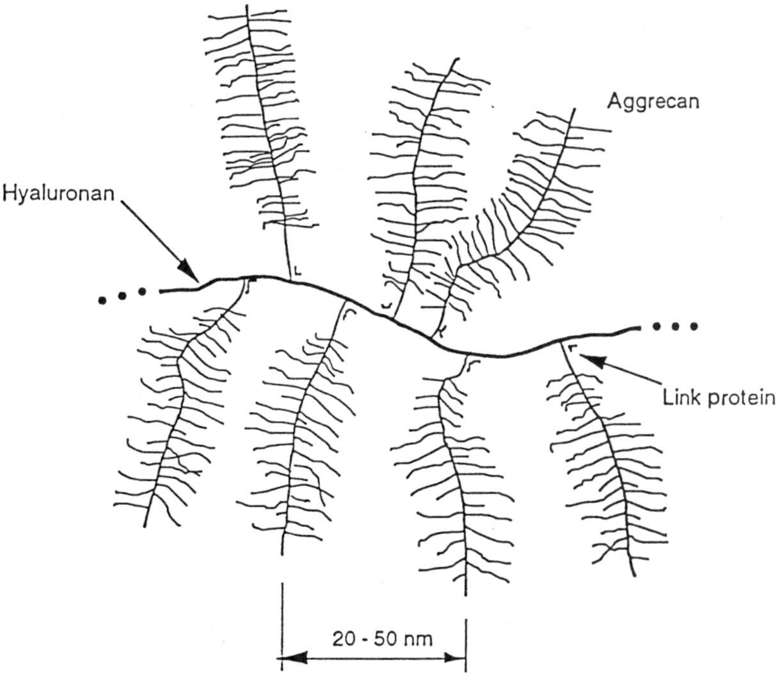

FIGURE 2–4 Model of aggrecan–hyaluran complex in articular cartilage. (From Knight MM: Deformation of Isolated Articular Chondrocytes Cultured in Agarose Constructs. PhD Thesis. London, University of London, 1997.)

charged ions, such as calcium, sodium, and hydrogen, can establish streaming potentials in cartilage that can alter cell metabolism.

BIOMECHANICAL CONSIDERATIONS

Load Carriage

The physicochemical interaction of the various components of the ECM is responsible for the mechanical properties of the healthy tissue. For example, in articular cartilage, there is a physicochemical equilibrium between the osmotic swelling pressure ($P_{swelling}$) of the proteoglycan gel, which is balanced by the hydrostatic pressures ($P_{elastic}$), owing to the tensile stresses generated within the collagen fiber network. This balance exists even in unloaded articular cartilage. It is altered when the tissue is loaded in compression by an applied hydrostatic pressure ($P_{applied}$), resulting in a net pressure differential (Δp) and fluid flow away from the compressed tissue. This may be represented as follows:

$$\Delta p = P_{applied} + P_{elastic} - P_{swelling}$$

All of these terms may be a function of time. This fluid flow results in an increased proteoglycan concentration within the tissue and a change in the relative magnitudes of the stresses in the two solid components of articular cartilage. If the compressive load remains constant, the rate of fluid flow decreases with time and eventually reduces to zero at a new state of equilibrium, as follows:

$$P'_{swelling} = P_{applied} + P'_{elastic}$$

This time-dependent creep behavior is characteristic of all viscoelastic soft tissues. If the applied force is suddenly released, the cartilage recoils almost instantaneously to a limited extent and then recovers gradually to its original thickness. This time-dependent component of recovery occurs as water is reimbibed into the cartilage matrix, until the original unloaded equilibrium position is reached. Cyclic loading produces similar behavior, although the extent of the recovery within each cycle depends on the form and frequency of the loading pattern.

The resultant forces transmitted through the major load-bearing joints of the lower limb are largely compressive, and the cartilages, with their inherently low frictional properties, are thus subjected mainly to compression perpendicular to the articular surface. In resisting these compressive forces, the collagen fibers experience tensile forces, and it is clear that the mechanical properties of cartilage in both compression and tension are important to the transmission of joint forces by the tissue. The magnitude of the resultant forces regularly reaches five times body weight, equivalent to about 3500 newtons (N), corresponding to the period just after the heel-strike of the gait cycle. In some cases involving vigorous sporting activities, joint forces can exceed 10,000 N. Taking into account the surface area of the supporting cartilage in major load-bearing joints, contact stresses of the order of 5 megapascals (MPa) are common in normal walking.

The behavior of the ECM may be modeled in terms of a biphasic material incorporating a *fluid phase* of interstitial water and a *solid phase,* the collagen–proteoglycan organic solid matrix, to represent the fluid-filled porous-permeable medium.[11, 12] Other phases have been introduced to accommodate the presence of interstitial ions within the matrix. These models are discussed later.

Biomechanical Studies

Articular cartilage has been tested in vitro using a range of loading modes, including compression, tension, shear, and torsion. This section concentrates on the studies that have examined compression and tension.

Compression

Specific test methods have been developed for testing cartilage in compression. The two most common methodologies are the *indentation test,* which uses an indenter to apply compression to discrete areas of the cartilage surface in situ, and the *uniaxial compression test,* which involves the use of a platen or large indenter to compress isolated cylinders of cartilage perpendicular to the articular surface. This test has been performed with the cartilage specimen in either a confined state or an unconfined state. The former test state employs porous platens to apply compression to cylinders whose sides are confined.

A critique of the two test methods is provided in Table 2–2. Both methods, however, produce a similar response after the application of a rapid load to the cartilage surface, using a damped mechanical testing system.[12, 13] Figure 2–5 demonstrates the characteristics of a typical viscoelastic material.

Many of these studies estimated the creep modulus 2 seconds after load application and related it to the chemical constituents of cartilage.[13] They found that this parameter, which as its name sug-

TABLE 2–2 **Appraisal of Testing Methods of Articular Cartilage in Compression**

METHOD	ADVANTAGES	DISADVANTAGES
Indentation	1. Provides normal physiologic constraints on deformation and fluid 2. Facilitates assessment of properties across joint surface	1. It is difficult to align the indenter perpendicular to the cartilage surface 2. Complex stress distribution under the indenter makes it difficult to determine material constants
Uniaxial compression (confined and unconfined)	1. Unidirectional stress allows the calculation of compressive stiffness 2. Specimen size permits controlled tests with surrounding media of different concentrations or incubation with biochemicals	1. Boundary conditions and fluid flow are different from those of intact joint

gests includes a degree of creep, was significantly correlated to total glycoaminoglycan content but was independent of the natural variation in the collagen content. Stress–relaxation tests have enabled a relaxation equilibrium modulus or relaxation modules (H_A) to be calculated. This parameter reflects the intrinsic stiffness of the solid components of the ECM. A summary of representative values of derived stiffness for the articular cartilage is presented in Table 2–3.[12–15] This table also shows some data from cartilage areas where the damage ranged from slight surface fibrillation to gross ulceration.

In the studies cited in Table 2–3, the short-term response of the tissue was partly determined by the dynamic characteristics of the test apparatus. This limitation was recognized by Woo and colleagues,[16] who found that the initial elastic stiffness of the articular cartilage continued to increase at very high loading rates and that its measurement is thus limited ultimately by the response of the measuring equipment. Indeed, some studies reported that when loaded rapidly in compression, cartilage displayed a transient oscillatory response that decayed to a steady creep less than 1 second after application of load.[16–18] The more recent study[18] addressed this response by using an underdamped mechanical system to test articular cartilage in unconfined compression. The resulting initial transient oscillatory response of cartilage, as seen in Figure 2–5, could be used to uncouple the elastic stiffness and the viscous damping in the tissue. This investigation examined the effects of two enzymes on the short-term compressive properties of cartilage. It demonstrated that the collagen component of cartilage largely influenced the elastic stiffness, whereas the damping term was influenced by the proteoglycan constituents. Examination of the data related to individual cartilage specimens revealed an inverse relation between the elastic stiffness of cartilage and the specimen thickness, t. This relation is consistent with the expression for the stiffness of an elastic prism, k, of constant cross-sectional area, A, and constant Young's modulus, E, as follows:

$$k = EA/t$$

The result implies that the initial "elastic" modulus of cartilage in compression is fairly constant in healthy joints, yielding a value of about 10 MPa.

TABLE 2–3 **Stiffness Values for Adult Human Articular Cartilage**

TEST MODEL	JOINT SURFACE	STIFFNESS MODULUS (MPA)	POISSON'S RATIO
Indentation	Femoral head	1.9–14.4	0.50
2-Second creep[13]	Normal areas (mean)	7.0–8.7	
Linear elastic	Damaged areas (mean)	3.1–6.4	
Compression unconfined	Femoral condyles	6.1–14.9	—
0.6 second[14]	Femoral head	5.3–19.7	
Compression confined Biphasic[12]	Patella	$0.79 < H_A < 1.91$	—
Indentation Biphasic[15]	Femoral condyles	$0.59 < H_A < 0.70$	$0.07 < v < 0.10$

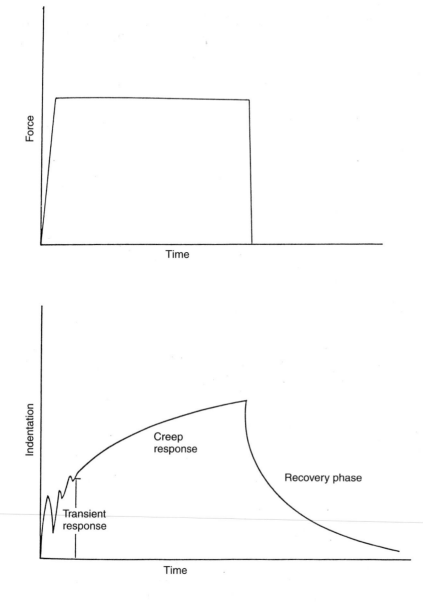

FIGURE 2–5 Typical response of articular cartilage to a compressive step-load input, with transient response indicative of an undamped mechanical loading system.

Tension

Collagen fibers are the main tension-resistant elements in connective tissues. Their presence in articular cartilage suggests that tensile stresses are present, even though the tissue is loaded predominantly in compression perpendicular to the articular surface.

Investigators have examined the tensile properties of thin slices of articular cartilage. When an isolated dumbbell-shaped specimen of cartilage is subjected to a tensile force in a plane parallel to the articular surface, a nonlinear relationship is produced. This response can be regarded as the continuous progression between three phases of behavior. Initially, at low levels of stress, the colla-gen fibers tend to become aligned in the direction of the tensile force. The tensile tangent modules in this phase depend on the initial orientation of the collagen fibers and the effective resistance of the proteoglycan gel for their alignment. With increasing alignment of the collagen fibers, the component of the applied stress along the fibers increases, and the stress–strain curve increasingly reflects the mechanical properties of the fibers. With increasing stress, therefore, the tangent modulus increases until specimen fracture occurs. The dependence on the relationship between the two main structural components and tensile properties can be demonstrated by the incubation of cartilage specimens in proteolytic enzymes.[14, 19]

There is also considerable variation in the tensile properties with orientation of the specimen with respect to the predominant direction of the superficial collagen fibers. Parallel-orientated specimens yield higher tensile stiffness and strength when compared with perpendicular-orientated specimens. Tensile properties also decrease with respect to distance from the articular surface. These results demonstrate both the anisotropic and nonhomogeneous nature of articular cartilage.

In two tensile fatigue studies, Weightman and colleagues[20, 21] demonstrated that human articular cartilage is prone to tensile fatigue failure in vitro. Tests on specimens from human femoral head cartilage revealed that the fatigue resistance decreased with age at a rate that was faster than that which could be explained by normal usage. The decrease in fatigue resistance was not related to either of the two major solid constituents of the specimens. By combining the observations, the following model was produced:

$$S = 23 - 0.1a - 1.83 \log (N)$$

where S is the stress in megapascals, a is the age in years, and N is the number of cycles to failure.

AGING AND CLINICAL FEATURES

During aging, changes occur in the composition of articular cartilage, including a decrease in total water content and an increase in the concentration of proteoglycan.[22] There are also alterations in the composition and size of the aggrecan, in particular a decrease in the proportion of the CS-rich region of the monomer and an increase in the proportion of the binding region.[22] In addition, there is a reported increase in the diameter of collagen fibrils with age. The stiffness of articular cartilage inevitably decreases with age and degeneration.[14]

Osteoarthritis is a degenerative condition that affects the synovial joint. The prevalence of the condition increases with age, reaching a maximum in the sixth and seventh decades. However, there is a growing number of younger patients who develop the disease subsequent to traumatic damage of major load-bearing joints, such as the knee. Some of the earliest detectable changes leading to osteoarthritis occur in the articular cartilage. Features of degenerative cartilage are a gradual softening and disruption of the articular cartilage from the bone surfaces. Small fissures appear in the superficial zone; the subsequent exposure and disruption of the collagen fibers is termed *fibrillation*. Not all cartilage fibrillation leads to a progressive form of degeneration, however—some mechanical weakening with age is a direct result

of the fatigue processes within the articular cartilage. Other manifestations of the disease condition include the formation of microfractures and subarticular cysts in the subchondral bone and gross geometric changes.

Recent interest has developed in devices designed to measure cartilage stiffness during clinical investigations. One such instrument used under arthroscopic control aims to measure cartilage stiffness objectively and to facilitate diagnosis of the softening of articular cartilage at an early stage.[23] If such an instrument proves reliable, it will enable the assessment of cartilage repair after surgery.

Treatment

Articular cartilage has limited intrinsic repair potential. Many options have been proposed for the repair of the soft tissues. These generally involve either synthetic or biologic materials. Synthetic materials have the advantage of providing a structure that is immunologically acceptable, with the mechanical integrity required of load-bearing structures. The polymeric nature of most synthetic options, however, leads to inherent instability in the body and thus poor long-term performance. Biologic solutions traditionally involve autografts, allografts, and xenografts. Each of these options has proved to be far from ideal; for example, autographs have led to donor site morbidity.

Other common solutions involve augmentation devices incorporating both synthetic structures and biologic grafts. These devices depend on tissue ingrowth and regeneration induced by the successful transfer of stress from the synthetic material to the natural tissues. This stress transfer process would need to change with time after implantation as the tissue regenerates. Clinical reports are not generally convincing because of, for example, the inadequate initial performance of the synthetic component of the augmentation device.

The relative failure of many synthetic and graft solutions has led to the growing interest in the development of cell-seeded repair systems for solving a number of clinical problems related to connective tissues, including articular cartilage, menisci, and ligaments. These systems have also been called *tissue-engineered repair systems*. Typically, autologous or allogenic cells are isolated from a tissue biopsy removed from an undamaged site remote to the injury. The cells are expanded in cell culture and seeded in suitable three-dimensional resorbable scaffold material, which when implanted into the defect site elicits a biologic repair. The potential advantages of these systems include a complete repair that effectively eliminates the problems of synthetic wear particles or prosthetic failure. In addition, the biologic nature of the system may ensure maintenance and turnover of the repaired tissue in the long term. Success depends, however, on the ability of the cells to synthesize a functional matrix at a rate sufficient to balance the loss of mechanical integrity of the resorbing scaffold material. Additionally, on implantation, those systems are subjected to normal physiologic forces. Thus, mechanotransduction pathways are activated that alter cell response in a manner that cannot be predicted in an unstrained cell culture environment. It is vital, therefore, to understand the effect of dynamic mechanical strain on cells within tissue-engineered systems to predict the success of the device in vivo. In addition, it has been proposed that the application of strain in vitro using cellular engineering techniques may be used to optimize device performance after implantation.[24]

A number of reports have described in vitro and in vivo evaluation of cell-engineered systems for repair of load-bearing cartilaginous tissues.[25–27] One such approach involving the injection of autologous chondrocytes beneath a periosteal graft has been evaluated with some success after a few years in clinical study. Most of the postimplantation analysis has involved histologic and biochemical analysis of repair tissue, with only a few reports assessing its biochmechanical integrity.[26–27] This integrity of the constructs both before and after implantation is crucial to assessing their long-term performance.

INTERVERTEBRAL DISK

GENERAL FEATURES

The intervertebral disk constitutes the primary connection between two adjacent vertebrae in the spinal column. It allows for motion in all directions while being guided and constrained by the uncovertebral and facet joints as well as the vertebral ligaments and muscles. Its main mechanical function is the transmission of loads from the upper body to the pelvis. This involves the transmission of the weights and resulting moments of the head and trunk and any additional masses lifted by the upper body. In addition, the disk serves as a shock absorber in rapidly increasing loads. By measuring the intradiskal pressure, it has been determined that the loads acting on a lumbar disk in sitting and standing with straight back amount to twice the whole body weight and as much as three times the body weight if a weight of 20 kg is held in the hands.[28, 29] In these positions, the major load on the spine is axial and mainly produces compression of the intervertebral disk. In normal daily activities, however, the disk is often loaded dynamically and in a complex manner, owing to combined bending, compression, and torsion of the spine. Consequently, the actual load on the intervertebral disk is much higher and produces increased compressive as well as tensile and shear stresses in the disk.

There are 23 intervertebral disks in the spinal column, amounting to one fourth to one third of the total height of the spinal column. No disks are found between the axis, atlas, and occiput (the base of the skull) or between the fused vertebrae of the pelvic region of the spine. The individual disks are roughly cylindrical, with a diameter of 2 to 4 cm and a thickness of about 1 cm.[30] Disk size and shape vary from cranial to caudal, with the largest disks being in the lumbar region and the most rounded ones in the cervical region of the spine. The ratio of disk height to the height of the vertebral body varies from 1:3 in the lumbar region to 1:5 in the thoracic region and 2:5 in the cervical region. Because of the greater proportional height of the disks, the lumbar and cervical regions of the spine have greater mobility than the thoracic spine. In the lumbar and cervical regions, the disks are also thicker anteriorly than posteriorly, resulting in anteriorly convex curvatures of the spine, known as the lumbar and cervical *lordoses*. The thoracic spine, on the other hand, exhibits a posteriorly convex curvature, known as thoracic *kyphosis*.

The mechanical function and load-bearing capacity of the intervertebral disk are dependent on its anatomy and chemical composition and are influenced by disk degeneration as a result of aging or disease. When a disk is loaded beyond its load-bearing capacity, structural damage may occur. Usually, damage occurs as a consequence of high-level, short-term loads that exceed load tolerance. Submaximal long-term and repeated loads may also cause disk failure. To understand the mechanisms of disk failure, a basic knowledge of the mechanical behavior of intervertebral disk tissue under normal and extreme loading conditions is crucial.

STRUCTURE AND COMPOSITION

The intervertebral disk is an avascular, fibrocartilaginous structure consisting of a gelatinous center, the *nucleus pulposus,* surrounded by the concentrically arranged fibrous layers or lamellae of the *anulus fibrosus,* and two cartilaginous *end plates* that cover the top and bottom of the nucleus and the anulus (Fig. 2–6).

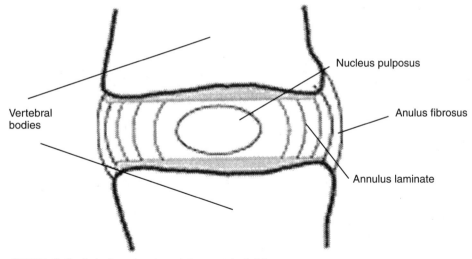

FIGURE 2–6   Sagittal section through intervertebral disk.

As a result of the presence of both randomly and aligned fiber networks, the structure of intervertebral disk tissue is anisotropic. Like articular cartilage, it consists of cells, at a low density of about 5800 cells/mm³, embedded in ECM. Most of the disk volume is taken up by the ECM, which consists mainly of water, collagen fibers, and proteoglycans. The relative proportions of the ECM components change with location in the disk; for example, the water content is highest in the gelatinous nucleus, whereas the collagen content is highest in the fibrous anulus (Table 2–4).[31–34] The different structures in the intervertebral disk are most conveniently described in separate sections.

Nucleus Pulposus

The gel-like nucleus pulposus is the stress-absorbing and load-distributing center of the intervertebral disk. It consists of highly hydrated proteoglycan ground substance with a few cells and randomly oriented loose collagen fibers. The cells are rounded with a spheroidal nucleus and occur either singly or in groups of four to six. The average density of cells is 4000 cells/mm³.[2] Like articular cartilage, most of the collagen in the nucleus is type II, but types IV, IX, and XI are also found.[35] The nucleus forms 25% to 50% of the sagittal cross-area of the disk. It is roughly located at the center of the disk, except in the large lumbar disks, where the nucleus is more posterior than central.

Because of the high proteoglycan content, the nucleus can attract water by means of osmosis and can mechanically be considered a highly hydrated, flattened, incompressible sphere that exerts pressure in all directions. In the unloaded disk, the hydrostatic intradiskal pressure is 70 kilopascals (kPa) and balances the tensile stresses in the anulus fibers and longitudinal spinal ligaments.[29]

Anulus Fibrosus

Although there are significant differences in their structural organizations, there is no clear boundary between the nucleus and the anulus: the nucleus

TABLE 2–4   **Relative Proportions of Noncellular Components in the Three Structures of the Adult Human Intervertebral Disk**

COMPONENT	NUCLEUS PULPOSUS		ANULUS FIBROSUS		END PLATES	
	WET WEIGHT (%)	DRY WEIGHT (%)	WET WEIGHT (%)	DRY WEIGHT (%)	WET WEIGHT (%)	DRY WEIGHT (%)
Collagen	5	25	20	65	28	60
Proteoglycan ground substance	10	50	3–6	10–20	2–8	5–18
Water	80	*	70	*	55	*

*Values not available.
Data from references 31 to 34.

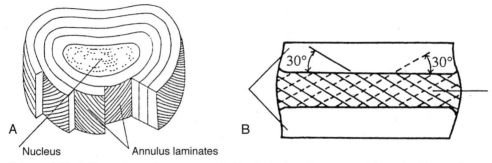

A   Nucleus   Annulus laminates   B

FIGURE 2–7   *A*, The nucleus pulposus surrounded by the laminated structure of the anulus fibrosus. Part of the anulus is removed to show the opposite direction of collagen fibers in the succeeding lamellae. *B*, The fibers run parallel at an angle of −30 to 30 degrees to the plane of the disk. (Adapted from Panjabi MM, White AA: Physical properties and functional biomechanics of the spine. *In* White AA, Panjabi MM [eds]: Clinical Biomechanics of the Spine. Philadelphia, JB Lippincott, 1990, p 3.)

simply merges into the anulus in the transitional zone or inner anulus. The outer anulus consists of 15 to 25 concentric laminated layers of collagen fibers, ground substance, a few elastin fibers, and narrow, elongated fibroblast-like cells (9000 cells/mm³). The elastin fibers play a role in recovery of the anulus after deformation.

In the circumferential direction, the anular layers, or lamellae, terminate, join, or split into two layers but do not form complete rings.[36] In the individual lamellae, the collagen fibers run parallel at an average direction of 30 degrees to the disk plane. In adjacent lamellae, however, they run in opposite directions and are therefore oriented at 120 degrees to each other (Fig. 2–7).[37] This arrangement is optimal for absorbing the centrifugal stresses generated by the nucleus pulposus in axial loading of the disk and is believed to play a role in restricting axial rotation of the spine.

The inner lamellae of the anulus fibrosus merge into the cartilage end plates of the vertebrae,

whereas the outer ones attach directly to the bone and are known as *Sharpey's fibers*. This latter connection is substantially firmer. On the outside, the lamellae are mutually connected by the anterior and posterior longitudinal ligaments (Fig. 2–8). From the transitional zone outward, the lamellae increase in thickness, and there is a steady increase in the proportion of collagen. The type of collagen also varies in the radial direction: the inner anulus contains mainly type I collagen that predominates in tendons and fibrous cartilage, whereas the outer anulus contains mainly type II collagen. Other collagen types found in the anulus are types III, V, VI, IX, and XI.[38] Contrary to the collagen content, the proteoglycan, and hence water content, decreases from the inner to the outer anulus.[39, 40]

End Plates

The end plates separate the nucleus and anulus from the vertebral bodies. They are mainly com-

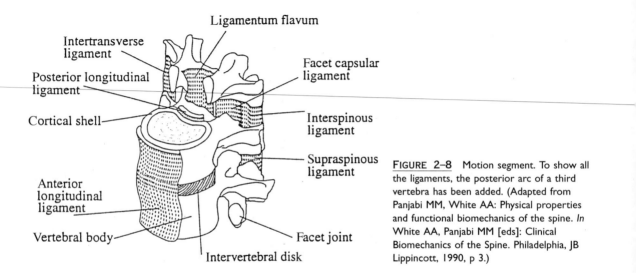

FIGURE 2–8   Motion segment. To show all the ligaments, the posterior arc of a third vertebra has been added. (Adapted from Panjabi MM, White AA: Physical properties and functional biomechanics of the spine. *In* White AA, Panjabi MM [eds]: Clinical Biomechanics of the Spine. Philadelphia, JB Lippincott, 1990, p 3.)

posed of hyaline cartilage, which lacks the distinctive fibrous appearance of the anulus and is more translucent. The plates have a mean thickness of 0.6 mm and are weakly attached to the vertebral bodies by a layer of calcified material.[34] At the side of the disk, they connect to the lamellae that form the inner one third of the anulus. The collagen fibers of these lamellae continue in the end plate, thereby enveloping the nucleus pulposus. Within the end plate, the collagen fibers are densely packed and run parallel to the surface.

The radial proteoglycan and water profiles show the same tendency as those in the nucleus and anulus: ratios are highest at the center and decrease toward the periphery of the end plate. The end plates are of major importance to the nourishment of the intervertebral disk. Small capillaries stretch from the bone marrow into the end plates and provide essential nutrients. This pathway accounts for 70% of the metabolic requirements; the other 30% is provided by the blood vessels on top of the exterior lamellae of the anulus fibrosus. Nutritional conditions and biochemistry of the intervertebral disk are crucial to its viability and mechanical functioning. Therefore, even minor disturbances in end plate structure and composition may lead to disk failure.

Motion Segment

Clarification of the biomechanical behavior and injury mechanisms of the intervertebral disk is largely facilitated by the introduction of the *motion segment,* first described in 1951.[41] A motion segment, or functional spinal unit (FSU), is a 6-degrees-of-freedom structure that comprises two adjacent vertebrae with the surrounding soft tissues: intervertebral disk, uncovertebral joints, facet joints, and ligaments (see Fig. 2–8). Its biomechanical behavior is similar to that of the entire spinal column, which may be considered as a series of connecting motion segments.

BIOMECHANICAL CONSIDERATIONS

Load Carriage

Similar to articular cartilage, the intervertebral disk exhibits time-dependent properties, such as viscoelasticity, characterized by load-rate sensitivity, hysteresis, creep, and relaxation, to deal with both short-term high-amplitude loads and long-term low-amplitude loads. Its mechanical behavior depends largely on the intrinsic viscoelasticity of the collagen network but is also highly influenced by the fluid flow inside the disk. In addition, the disk possesses anisotropy owing to the lamellar

arrangement of the anulus fibrosus. Thus, its mechanical behavior is influenced by the type and direction of the applied load.

As emphasized by Panjabi and White,[37] it is important to distinguish between the global, external loads applied to the disk as a whole and the internal stresses and strains within the disk structures. Normal axial loading produces complex stresses and a distribution of forces within the disk. As a result, the anular fibers are radially and circumferentially stretched as they are pushed outward (see Figs. 2–2 to 2–4). During compression, fluid is expelled from the disk in a manner similar to that with articular cartilage. As a result of the loss of water, the proteoglycan content and hence osmotic pressure increase, whereas the tension in the collagen–proteoglycan network decreases. The fluid flow continues until the external load is balanced. Removal of the compressive load results in an uptake of fluid by the tissue, leading to a decrease in the osmotic pressure and an increase in tension of the network. It has been experimentally determined that the intranuclear fluid pressure during axial compression on the disk is 1.5 times the externally applied load. The tensile stresses are much higher: in the dorsal part of the anulus, they can reach values up to 5 times the applied load.[42, 43]

During flexion, extension, and lateral bending of the spine, one part of the disk is subjected to compression while the other part is loaded in tension (Fig. 2–9). There is associated bulging of the anulus fibrosus on the pressure side and retraction on the traction side. As a consequence, part of the anular fibers are stretched, whereas other parts are relaxed. Axial rotation of the spine produces torsional loads that result in shear stresses inside the disk. Pure shearing forces acting on the disk as a whole do not occur in vivo. Usually, they are combined with flexion and rotation.

Biomechanical Studies

The mechanical properties of the intervertebral disk are generally estimated from the viscoelastic behavior during load-displacement experiments. Typically, such experiments have concentrated on uniaxial loading because mechanical characterization during more physiologic simulations of combined, or coupled, movements (e.g., bending and rotation) is extremely difficult to achieve. Test specimens are usually single or multisegmental cadaveric motion segments. Isolated disks, or specimens from disk tissue, are less frequently studied.

The properties of test specimens are presented by means of structural, load-displacement, stiff-

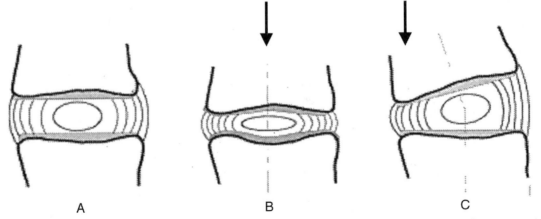

A   B   C

FIGURE 2–9   Schematic representation of the intravertebral disk in unloaded condition (A); in pure axial loading (B); and in flexion or extension (C). During axial loading, the anulus fibrosus is pushed outward and the anular fibers are stretched. Bending causes bulging of the disk on the pressure side and retraction on the traction side. Some of the anular fibers are stretched, whereas others are relaxed.

ness–flexibility, or material (i.e., stress–strain) relationships. The load-displacement curve of the intervertebral disk has the typical nonlinear, sigmoidal shape of viscoelastic materials. At low loads, the disk provides little resistance and remains relatively flexible (neutral zone). At higher loads, it becomes stiffer and more resistant, providing greater stability (elastic zone). Owing to this viscoelasticity, as well as to the anisotropic structure of the disk, load-displacement curves and related mechanical properties vary with strain rate and loading direction. In addition, the nonlinear nature of the load-displacement curve gives rise to difficulties when mechanical properties, such as stiffness or relaxation, are represented by a unique value.[44] Hence, differences in experimental conditions and setup, as well as the representation of experimental data, may lead to considerable variations in mechanical properties. These factors, together with the inherent biologic variation of disk properties and the limited accuracy of the complicated experiments, are responsible for the large differences between mechanical properties reported in the literature.

For clarity, only average values and general conclusions are presented here, but the obvious variation in mechanical properties should be kept in mind when interpreting the quoted values.

Mechanical Properties of Motion Segments

The experimental arrangement for the mechanical characterization of a motion segment is shown in Figure 2–10. The lower vertebra is fixed to a test frame, whereas the upper vertebra is free to move in all directions in response to the applied loads.

The origin of a three-dimensional coordinate system has been placed at the geometric center of the upper vertebral body. The signs for the directions of force (F) and moment (M) and the corresponding translations (t) and rotations (ϕ) need to be defined to reflect the different mechanical behavior for positive and negative displacements around and along the same axis. Assuming symmetry with respect to the midsagittal plane, the mechanical behavior for left and right lateral shear ($\pm F_y$), left

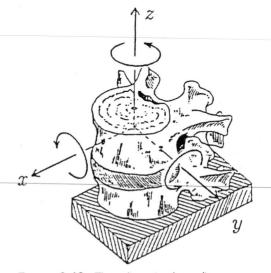

FIGURE 2–10   Three-dimensional coordinate system associated with the center of the upper vertebral body of a motion segment. (Adapted from Panjabi MM, White AA: Physical properties and functional biomechanics of the spine. In White AA, Panjabi MM [eds]: Clinical Biomechanics of the Spine. Philadelphia, JB Lippincott, 1990, p 3.)

and right lateral bending ($\pm M_x$), and left and right axial rotation ($\pm M_z$) is identical.

In most studies, the motion segment is placed in a universal testing machine and subjected to controlled loads, whereas load and deformation are recorded simultaneously. Generally, loads are applied statically, with the load increasing in small increments, after which the specimen is given adequate time to relax before the displacement is measured. Consequently, viscous effects are minimized, and the relaxed elastic characteristics are obtained. In few cases, loads are applied quasistatically or dynamically, with the load continuously increasing at prescribed rates and the viscoelastic characteristics subsequently estimated.

Almost all research on the mechanical properties of motion segments has been carried out on lumbar segments. Many of these properties, however, are relatively consistent throughout the spine and are merely dependent on loading direction rather than spinal level. Therefore, mechanical properties of motion segments, whether in the cervical, thoracic, or lumbar spine, are included as average values or ranges with respect to loading direction. Properties that might be expected to vary with spinal level are described separately.

The displacement of a motion segment in the flexible neutral zone of the load-displacement curve is on average 0.3 mm for tension and compression and 0.8 mm for shear.[45] It ranges between 1.7 and 3.2 degrees for lateral bending, flexion, extension, and axial rotation.[46] The physiologic range of motion, covering the neutral zone and the subsequent linear elastic zone of the load-displacement curve, ranges between 0.1 and 1.9 mm for tension, compression, and shear,[45, 47] whereas values ranging from 1 to 17 degrees have been reported for lateral bending, flexion, extension, and axial rotation.[46, 48, 49]

Several authors have presented an overview of stiffness coefficient, or reciprocal flexibility coefficients, of motion segments for different modes of loading.[37, 44] On average, stiffness increases from the cervical to lumbar regions of the spine for all loading directions; the cervical spine is more flexible, whereas the lumbar spine is more resistant to the relatively high-amplitude loads in this region. A summary of average values and ranges reported from a selected number of studies is provided in Table 2–5.[45, 46, 50–58]

It is clear that there is little difference in stiffness for bending, flexion and extension, and axial rotation of the spine. Also, the resistance to shear is about equal in all directions. Shearing forces are less well resisted than forces in the axial direction, the stiffness being about 10% of the resistance to compression. The highest stiffness of the disk is seen during compression, probably because of the increased nuclear pressure seen with compression of the disk.

After periods of sustained loading of the motion segment, the intervertebral disk shows creep. In quasi-static compression, disk creep is five to seven times higher in magnitude than creep in the bony structures of the segment.[59] A 3-hour period of compressive loading at 1200 N, comparable to unsupported sitting with anterior flexion, results in a 10% decrease in disk height and a 5% to 13% increase in sagittal disk diameter,[60] which is of the same order of magnitude as that for diurnal variation seen in vivo. Higher compressive loads produce greater deformation and a higher creep rate. A significant fraction of creep under compression is due to fluid loss,[61] but creep and recovery characteristics of the disk are also influenced by the viscoelasticity of the anulus fibrosus.[62] Creep causes the intranuclear pressure to fall and the anular stresses to rise. The disk becomes stiffer in

TABLE 2–5 Mean Stiffness Values and Ranges of Spinal Motion Segments

DIRECTION OF LOAD	NAME	MEAN STIFFNESS	STIFFNESS RANGE
		N/mm	N/mm
$+F_x$	Anterior shear	105	34–183
F_x	Posterior shear	105	49–189
$\pm F_y$	Lateral shear	150	53–385
$+F_z$	Tension	417	53–1000
F_z	Compression	1065	141–2500
		N m/deg	N m/deg
$\pm M_x$	Lateral bending	1.6	0.01–7.7
$+M_y$	Flexion	1.2	0.1–2.2
M_y	Extension	1.2	0.1–2.8
$\pm M_z$	Axial rotation	1.3	0.2–5.0

Data from references 45, 46, and 50 to 58.

compression and more flexible in bending.[63] Thus, the loading history is important for both the mechanical behavior and the load-bearing capacity of the disk.

Hysteresis of disk tissue in motion segments was first described by Virgin,[58] who noted that hysteresis was most marked in the lower lumbar spine and increased with the applied load. Hysteresis decreased when the same segment was loaded for the second time. This may explain why the intervertebral disk is less resistant to repetitive or vibrational loads than to sustained or single-impact loads. The number of load repetitions that can be tolerated before disk damage occurs has been extensively studied in fatigue tests of motion segments.[51, 61, 64, 65] Although there is little agreement between the different studies and experimental outcomes, it is generally concluded that risk of disk damage increases with load and number of cycles. Furthermore, major damage is inflicted by cyclic axial compressive loads, whereas cyclic flexion and extension and axial rotation may not be capable of producing any serious damage to the disk because of the protection provided by the ligaments and associated muscles.[66]

Mechanical Properties of Disk Tissue

Relatively few studies have been completed on the mechanical properties of disk tissue, with the exception of investigations involving the anulus fibrosus[39, 67, 68] and the cartilage end plates.[69] Because of the anisotropy and inhomogenicity of its structure, the mechanical properties of the anulus fibrosus vary with region and direction of applied load. To date, experiments have been performed to determine mechanical properties of single or multilayer samples of anulus fibrosus. Cylindrical or dumbbell-shaped samples are cut from different regions of the anulus and loaded in compression or tension, respectively. Samples are mounted and tested in universal testing machines to study tensile properties. Compressive properties are studied in uniaxial confined or unconfined compression, the characteristics of which are discussed later.

Figure 2–11 shows an example of a confined compression experiment.[70] A cylindrical sample is uniaxially confined with a load of 0.2 MPa, and its height variation is plotted as a function of time. To stabilize the hydration of tissue, the sample is bathed in physiologic saline solution.

In general, studies on anular mechanical properties have shown that axial compressive stiffness varies with location, being higher in outer regions and the posterior part than in the inner regions and anterior part.[39] Tensile stiffness shows higher values in the anterior and posterior parts as compared with the lateral parts and outer regions, which are stiffer than the inner regions.[68, 71] Thus, the central region near the nucleus pulposus appears to be the weakest area of the anulus, whereas

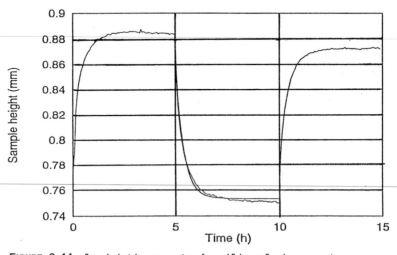

FIGURE 2–11   Sample height versus time for a 15-h confined compression experiment on anulus fibrosus tissue. The sample was taken from the outer region of the anulus and compressed with a load of 0.2 MPa. The gradual increase in sample height at the beginning of the experiment represents the swelling of the sample when it was placed in saline solution. The solid line indicates the mechanical behavior during the compression phase as predicted by a finite element model of the tissue. (Adapted from Houben GB, Drost MR, Huyghe JM, et al: Nonhomogeneous permeability of canine anulus fibrosus. Spine 22:7, 1997.)

the strongest parts are found on the anterior and posterior sides of the disk. With respect to the orientation of the anular samples tested in tension, Galante[42] has demonstrated that anulus layers are weakest when loaded in the axial direction and strongest when loaded along the major fiber direction.

Setton and colleagues[69] studied creep behavior of cartilaginous end plates in confined compression experiments. They found that creep rates of the end plates were significantly higher than those observed for articular cartilage. Possible changes in mechanical behavior with relation to biochemical composition and location within the end plate were not studied.

Modeling

To achieve more insight into the mechanical properties of the intervertebral disk, and in particular into the internal stresses and strains inside the disk, various mathematical models have been developed. The recent application of biphasic mixture models, describing a solid component and a fluid component in their formulation, is popularly used to predict the mechanical behavior of the disk.[39, 69, 72] These models are based on assumptions of elastic or viscoelastic material behavior and incorporate the movement of interstitial fluid. Hence, they are capable of predicting flow-dependent mechanical behavior. A third or fourth phase or component is added to reflect further the complicated interaction between the biochemical constituents and the mechanical behavior of the disk.[73, 74] With the increasing complexity of these models, however, experimental validation is also more difficult.[75] Furthermore, considering the increasing number of assumptions and simplifications, care should be taken to avoid overgeneralizing the numerical solutions of the models. Nevertheless, mathematical modeling is a helpful and necessary tool to study the biomechanics and related injury mechanisms of the intervertebral disk.

CLINICAL FEATURES AND AGING

Many spinal injuries are associated with disk failure; for example, up to 30% are directly or indirectly related to disk herniation.[76, 77] In addition, disk ruptures or degenerative changes in nonherniated disks are associated with low-back pain and whiplash injuries, which may lead to severe limitation in activity and constitute the most common cause of sick leave in industrialized countries.[78] Short-term, high-amplitude loads cause irreparable structural damage to the intervertebral disk when a stress higher than the ultimate failure stress is generated at a given point. The mechanism of failure during long-term, low-amplitude loads and repetitive loading of relatively low magnitude is entirely different and is due to fatigue failure: a tear develops at a point where the nominal stress is relatively high and enlarges, eventually leading to complete disk failure. Although exact load tolerance levels cannot be given, especially in the case of fatigue failure, it is clear that they are highly dependent on the chemical and structural composition of the disk, which changes with age and disease. Age-related changes in structure and composition of the intervertebral disk are responsible for a more than two-fold increase in the incidence of disk-related back problems in people 45 to 65 years of age, compared with those 18 to 44 years of age.[79] In addition, diseases such as osteoporosis and metabolic disorders such as ochronosis accompanied by disk calcification influence the composition of the disk and hence increase its sensitivity.[59]

With increasing age, the metabolic exchange in the tissues of the intervertebral disk retards, so that the tissues simultaneously change in biochemical quality and fluid content. The water content of the nucleus decreases from more than 80% in young adults to about 70% after the fifth decade.[80] The proteoglycan concentration and thus the water-binding capacity in the nucleus also decrease; by the age of 60 years, these measure one half the value of those in the young adult.[32] On the other hand, the concentration and diameter of collagen fibers increase, accompanied by an increase in collagen–proteoglycan binding. The relative concentration of type I fibers to type II fibers decreases. In contrast, the concentration and diameter of collagen fibers in the anulus fibrosus decreases,[36] and the ratio of type I to type II collagen increases.[81] As a result, the parallel fiber arrangement is gradually lost, and the distinction between the anulus and the nucleus vanishes. There is also evidence of a decrease in proteoglycan and water content of the anulus, but the influence of these changes on both the swelling pressure and the mechanical behavior of the anulus is unclear.[68] Age changes in the fibrocartilaginous end plates result in irregularly arranged cartilage tissue, which disappears with time and is replaced by bone.[82]

All these changes together lead to a biochemical and thus biomechanical compromise to the intervertebral disk, which eventually limits its ability to perform the required mechanical function. As disks degenerate, they become stiffer and less viscoelastic, with associated decreases in both creep and hysteresis.[62, 83] Consequently, the disks exhibit a diminished tolerance to normal loading. Load tolerance levels have been experimentally determined for whole-body segments under compression, tension, shear, and axial rotation. These values are summarized in Table 2–6[84] for different spinal levels. Generally, stress tolerance levels result from quasi-static, uniaxial tests and therefore cannot be extrapolated to more physiologic conditions. From Table 2–6, it can be concluded, however, that the larger lumbar motion segments can tolerate higher loads than the smaller and more cranial motion segments.

From the experiments on motion segments, it has been generally accepted that pure compressive loads do not directly cause disk failure. Virgin[58] observed that after compressing lumbar disks under loads severe enough to deform the anulus permanently, there was no evidence of herniation of nuclear material. He found that disks could support more than 4400 N. Even when an incision was made in the postolateral part of the anulus and the disk was loaded in compression, there was still no herniation. Brown and colleagues[51] found that the first component to fail under axial compression was the vertebra, in particular involving a central fracture of the end plates. Under further loading, the gelatinous material of the nucleus pulposus or even parts of the anulus fibrosus can enter the vertebral body.

The degeneratively altered disk shows another injury mechanism during compression. The dehydrated nucleus cannot absorb and laterally distribute any load. Hence, the axial load is transmitted by the anulus alone, so that the outer zones of the end plates are stressed relatively more than the central parts. Fractures of the outer zones of the end plate, therefore, become more probable with increasing degeneration of the intervertebral disk.

Tension experiments have demonstrated a relatively high vulnerability of the disk. Under tensile loading, the intervertebral disk is damaged before the adjacent vertebrae suffer any injury. As mentioned previously, mechanical properties and hence tensile strength of the intervertebral disk vary with the location in the disk, the anterior and posterior sides being the strongest parts. Values as high as 1.4 MPa have been reported as the maximal stresses tolerated by these areas, whereas the central region of the disk can tolerate tensile stresses up to 0.3 MPa.[51] Under normal physiologic loading conditions, the disk is seldom subjected to pure tensile loads, but local tensile stresses can occur in the anulus fibrosus in various conditions. Damaging tensile stresses are associated with the hyperextension, hyperflexion, and lateral inclination of the spine. Under these conditions, the disk ruptures near the end plate, and disk fragments can extrude from the intervertebral space.

With regard to axial rotation, the intervertebral disk is more resistant than the vertebral bones. Farfan and colleagues[52] tested the torsional characteristics of lumbar motion segments. They were unable to produce any radial tears in the disk, but circumferential separations of annular lamellae were observed. About 16 degrees of rotation was generally required to produce this type of damage. For degenerated disks, the angle of failure was somewhat smaller, that is, 14.5 degrees. The average failure torque for nondegenerated disks was 25% higher than that for the degenerated disks. When the tolerance for rotational loads was exceeded, ruptures in the external layer of the annulus fibrosus were observed near the end plate. Such tears may be the precursors of dorsolateral extrusion of the intervertebral disk.[59]

With shear, the periphery of the disk always experiences the greatest stress, and disk damage is usually seen in this area. It is relatively rare, however, for the disk to fail clinically from pure shear loading. Similarly, disk failure due to pure compressive, tensile, or rotational loading is a rare phenomenon. Clinical evidence of disk failure implies that the intervertebral disk most likely fails because of some combination of bending, tension, and torsion. For instance, pure compression experiments indicate that some factor other than compression must be involved in the production of acute herniation in healthy disks. It has been suggested that a combination of bending and

TABLE 2–6   Average Load Tolerance Values of Motion Segments of Different Spinal Levels Under (Quasi) Static Loading

SPINAL LEVEL	COMPRESSION (N)	TENSION (N)	SHEAR (N)	AXIAL ROTATION (N m)
Cervical spine	1700	1400	20	2
Thoracic spine	2800	2000	150	3
Lumbar spine	5000	2800	150	20

Data from references 47, 52, 54, 58, 66, 83, and 84.

torsional loads is necessary to produce this type of injury.[85] Similarly, rupture of the disk has been associated with coupled movements, namely, flexion or extension, both with a rotational component.

Only a few studies have investigated the fatigue tolerance levels of the intervertebral disk. By definition, fatigue tolerance may result from cyclic loads of relatively low amplitude, well within physiologic limits.[37] By subjecting lumbar motion segments to cyclic compressive loads, up to 80% of the ultimate failure load, at 0.5 Hz, Liu and others[64] reported end-plate failure after about 1000 cycles. From a compression fatigue study,[86] it can be concluded that the number of cycles to failure is inversely related to the applied compressive cycle stress raised to a power of 14. Thus, even a small increase in stress considerably decreases the number of cycles needed to produce disk failure.

As a result of the lack of adequate capillary perfusion, the intervertebral disk has a limited capacity for regeneration, even after extensive therapy and other clinical interventions. Extensive studies are being performed to develop intervertebral disk prostheses as a replacement for nonhealing and irreparable disks. So far, these studies have focused on fully artificial disks, mainly consisting of fiber-reinforced composites,[87] and on the development of cell-seeded structures. The latter alternative offers great possibilities considering biocompatibility, whereas the former can be more easily adapted to the required mechanical properties. However, complete experimental validation must be performed before these alternatives become available for application in the clinical field.

LIGAMENTS

GENERAL FEATURES

Skeletal ligaments are passive bands of fibrous tissue that connect the bony parts of articulating joints at two ligament–bone junctions. There is minimal stress concentration at the insertions of the ligament into the stiffer bone, owing to the presence of functionally graded materials, involving fibrocartilage with varying degrees of mineralization. The ligaments are constructed to resist tensile forces without considerable elongation. Hence, they are composed of densely packed fiber bundles, which run mostly parallel along the longitudinal axis of the tissue. The primary functions of the passive ligaments are to stabilize the joints and to guide and restrict articular movements. In addition, they function as a signal source for reflexes and provide proprioceptive information about movements and postures.

Ligaments have a number of gross forms. In the hip and shoulder joints, some ligaments are local reinforcements of the joint capsule that primarily act to stabilize the joint. Extraarticular ligaments, such as the medial collateral ligament (MCL) of the knee, or intraarticular ligaments, such as the anterior cruciate ligament (ACL) in the knee, on the other hand, are distinct structures that guide movements and restrain the joint from abnormal excursions. In general, extraarticular and intraarticular ligaments are relatively long, cord-like structures, whereas capsular ligaments are broad, bandlike structures, in which different fiber bundles are loaded during different types of movements. Because of the high incidence of injuries to the ligaments in the knee, such as the ACL or MCL, these structures have been studied intensively and have been described widely in the literature.

STRUCTURE AND COMPOSITION

Most ligaments consist of nearly parallel-fibered bundles of collagen. There are two exceptions: the ligamentum nuchae and the ligamenta flava along the spinal column, which contain large amounts (almost 75% of the dry weight) of elastic fibers. In normal ligaments, however, collagen predominates and constitutes between 70% and 80% of the dry weight.[88] Normal ligaments contain more than 90% type I collagen with less than 10% type III collagen. Type IV collagen is present in smaller quantities. Other constituents of ligament tissue are fibroblasts (3% to 6%), proteoglycans, water, and elastin. The noncellular composition of ligaments is included in Table 2–7.[89]

Both collagen and elastic fibers influence the mechanical function of ligaments. The structure and mechanical behavior of collagen fibers was described previously. Contrary to collagen fibers, elastic fibers can be easily stretched to a considerable length—up to 200% of their unloaded length—at relatively low loads. At higher loads, they rupture suddenly. Elastic fibers are of great importance to the recovery of tissues after loading.

TABLE 2–7   **Proportion of Noncellular Components in a Normal Ligament**

COMPOSITE	WET WEIGHT (%)	DRY WEIGHT (%)
Collagen	25–32	70–80
Elastin	1–4	2–9
Proteoglycans	0.3	1
Water	60–65	—

Their function in recovery, however, reduces toward maximal loading levels because their maximum strength is about five times lower than that of collagen.[90]

Elastic fibers are composed mainly of elastin, a hydrophobic, nonglycosylated protein composed of about 830 amino acid residues. Elastin molecules are secreted by the fibroblasts in the ECM, where they form filaments and sheets in which the elastin molecules are highly cross-linked to one another to generate an extensive network. The cross-links are formed between lysine residues by the same mechanism that operates in cross-linking collagen molecules. Elastin molecules are unlike most other proteins in that their function requires their polypeptide backbone to remain unfolded as "random coils." It is the cross-linked, random-coil structure of the elastic fiber network that allows the network to stretch and recoil. Sheaths constituted by type I, III, and IV collagens surround elastic and collagen fibers, fiber bundles, and whole ligaments. The individual fibers attach either to the periosteum or directly to the bone, where they join the collagen of the bone in Sharpey's fibers.

The structural organization of fiber bundles in ligaments is less well organized than in tendinous tissue. In most cordlike ligaments, nearly all fibers run in parallel. Some fibers, however, run crisscross through the ligament (Fig. 2–12). Therefore, not all fiber bundles are stretched when loaded along the main fiber axis. Consequently, ligaments are less strong than tendons. In broad bandlike ligaments, different portions of the structure have different fiber directions, with the main fiber direction dependent on the function and working range of the particular portion. In the cruciate ligaments of the knee, fiber organization is even more complex. The fibers are twisted between 90 and 180 degrees from the femoral to the tibial attachment sites, and as a result, different portions of the cruciate ligaments function at different rotation and knee flexation angles.[91, 92]

As with other tissues in the human body, ligaments exhibit remodeling behavior. The metabolism of the fibroblasts within the tissue responds to environmental stimuli and functional needs and alters the ultrastructure, chemistry, and physical properties of the ligament. In this way, ligaments are capable of hypertrophy, atrophy, and healing responses. Carefully conducted training protocols may increase tensile strength and stiffness of ligaments,[93] whereas controlled, functional stresses applied to a damaged ligament stimulate the healing process by increasing fibril diameters.[94] During immobilization or disuse, on the other hand, ligament structure deteriorates, and mechanical properties are drastically decreased.[95] Although this effect is not irreversible, it may be present for a considerable period of time. In primates immobilized for 8 weeks, the ultimate tensile strength of the ACL fell to 60% of the original strength. After 5 months of recovery, only 80% of the original strength was restored, and 12 months of recovery were needed to regain 90% of the original strength.[96]

BIOMECHANICAL CONSIDERATIONS

Like other soft connective tissue, ligaments display time and loading history–dependent viscoelastic behavior.[97, 98] These mechanical characteristics are influenced by the structural organization of the fiber bundles; the relative amount of collagen, elastin, and proteoglycans; and the interactions between tissue constituents.

The primary role of ligaments is to resist tensile loading; hence, their mechanical properties are commonly measured in tensile loading experiments. Usually, isolated cadaveric bone–ligament–bone complexes of human or animal origin, such as the rabbit femur–MCL–tibia complex, are used for this purpose. The ligament is tested with the bones affixed to clamps to produce uniform stress distributions across the ligament. Load can be measured, for instance, with load cells[99] or omega-shaped strain gauges,[100] whereas elongation can be determined using displacement transducers[101] or optical techniques, such as the video dimensional analyzer system.[102] The resulting load-elongation relations and parameters, such as stiffness, ultimate load, ultimate elongation, and energy absorbed to failure, are representative of the whole bone–ligament–bone complex. Geometric cross-

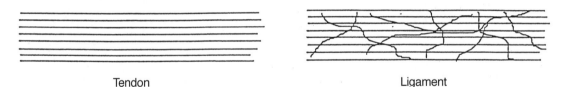

Tendon   Ligament

FIGURE 2–12   Structural organization of fibers in a normal tendon compared with that of fibers in a ligament.

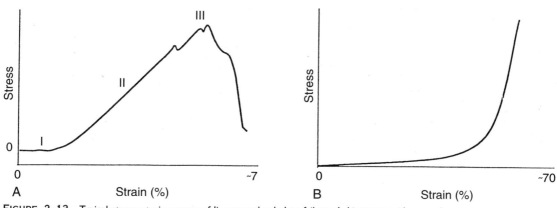

FIGURE 2–13   Typical stress–strain curves of ligaments loaded to failure. A, Ligament with normal composition. B, Ligament with high concentration of elastin.

sectional data for the ligament tissue and strain data are required to obtain a stress–strain curve of the ligament alone, which can be used to calculate, for instance, modulus, ultimate tensile strength, and ultimate strain of the ligament tissue.[103] Indirect methods using a mass measure divided by specimen length, as well as direct methods such as laser micrometer systems, have been employed to determine the cross-sectional shape and area of a ligament.[104, 105] In the laser micrometer method, the widths of the tissue are measured as the specimen is rotated about its longitudinal axis.

A typical stress–strain curve for most ligaments in uniaxial tension is shown in Figure 2–13A. This curve starts with a nonlinear toe region (region I), where the resulting stress per unit strain gradually increases. The toe region is believed to reflect uncrimping of collagen fibers and is followed by a rather linear segment of the curve (region II) when the fiber bundles are optimally aligned in parallel and the collagen triple helix is stretched. Toward the end of the linear segment, interfibrillar slippage occurs, and individual fibers start to rupture.[106] Finally, the curve begins to bend toward the strain axis (region III) and reaches a point of ultimate stress; the stress then decays while more and more fibers rupture.[96] The stress–strain curve of ligaments with a high concentration of elastin, like the ligamenta flava, is entirely different and resembles the stress–strain curve of elastin (Fig. 2–13B). Here, considerable elongation is possible before stiffness increases. At this point, the stiffness increases sharply, and the ligament ruptures suddenly thereafter.[90]

Numerous studies have been performed to determine the biomechanical properties of various ligaments and to assess the effects of several physiologic factors, including aging and exercise, on the biomechanical properties. Table 2–8 provides

data from a range of studies that have focused on stress–strain properties of ligament tissue as determined from the uniaxial tension tests on bone–ligament–bone complexes.[107–114] As can be observed, the reported mechanical properties of ligaments have been widely divergent. For example, ultimate strains at failure range from 5% to more than 40%. One study reports strain to failure as high as 93%.[115] As with the other soft tissues, the variability of data can be attributed to specimen considerations such as age, species, and anatomic location, and to experimental factors, such as testing method, loading history, and accuracy of applied techniques.

Mechanical properties of ligaments are generally determined in vitro because the measurement of loads, ligament length, and cross-section in vivo is extremely difficult. Tipton and colleagues[116] determined the uniaxial load-elongation properties of the femur–MCL–tibia complex of anaesthetized rats in vivo and compared the results with those obtained in vitro. Linear stiffness and ultimate load at failure for the in vivo specimens were 6% and 4% lower, respectively, whereas the ultimate elongation was 12% higher. The major drawback of these in vivo experiments[116] is that during uniaxial tensile testing of the bone–ligament–bone complexes, nearly all fibers along the loading axis are stretched simultaneously. This situation is very unlike the normal physiologic situation and may provide a false impression of the functional properties of ligament. Thus, care should be taken when interpreting the properties listed in Table 2–8.

Modeling

Various mathematical and numerical models have been developed to study mechanical properties of

TABLE 2–8   **Tensile Properties of a Range of Ligaments From Various Sources**

LIGAMENT AND SOURCE	ULTIMATE STRESS (MPa)	ULTIMATE STRAIN (%)	MODULUS* (MPa)	STRAIN RATE (%/S)	REFERENCE NO.
Monkey ACL	66.1 ± 8.4	47 ± 5.6	186 ± 26	66	115
Human young adult ACL	66.1 ± 8.4	44.3 ± 8.5	111 ± 26	100	115
Human lateral collateral ligament	32–44	10–17	360–410	100	116
Human ACL	30–40	14–16	280–330	100	116
Human PCL	35–43	14–18	280–440	100	116
Human lateral collateral ankle	24.2–46.2	13–17	217–512	0.13	117
Human medial collateral ankle	15.6–34	10–33	100–321	0.13	117
Sheep ACL	60–124	45–93	180–437	(8.3 mm/s)	107
Rabbit mature MCL	75.2 ± 2.4	9.5 ± 0.5	700 ± 70	0.01	118
	106.7 ± 6.8	13.0 ± 1.0	760 ± 160	222	
Human wrist joint ligaments	—	—	22.6–119.3	66	119
Rabbit ACL	42	8	711	0.016	120
	50	10	674	1.3	
	68	9	930	381	
Human older PCL	24–36	18.0–19.5	145–248	50	121
Human coracoacromial ligament	25.3 ± 8.7	5.1 ± 1.2	658.4 ± 261.3	0.1	122

*The modulus was generally estimated from the linear region of the stress–strain curve.
ACL, anterior cruciate ligament; MCL, medial collateral ligament; PCL, posterior cruciate ligament.

ligaments. For example, Fung[117, 118] used advanced theories of viscoelasticity to characterize time- and history-dependent properties of a range of soft tissues. Numerical models have also been developed, using combinations of ideal elastic, viscous, and plastic elements in parallel and in series with each other.[119] Three-dimensional, computer-simulated models of whole joints (e.g., the knee joint) permit the analysis of the relations between various ligament properties and ligament function.[120, 121] In addition, computer-simulated conditions may provide clinically relevant data that cannot be obtained otherwise. For example, application of computer models to ACL replacement can help determine the ideal anatomic insertion points for reconstruction.[122] Experimental validation of model predictions, however, is difficult owing to lack of realistic in vivo data.

CLINICAL FEATURES OF AGING

The most common injuries to the ligaments are acute ruptures caused by high strain rate supramaximal tensile loads. For example, ACL and MCL ruptures account for as much as 77% of all acute injuries to the knee.[123] Other ligament injuries are overload injuries due to repetitive submaximal loading. These injuries result in microtears, followed by inflammation reactions and sometimes calcification of the ligament tissue. Both types of injuries frequently occur as a consequence of sports activities, with American football, soccer, and skiing accounting for many of

the acute ligament ruptures in athletics, pitching, racquet sports, and swimming being responsible for most of the overload injuries. Tensile failure of a ligament, resulting either in acute rupture or in microtears, is a result of the weakest link in the bone–ligament–bone complex. It can occur at the insertion sites, which is known as *avulsion;* within the ligament itself (substance tear); or as a combination of both. Some investigators reason that the failure mode is strain rate dependent in that avulsion failures result primarily from slow extension rates, whereas ligament substance tears result from high extension rates.[107, 124] This suggests that with increasing strain rate, the increase in tissue strength is higher at the bone–ligament junction than in the ligament itself. Other investigators have shown that failure modes are independent of strain rate and merely depend on the maturation of the loaded bone–ligament–bone complex. In a study of rabbits grouped by age ranging from 1.5 to 15 months, Woo and associates[125] showed that the ligament substance matured earlier than the ligament–bone junction. Therefore, in the immature animals, ligaments failed by avulsion, whereas in the mature animals, ligaments failed by substance tear.[126] Ligament mechanical properties change considerably with maturation and aging. Stiffness, strength, and energy required to rupture the tissue peak during late maturity and then decline.[127, 128] In the ACL, for example, stiffness and ultimate load of bone–ligament–bone specimens obtained from subjects at old age are two to three times lower than

ACL specimens obtained from young adults.[107, 129] Similar to mature bone–ligament–bone complexes, aged bone–ligament–bone complexes fail by ligament substance tear.

Ligament Healing and Repair

It has been recognized that extraarticular ligaments, such as the MCL, can generally heal effectively when injured,[130, 131] whereas intraarticular ligaments, such as the ACL, do not heal effectively.[132] Ruptured ACL ligaments do not heal because the torn ends do not meet and new tissue does not fill the gap,[133] even if the ends are appositioned by sutures or wires.[134] Therefore, surgical repair of the ACL usually aims at reconstruction of the ruptured ligament by grafts. Most commonly used are autografts, such as the patellar tendon or semitendinosus tendon, but in recent years, allografts or synthetic polymeric materials have also been used.[89] In the United States, about 50,000 ligament reconstructions are performed each year, most of which are performed to reconstruct a ruptured ACL.[135] The aim of reconstructive surgery is to restore normal passive function of the ligaments and the laxity characteristics of the knee joint. Whether a reconstruction is successful depends on the mechanical properties of the graft, its pretension,[136] and its position in the knee.[91, 136]

Functional and mechanical tests on reconstructed ligaments indicate that grafts that mimic closely the structure and mechanics of the natural knee ligament have a higher chance of success. For example, the use of two distinct segments with separate insertion sites and pretension, unlike a graft consisting of one individual bundle, gives more stability during flexion of the knee.[137] Extensive evaluations of reconstructed ACLs, however, show that the rate of success is less than perfect.[138, 139] Generally, there is a marked, prolonged postoperative weakening of ligament replacements. After 1 year, autografts have less than 80% of the tensile strength and 50% of the ultimate load that they had before transfer.[140] This weakening is caused partly by the inability to reproduce in the graft the stresses and strains of the collagen fibers found in the original ligament. Moreover, ligament replacements may not achieve normal strength and normal morphology, including collagen fiber diameter, because of the abnormal loading states in those replacements.[122] As with other connective tissues, tissue-engineered equivalents of ligaments are being developed for repair and healing of irreversibly damaged structures or as a model to study environmental factors on ligament healing.[141, 142] With time, this development may lead to a new generation of ligament replacements with optimized morphology and properties.

TENDONS

GENERAL FEATURES

Tendons, like ligaments, are highly fibrous regular connective tissues, in which the fibers are regularly orientated with respect to one another to form thicker bundles. Tendons connect muscles to structural elements such as bone, adopting the form of cords or straps, and are round, oval, or elongated in cross-section. Tendons are highly resistant to extension but are relatively flexible and can therefore be angulated around bone surfaces or deflected beneath retinacula to alter the direction of the muscular pull. Tendons consist of fascicles of collagen fibers largely running parallel to the long axis of the tendon. Their surface is generally smooth, although longitudinal ridging due to the arrangement of coarse fasciculi is common in larger tendons. Bundles of collagen fibrils, each 0.02 to 0.20 μm in diameter, assemble into fibers 1 to 20 μm in diameter. These fibers bundle into the fascicles, within which the fibers are more or less longitudinally orientated. Within the fascicles, the fibers are bound by a small amount of an amorphous mucoprotein cement. It is well established that the fibers demonstrate a planar crimping, of wavelength between 100 and 300 μm.

The areolar connective tissue that permeates the tendon between its fascicles provides a route for vessels and nerves. The blood supply of tendons is provided by a relatively sparse array of small arterioles, which run longitudinally from the adjacent muscular tissues. These arterioles ramify in the interfascicular spaces, where they intercommunicate freely and are accompanied by veins. The longitudinal network in the tendon is augmented by small vessels from the surrounding areolar connective tissue or, where present, the synovial sheaths. Because vascular networks are of low density, tendons appear white.

The nerve supply of tendons appears to be mainly afferent, with no clear evidence of vasomotor control. Specialized afferent receptors, neurotendinous endings known as Golgi tendon organs, exist particularly near the tendinomuscular junction. Each is about 500 μm long and 100 μm in diameter and consists of a small bundle of tendon fibers enclosed in a delicate capsule. When tendons are stretched, these neurotendinous endings activate and initiate myotactic reflexes, which inhibit the development of excessive tension during muscular contraction.

STRUCTURE AND COMPOSITION

Tendons may be considered unidirectional fiber-reinforced composites, as indicated in Figure 2–12. The building block of the fibrous phase consists of tropocollagen molecules, which reinforce a matrix made up of a hydrated proteoglycan gel. Collagen constitutes at least 30% of the wet weight of tendons. The collagen fibers may be considered largely independent, although stress can be transferred from one fiber to its neighbor by shear in the matrix or by more specific cross-links. The tendons are surrounded by some loose connective tissue, the epitendon, which facilitates gliding of the tendon over extratendinous tissues as well as through synovial sheaths at the digits. The epitendon contains tendon cells that are physically joined to tendon fibroblasts inside the tendon. Both cell types are subjected to a combination of shear stresses during gliding as well as tension as a result of muscle contraction. In general, the cellular material occupies about 20% of the tissue volume, whereas the ECM accounts for the remaining 80%.

BIOMECHANICAL CONSIDERATIONS

Load Carriage

Tendons act as linking elements connecting muscles to bones, thus transmitting muscular pulls and external loads. In slow concentric activities, in which the inertial effects may be neglected, the maximal load to which the tendon may be subjected is the muscle isometric tetanic contraction, about equal to 0.35 N/mm² of muscle belly.[143] As an example, the isometric stress in the patellar tendon can be estimated at 29 MPa, based on the cross-sectional areas of 125 mm² and 10,300 mm² for the tendon and the quadriceps femoris muscle, respectively. Most daily activities, however, consist of quick eccentric movements, in which inertial effects play an important role. Experimental studies have indicated that these dynamic activities are associated with tendon stresses in the range of 42 to 110 MPa, the latter exceeding the established values of the ultimate tensile strength.[144, 145] In most cases, however, human tendons are so thick that there is no possibility of rupture by a single application of maximum load.

Healthy people are estimated to walk about 1 to 1.5 million strides per year.[21, 146] During locomotion, the musculoskeletal system is subjected to a constant external load, the body weight. Movement is achieved by muscular contraction and the consequent production of torque around the joints of the lower limbs. Evidently, any specific muscle–tendon unit produces a cyclic force with a constant maximal value, which is proportional to the external load. Because of muscle tone, a small amount of tension is always present, ensuring that the muscle–tendon units are taut even when the muscle is relaxed. Moreover, any possible slackening due to creep of the tendon would be eliminated by a reduction in the length of the muscle. Therefore, the in vivo repetitive loading pattern of tendons in the lower limbs may be broadly classified as a tension–tension square wave, as observed in the in vivo tensile load pattern in the Achilles tendon during various forms of locomotion.[145]

Biomechanical Studies

The load-bearing function of functional collagenous tissues prompted a plethora of biomechanical studies over several decades. The uniaxial tensile testing of animal and human tendons has been performed over many decades.[147–149] In vitro testing is fraught with practical difficulties associated with specimen preparation, gripping, and local strain measurements. When these are overcome, however, the resulting stress–strain curves for tendons are nonlinear, with a characteristic toe-in region followed by a linear region before failure. This is very similar to the form for ligaments (see Fig. 2–13A), which can be related to the structural aspects of the tissue, with the toe-in region at low stress levels producing a straightening of the crimped collagen fibers with an associated increase of the tangent modulus. A quasi-static test produces an ultimate tensile strength (UTS) of about 100 MPa and a failure strain of about 15%. The material properties are clearly dependent on the rate of tensile testing, with values for elastic modulus quoted within the range of 1 to 2 giga-pascals (GPa). More recently, dynamic characterization of human tendons has been performed.[150, 151] These tests emphasize the viscoelastic nature of these collagenous tissues.

A recent study addressed the in vitro fatigue behavior of human tendons.[152, 153] A linear model based on the median value, equivalent to a 50% probability of failure (or survival), was employed as illustrated in Figure 2–14. The relation of stress level against the median fatigue life produced a statistically significant linear model of the following form:

$$S = 101.25 - 14.83 \log (N)$$

where S is the normalized stress expressed as a percentage of the UTS, and N is the number of cycles to failure.

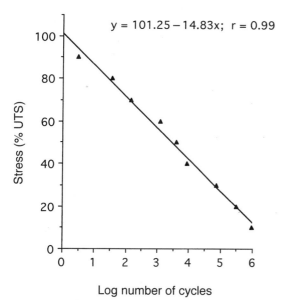

$y = 101.25 - 14.83x; \quad r = 0.99$

FIGURE 2–14   Fatigue life of human tendons. Normalized stress versus logarithm of median number of cycles to failure. UTS, ultimate tensile strength. (From Schechtman H: Mechanical Characterisation of Fatigue Failure in Human Tendons. PhD Thesis. London, University of London, 1995.)

This model predicted a static strength of 101.3 MPa, which was clearly within 1 standard deviation of the experimental data obtained in the quasistatic tensile tests. The linear model also suggested the absence of an endurance limit. Some analysis that takes into account in vivo healing was proposed. This analysis was able to explain the presence of intact tendons throughout the lifetime of a patient. The results implied a finite fatigue behavior with no apparent endurance limit. To explain the presence of intact tendons throughout the lifetime of a patient, the authors postulated the importance of remodeling processes in vivo.

CLINICAL FEATURES AND AGING

During aging, changes occur in the composition of tendon. In particular, the collagen content decreases with age, with an associated decrease in the mechanical strength, stiffness, and ability to withstand deformation.

Tissue trauma or injury can result from two basic mechanisms. A single-impact macrotrauma, such as a blow to a leg or a twisting injury of a joint, injures bone, muscle, tendon, ligament, and even neurovascular elements. The other mechanism of injury is repetitive microtrauma caused by the repeated exposure of tissue to low-magnitude force, which itself does not result in tissue injury.[154] The frequency of overuse injuries is esti-

mated to be about 30% to 50% of all sports-related injuries in the United States.[155] Tendon injuries are common examples of such injuries because during physical activity, much of the force is focused on the tendon component of the muscle–tendon–bone unit. Thus, rapid elongation of this unit with maximum uncoordinated muscle contraction may rupture healthy tendons.

Adult tendons have a low metabolic rate and vascularity. Increasing intratendinous tension causes a decrease in blood perfusion. As a result of persistent hypoxia, parts of the tendon may undergo fibrocartilaginous metaplasia.[156] In these cases, chondrocytes may mediate calcium deposition, which may proceed to the formation of discrete nodules within the tendons. This alters the biomechanical properties of the whole tendon.

Tendon Healing and Repair

Tendons, like ligaments, remodel in response to the mechanical demands placed on them.[157] This manifests as an increase in strength and stiffness when subjected to enhanced activity levels such as occur during physical training. By contrast, reducing the stress below normal levels, such as by stress shielding or immobilization, produces a decrease in strength and stiffness of the tendons.

It is well established that tendons are not well vascularized or well innervated; therefore, the healing response is limited. Much effort has been directed toward understanding the mechanisms associated with the stimulation of tendon healing. One such study has investigated the potential for mechanical stimulation in conjunction with growth factors to stimulate tendon cell activity in vitro. Banes and colleagues[158] applied loading by means of a commercial strain unit (Flexercell, Flexcell International, McKeesport, PA), in which cells were attached to a collagen substrate at the base of culture plates. Negative pressure was applied in a cyclic manner to provide deflection of the base of the plate. Results highlighted the complex mechanisms involved in the mechanical control of cell division and maintenance of matrix in tissue required to resist high tensile strains.

CONCLUSIONS

Certain features are common to the discussion of the biomechanics of all types of soft tissues:

- The complex microstructure, which varies with site, age, and so forth, and the lack of standard test methods have led to the diversity of biomechanical data in the literature. To date, there has been little consensus regarding a set of material constants that can uniquely characterize the properties of healthy soft tissues. This presents a major obstacle in producing a design template for replacement tissues.

- Biomechanical changes are apparent in soft tissues as a result of aging and disease. In addition, deviation from normal biomechanical loading, such as with joint immobilization, affects the structure and biomechanical integrity of the tissues.
- Synthetic options for the repair of soft tissues have limited success. More recent options, incorporating cell-engineering principles, might be effective in the future in creating tissue implants with mechanical integrity.

References

1. Materials Technology Foresight in Biomaterials. London, Institute of Materials, 1995.
2. Maroudas A, Stockwell RA, Nachemson A, Urban JP: Factors involved in the nutrition of the human lumbar intervertebral disc: Cellularity and diffusion of glucose in vitro. J Anat 120:113, 1975.
3. Mayne R: Cartilage collagens. Arthritis Rheum 32(3):241, 1989.
4. Weiss C, Rosenberg L, Helfet AJ: An ultrastructure study of normal young adult human articular cartilage. J Bone Joint Surg 50A:663, 1968.
5. Balazs EA, Bloom GD, Swann DA: Fine structure and glycosaminoglycan content of the surface layer of articular cartilage. Fed Proc Fed Am Soc Exp Biol 25:1813, 1966.
6. Broom N: The altered biomechanical state of human femoral osteoarthritic articular cartilage. Arthritis Rheum 27:1028, 1984.
7. McCall JG: Scanning electron microscopy of articular surface. Lancet 2:1194, 1968.
8. Bullough P, Goodfellow JG: The significance of the fine structure of articular cartilage. J Bone Joint Surg 50B:852, 1968.
9. Knight MM: Deformation of isolated articular chondrocytes cultured in agarose constructs. PhD Thesis. London, University of London, 1997.
10. Maroudas A: Physicochemical properties of articular cartilage. *In* Freeman MAR (ed): Adult Articular Cartilage. London, Pitman, 1979, p 215.
11. Mak AF, Lai WM, Mow VC: Biphasic indentation of articular cartilage. I Theoretical solution. J Biomech 20:703, 1987.
12. Armstrong CG, Mow VC: Variations in the intrinsic mechanical properties of human articular cartilage with age, degeneration and water content. J Bone Joint Surg 64(A):88, 1982.
13. Kempson GE: Mechanical properties of articular cartilage. *In* Freeman (ed): Adult Articular Cartilage. London, Pitman, 1979, p 281.
14. Bader DL: The relationship between the mechanical properties and the structure of adult human articular cartilage. PhD Thesis. Southampton, UK: University of Southampton, 1985.
15. Athanasiou KA, Rosenwasser MP, Buckwalter JA, et al: Interspecies comparisons of in situ intrinsic mechanical properties of distal femoral cartilage. J Orthop Res 9:330, 1991.
16. Woo SL-Y, Simon BR, Kuei SC, Akeson WH: Quasi-linear viscoelastic properties of normal articular cartilage. J Biomech Eng 102:85, 1980.
17. Coletti JM, Akeson W, Woo SL-Y: A comparison of the physical behaviour of normal articular cartilage and the arthroplasty surface. J Bone Joint Surg 54(A):147, 1972.
18. Bader DL, Kempson GE: The short-term compressive properties of adult human articular cartilage. Biomed Mater Eng 4:245, 1994.
19. Bader DL, Kempson GE, Barrett AJ, Webb W: The effects of leukocyte elastase on the mechanical properties of adult human cartilage in tension. Biochim Biophys Acta 677:103, 1981.
20. Weightman B: Tensile fatigue of human articular cartilage. J Biomech 9:192, 1976.
21. Weightman B, Chappell DJ, Jenkins EA: A second study of tensile fatigue properties of human articular cartilage. Ann Rheum Dis 37:58, 1978.
22. Wachtel E, Maroudas A, Schneiderman R: Age-related changes in collagen packing of human articular cartilage. Biochim Biophys Acta 1243, 239, 1995.
23. Lyrra T, Jurvelin J, Pitkanen P, et al: Indentation instrument for the measurement of cartilage stiffness under arthroscopic control. Med Eng Phys 17:395, 1995.
24. Lee DA, Bader DL: Compressive strains at physiological frequencies influence the metabolism of chondrocytes seeded in agarose. J Orthop Res 15(2):181, 1997.
25. Brittberg M, Lindahl A, Nilsson A, et al: The treatment of deep cartilage defects in the knee with autologous chondrocyte transplantation. N Engl J Med 331:889, 1994.
26. Kim WS, Vacanti JP, Cima LG, et al: Cartilage engineered in predetermined shapes employing cell transplantation on synthetic biodegradable polymers. Plast Reconstr Surg 94(2):233, 1994.
27. Paige KT, Cima LG, Yaremchuk MJ, et al: De novo cartilage generation using calcium alginate-chondrocyte constructs. Plast Reconstr Surg 97(1):168, 1996.
28. Andersson GBJ, Ortengren R, Nachemson A, Elfstrom G: Lumbar disc pressure and myoelectric back muscle activity during sitting. I. Studies on an experimental chair. Scand J Rehabil Med 3:104, 1974.
29. Nachemson A, Morris JM: In vivo measurement of intradiscal pressure: Discometry, a method for

the determination of pressure in the lower lumbar discs. J Bone Joint Surg 46A:1077, 1964.

30. Hukins DWL: Disc structure and function. *In* Ghosh P (ed): The Biology of the Intervertebral Disc, vol 1. Boca Raton, FL, CRC Press, 1988, p 1.

31. Eyre DR: Biochemistry of the intervertebral disc. Int Rev Connect Tissue Res 8:227, 1979.

32. Gower WE, Pedrini V: Age related variations in protein-polysaccharide from human nucleus pulposus, annulus fibrosus, and costal cartilage. J Bone Joint Surg 51 A:1154, 1969.

33. Lyons G, Eisenstein SM, Sweet MB: Biochemical changes in intervertebral disc degeneration. Biochim Biophys Acta 673:443, 1981.

34. Roberts S, Menage J, Urban JP: Biochemical and structural properties of the cartilage end plate and its relation to the intervertebral disc. Spine 14:166, 1989.

35. Ghosh P, Bushell GR, Taylor TKF, Akeson WK: Collagens, elastin and non-collagenous protein of the intervertebral disc. Clin Orthop Relat Res 129:124, 1977.

36. Marchand F, Ahmed AM: Investigation of the laminate structure of lumbar disc annulus fibrosus. Spine 15:402, 1990.

37. Panjabi MM, White AA: Physical properties and functional biomechanics of the spine. *In* White AA, Panjabi MM (eds): Clinical Biomechanics of the Spine. Philadelphia, JB Lippincott 1990, p 3.

38. Eyre DR: Collagens of the disc. *In* Ghosh P (ed): The Biology of the Intervertebral Disc, vol 1. Boca Raton, FL, CRC Press, 1988, p 171.

39. Best BA, Guilak F, Setton LA, et al: Compressive mechanical properties of the human annulus fibrosus and their relationship to biochemical composition. Spine 19:212, 1994.

40. Johnstone B, Urban JPG, Roberts J, Menage J: The fluid content of the human intervertebral disc. Spine 17:412, 1992.

41. Junghanns H: Die functionelle Pathologie der Zwischenwirbelscheiben als Grundlage fur klinische Betrachtungen. Arch Klin Chir 267:393, 1951.

42. Galante JO: Tensile properties of the human lumbar annulus fibrosus. Acta Orthop Scand Suppl 100:1, 1967.

43. Nachemson A: Lumbar intradiscal pressure. Acta Orthop Scand Suppl 43:1, 1960.

44. De Jager M: Mathematical modelling of the human cervical spine: A survey of the literature. *In* Proceedings of the International Conference on the Biomechanics of Impacts (IRCOBI). 1993, p 213.

45. Panjabi MM, Summers DJ, Pelker RR, et al: Three-dimensional load-displacement curves due to forces on the cervical spine. J Orthop Res 4:152, 1986.

46. Panjabi MM, Lydon C, Vasavada A, et al: On the understanding of clinical instability. Spine 19:2642, 1994.

47. Moroney SP, Schultz AB, Miller JAA, Andersson GBJ: Load-displacement properties of lower cervical spine motion segments. J Biomech 21:769, 1988.

48. Goel VK, Goyal S, Clark CR, et al: Kinematics of the whole lumbar spine: Effect of discectomy. Spine 10:543, 1985.

49. Goel VK, Clark CR, Harris KG, Schulte KR: Kinematics of the cervical spine: Effect of multiple total laminectomy and facet wiring. J Orthop Res 6:611, 1988.

50. Berkson MH, Nachemson A, Schultz AB: Mechanical properties of human lumbar spine motion segments. 2. Responses in compression and shear, influence of gross morphology. J Biomech Eng 101:53, 1979.

51. Brown T, Hanson R, Yorra A: Some mechanical tests on the lumbo-sacral spine with particular reference to the intervertebral disc. J Bone Joint Surg 39A:1135, 1957.

52. Farfan HF, Cossette JW, Robertson GH, et al: The effects of torsion on the lumbar intervertebral joint: The role of torsion in the production of disc degeneration. J Bone Joint Surg 52A:468, 1970.

53. Goel VK, Clark CK, McGowan D, Goyal S: An in-vitro study of the kinematics of the normal, injured and stabilized cervical spine. J Biomech 17:363, 1984.

54. Hirsch C, Nachemson A: A new observation on the mechanical behavior of lumbar disc. Acta Orthop Scand 23:254, 1954.

55. Miller JAA, Schultz AB, Andersson GBJ: Load-displacement behaviour of sacroiliacal joints. J Orthop Res 5:92, 1987.

56. Shea M, Edwards WT, White AA., Hayes WC: Variations in stiffness and strength along the human cervical spine. J Biomech 24:95, 1991.

57. Tencer A, Ahmed A, Burke D: Some static mechanical properties of the lumbar intervertebral joint, intact and injured. J Biomech Eng 104:193, 1982.

58. Virgin W: Experimental investigations into physical properties of intervertebral disc. J Bone Joint Surg 33B:607, 1951.

59. Junghanns H: Clinical Implications of Normal Biomechanical Stresses on Spinal Function. Aspen, CO, 1990.

60. McNally DS, Adams MA: Internal intervertebral disc mechanics as revealed by stress profilometry. Spine 17:66, 1992.

61. Adams MA, Hutton WC: The effect of posture on the fluid content of intervertebral discs. Spine 8:665, 1983.

62. Broberg KB: Slow deformation of intervertebral discs. J Biomech 26:501, 1993.

63. Adams MA, Dolan P, Hutton WC, Porter RW: Diurnal changes in spinal mechanics and their clinical significance. J Bone Joint Surg 72:266, 1990.

64. Liu YK, Njus G, Buckwalter J, Wakano K: Fatigue response of lumbar intervertebral joints under axial cyclic loading. Spine 6:857, 1983.

65. Goel VK, Voo L-M, Weinstein JN, et al:

Response of the ligamentous lumbar spine to cyclic bending loads. Spine 13:294, 1988.

66. Goel VK, Weinstein JN: Time-dependent biomechanical response of the spine. *In* Goel VK, Weinstein JN (eds): Biomechanics of the Spine: Clinical and Surgical Perspective. Boca Raton, FL, CRC Press, 1990.

67. Drost MR, Willems P, Snijders H, et al: Confined compression of canine annulus fibrosus under chemical and mechanical loading. J Biomech Eng 117:390, 1995.

68. Ebara A, Iatridis JC, Setton LA, et al: Tensile properties of nondegenerate human lumbar annulus fibrosus. Spine 21:452, 1996.

69. Setton LA, Zhu WB, Mow VC: Compressive properties of the cartilage endplate of the baboon lumbar spine. J Orthop Res 11:228, 1993.

70. Houben GB, Drost MR, Huyghe JM, et al: Nonhomogeneous permeability of canine annulus fibrosus. Spine 22:7, 1997.

71. Skaggs DL, Weidenbaum M, Iatridis JC, et al: Regional variation in tensile properties and biochemical composition of the human lumbar annulus fibrosus. Spine 19:1310, 1994.

72. Simon BR, Gaballa M: Poroelastic finite element models for the spinal motion segment in including ionic swelling. *In* Spilker RL, Simon BR (eds): Computational Methods in Bioengineering. ASME, 1988, p 93.

73. Snijders J, Huyghe J, Janssen J: Triphasic finite element model for swelling porous media. Int J Num Meth Fluids 20:1039, 1997.

74. Huyghe JM, Janssen JD: Quadriphasic mechanics of swelling incompressible porous media. Int J Eng Sci 35:793, 1997.

75. Oomens CWJ, Heus HJ, Huyghe et al: Validation of the triphasic mixture theory for a mimic of intervertebral disk tissue. Biomimetics 3:171, 1995.

76. Kalfas I, Wilberger J, Goldberg A, Protsko ER: Magnetic resonance imaging in acute spinal cord trauma. Neurosurgery 23:295, 1988.

77. Mirvis SE, Geisler FH, Jelinek JJ, et al: Acute cervical spine trauma: Evaluation with 1.5 T MR imaging. Radiology 166:807, 1988.

78. Andersson GBJ; Epidemiology. *In* Weinstein JN, Rydevik BL, Sonntag VKH (eds): Essentials of the Spine. New York, Raven 1995, p 1.

79. Praemer A, Furner S, Rice DP: Musculoskeletal conditions in the United States. Park Ridge, IL, American Academy of Orthopaedic Surgeons, 1992, p 26.

80. Panagiotacopulos ND, Pope MH, Block R, Krag MH: Water content in human intervertebral discs. II. Viscoelastic behaviour. Spine 12:918, 1987.

81. Pearce RJ: Morphologic and chemical aspects of aging. *In* Buckwalter JA, Goldberg VM, Wood SLY (eds): Musculoskeletal Soft-Tissue Aging: Impact on Mobility. Rosemont, IL, American Academy of Orthopaedic Surgeons, 1993, p 363.

82. Bernick S, Cailliet R: Vertebral end-plate changes with aging of human vertebrae. Spine 7:97, 1982.

83. Markoff KL: Stiffness and damping characteristics of the thoracic lumbar spine. *In* Proceedings of the NIH Workshop on Bioengineering Approaches to the Problems of the Spine, 1970.

84. Sonoda T: Studies on the strength for compression, tension and torsion of the human vertebral column. J Kyoto Prof Med 71:659, 1962.

85. Farfan HF: Hypothesis of degenerative process. *In* Farfan HF (ed): Mechanical Disorders of the Low Back. Philadelphia, Lea & Febiger, 1973, p 201.

86. Hansson TH, Keller TS, Spengler DM: Mechanical behaviour of the lumbar spine. II. Fatigue strength during dynamic compressive loading. J Orthop Res 5:479, 1987.

87. Lee CK, Langrana NA, Parsons JR, Zimmerman MC: Development of a prosthetic intervertebral disc. Spine 16:S253, 1991.

88. Amiel D, Frank C, Harwood F, et al: Tendons and ligaments: A morphological and biochemical comparison. J Orthop Res 1:257, 1984.

89. Silver FH: Biomaterials, medical devices, and tissue engineering. London, Chapman & Hall, 1994.

90. Nachemson AL, Evans JH: Some mechanical properties of the third human lumbar interlaminar ligament (ligament flavium). J Biomech 1:211, 1968.

91. Blankevoort L, Huiskes R, DeLange A: Recruitment of knee-joint ligaments. J Biomech Eng 113:94, 1991.

92. Amis AA, Dawkins GPC: Functional anatomy of the anterior cruciate ligament-fibre bundle actions related to ligament replacements and injuries. J Bone Joint Surg 73B:260, 1991.

93. Tipton CM, Vailas AC, Matthes RD: Experimental studies on the influences of physical activity on ligaments, tendons, and joints: A brief review. Acta Med Scand Suppl 771:157, 1986.

94. Williams IF, McCullagh KG, Silver IA: The distribution of types I and III collagen and fibronectin in the healing equine tendon. Connect Tissue Res 12:211, 1984.

95. Viidik A: Structure and function of normal and healing tendons. *In* Mow VC, Ratcliffe A, Woo SL-Y (eds): Biomechanics of Diarthrodial Joints, vol 1. New York, Springer-Verlag, 1990, p 3.

96. Noyes FR: Functional properties of knee ligaments and alterations induced by immobilization. Clin Orthop 123:210, 1977.

97. Johnson GA, Tramaglini DM, Levine RE, et al: Age related changes in the tensile and viscoelastic properties of the human patellar tendon. J Orthop Res 12:796, 1994.

98. Weisman G, Pope MH, Johnson RJ: The effect of cyclic loading on knee ligaments. Trans Orthop Res Soc 4:24, 1979.

99. Amiel D, Woo SL-Y, Harwood FL, Akeson WH: The effect of immobilization on collagen turnover in connective tissue: A biochemical-

biomechanical correlation. Acta Orthop Scand 53:325, 1982.

100. Durselen L, Claes L: Ligament strain measurements using strain gauge equipped omega transducers. Workshop on Biomechanics of Human Knee Ligaments. Ulm, Germany, 1987.

101. Arms SW, Pope MH, Boyle JB: Knee medial collateral ligament strain. Trans Orthop Res Soc 7:47, 1982.

102. Woo SL, Gomez MA, Seguchi Y, et al: Measurement of mechanical properties of ligament substance from a bone-ligament-bone preparation. J Orthop Res 1:22, 1983.

103. Woo SL, Chan SS, Yamaji T: Biomechanics of knee ligament healing, repair and reconstruction. J Biomech 30:431, 1997.

104. Lee TQ, Woo SL-Y: A new method for determining cross-sectional shape and area of soft tissues. J Biomech Eng 110:110, 1988.

105. Woo SL, Danto MI, Ohland KJ: The use of a laser micrometer system to determine the cross-sectional shape and area of ligament: A comparative study with two existing methods. J Biomech Eng 112:426, 1990.

106. Mosler E. Folkhard W, Knorzer E, et al: Stress-induced molecular rearrangement in tendon collagen. J Mol Biol 182:589, 1985.

107. Noyes FR, Grood ES: The strength of the anterior cruciate ligament in humans and rhesus monkeys. J Bone Joint Surg 58B: 1074, 1976.

108. Butler DL, Kay MD, Stouffer DC: Comparison of material properties in fascicle bone units from human patellar tendon and knee ligaments. J Biomech 19:425, 1986.

109. Siegler A, Block J, Schneck CD: The mechanical characteristics of the collateral ligaments of the human ankle joint. Foot Ankle 8:234, 1988.

110. Woo SL-Y, Peterson RH, Ohland KJ, et al: The effects of strain rate on the properties of the medial-collateral ligament in skeletally immature and mature rabbits: A biomechanical and histological study. J Orthop Res 8:712, 1990.

111. Savelberg HHCM, Kooloos JGM, Huiskes R, Kauer JMG: Stiffness of the ligaments of the human wrist joint. J Biomech 25:369, 1992.

112. Danto MI, Woo SL-Y: The mechanical properties of skeletally matured rabbit anterior cruciate ligament and patellar tendon over a range of strain rates. J Orthop Res 11:58, 1993.

113. Race A, Amis AA: The mechanical properties of the two bundles of the human posterior cruciate ligament. J Biomech 27:13, 1994.

114. Soslowsky LJ, An CH, Johnson SP, Carpenter JE: Geometric and mechanical properties of the coracoacromial ligament and their relationship to rotator cuff disease. Clin Orthop Relat Res 304:10, 1994.

115. Rogers GJ, Milthorpe BK, Muratore A, Schindhelm K: Measurement of the mechanical properties of the ovine anterior cruciate bone-ligament-bone complex: A basis for prosthetic evaluation. Biomaterials 11:89, 1990.

116. Tipton CM, Matthes RD, Sandage MS: In situ measurement of junction strength and ligament elongation in rats. J Appl Physiol 37:758, 1974.

117. Fung YCB: Elasticity of soft tissues in simple elongation. Am J Physiol 213:1544, 1967.

118. Fung YCB: Biomechanics: Mechanical Properties of Living Tissues. New York, Springer-Verlag, 1981.

119. Viidik A: Mechanical properties of parallel-fibred collagenous tissues. In Viidik A, Vuust J (eds): Biology of Collagen. London, Academic Press, 1980, p 237.

120. Huiskes R: Mathematical modeling of the knee. In Finerman GAM, Noyes FR (eds): Biology of the Traumatized Synovial Joint: The Knee as a Model. Park Ridge, IL, American Academy of Orthopaedic Surgeons, 1992, p 419.

121. Hirokawa S: Biomechanics of the knee joint: A critical review. Crit Rev Biomed Eng 21:79, 1993.

122. Finerman GAM, Noyes FR (eds): Biology of the Traumatized Synovial Joint: The Knee as a Model. Park Ridge, IL, American Academy of Orthopaedic Surgeons, 1992.

123. Hirschman HP, Daniel DM, Miyasaka K: The fate of unoperated knee ligament injuries. In Daniel DM, Akeson WH, O'Conner JJ (eds): Knee Ligaments: Structure, Function, Injury and Repair. New York, Raven, 1990, p 481.

124. Crowinsheild RD, Pope MH: The strength and failure characteristics of rat medial collateral ligaments. J Trauma 16:99, 1976.

125. Woo SL-Y, Orlando CA, Gomez MA, et al: Tensile properties of the medial collateral ligaments as a function of age. J Orthop Res 4:133, 1986.

126. Peterson RH, Gomez MA, Woo SL-Y: The effects of strain rate on the biomechanical properties of the medial collateral ligament: A study of immature and mature rabbits. Trans Orthop Res Soc 12:127, 1987.

127. Viidik A: Age-related changes in connective tissues. In Viidik A (ed): Lectures on Gerontology; vol I: On Biology of Aging. London, Academic Press, 1982, p 173.

128. Woo SL-Y, Ohland KJ, Weiss JA: Aging and sex-related changes in the biomechanical properties of the rabbit medial collateral ligament. Mech Ageing Dev 56:129, 1990.

129. Woo SL-Y, Hollis JM, Adams D, et al: Tensile properties of human femur-anterior cruciate-tibia complex: The effects of specimen age and orientation. Am J Sports Med 19:217, 1991.

130. Fetto JF, Marshall JL: Medial collateral ligament injuries of the knee: A rationale for treatment. Clin Orthop 132:206, 1978.

131. Jones RE, Henley MB, Francis P: Nonoperative management of isolated grade III collateral ligament injury in high school football players. Clin Orthop 213:137, 1986.

132. O'Donoghue DH, Rockwood CA, Frank GR, et al: Repair of the anterior cruciate ligaments in dogs. J Bone Joint Surg 48A:503, 1966.

133. Hawkins RJ, Misamore GW, Merritt TR: Followup of the acute nonoperated isolated anterior cruciate ligament tear. Am J Sports Med 14:205, 1986.

134. O'Donaghue DH, Frank GR, Jeter GL, et al: Repair and reconstruction of the anterior cruciate ligament in dogs. J Bone Joint Surg 53A: 710, 1971.

135. Daniel DM, Teiege RA, Grana WA: Knee and leg: Soft-tissue trauma. *In* Orthopaedic Knowledge Update. Park Ridge, IL, American Academy of Orthopaedic Surgeons, 1990, p 557.

136. Fleming B, Beynnon BD, Johnson RJ, et al: Isometric versus tension measurements: A comparison for the reconstruction of the anterior cruciate ligament. Am J Sports Med 21:82, 1993.

137. Radford WJP, Amis AA: Biomechanics of a double prosthetic ligament in the anterior cruciate deficient knee. J Bone Joint Surg 72B:1038, 1990.

138. Daniel DM, Stone ML, Dobson BE, et al: Fate of the ACL-injured patient: A prospective outcome study. Am J Sports Med 22: 632, 1994.

139. Gillquist J: Repair and reconstruction of the ACL: Is it good enough? Arthroscopy 9:68, 1993.

140. Clancy WG, Narechania RG, Rosenberg TD, et al: Anterior and posterior cruciate ligament reconstruction in rhesus monkeys. J Bone Joint Surg 63A:1270, 1981.

141. Eastwood M, Rayfield EJ, McGrouther DA, Brown RA: Cellular alignment and collagen production in ligament equivalent constructs. *In* Proceedings of the 3rd International Conference on Cellular Engineering. San Remo, Italy, September 1997.

142. Woo SL-Y, Smith DW, Allen CR, et al: Engineering and healing of the rabbit medial collateral ligament. *In* Proceedings of the 3rd International Conference on Cellular Engineering. San Remo, Italy, September 1997.

143. Guyton AC: Textbook of Medical Physiology, 7th ed. Philadelphia, WB Saunders, 1986.

144. Wahrenberg H, Lindbeck L, Ekholm J: Knee muscular moment, tendon tension force and EMG during a vigorous movement in man. Scand J Rehabil Med 10:99, 1978.

145. Komi PV, Fukashiro S, Jarvinen M: Biomechanical loading of Achilles tendon during normal locomotion. Clin Sports Med 11:521, 1992.

146. Wallbridge N, Dowson D: The walking activity of patients with artificial hip joints. Eng Med 11:95, 1982.

147. Abrahams M: Mechanical behavior of tendon in vitro: A preliminary report. Med Biol Eng 5:433, 1967.

148. Benedict JV, Walker LB, Harris EH: Stress-strain characteristics and tensile strength of unembalmed human tendons. J Biomech 1:53, 1968.

149. Butler DL, Grood, ES, Noyes FR, et al: Effects of structure and strain measurement technique on the material properties of young human tendons and fascia. J Biomech 17:579, 1984.

150. Bennett MB, Ker RF, Dimery NJ, Alexander RM: Mechanical properties of various mammalian tendons. J Zool Lond (A) 209:537, 1986.

151. Schechtman H, Bader DL: Dynamic characterisation of human tendons. Eng Med 208:241, 1994.

152. Schechtman H, Bader DL: In vitro fatigue of human tendons. J Biomechanics 30:829, 1997.

153. Schechtman H: Mechanical characterisation of fatigue failure. *In* Human Tendons. PhD Thesis. London, University of London, 1995.

154. Micheli LJ: Lower extremity overuse injuries. Acta Med Scand Suppl 711:171, 1986.

155. Jarvinen M: Epidemiology of tendon injuries in sports clinics. Sports Med 11:493, 1992.

156. Uhthoff HK, Sarkar K, Maynard JA: Calcifying tendinitis: A new concept of its pathogenesis. Clin Orthop Relat Res 118:164, 1976.

157. Hayashi K: Biomechanical studies of the remodelling of knee joint tendons and ligaments. J Biomech 29:707, 1996.

158. Banes AJ, Tsuzaki M, Hu P, et al: PDGF-BB, IGF-1 and mechanical load stimulate DNA synthesis in avian tendon fibroblasts in vitro. J Biomech 28:1505, 1995.

CHAPTER 3

BIOMECHANICS OF BONE

John Behiri and Deepak Vashishth

Because bone is the major component of the skeleton, associated with sustaining and distributing a range of applied forces to the supporting surface of the body, the mechanical behavior of this system has become one of the most extensively investigated when compared with those of any other biologic tissue material, with both its mechanical properties and its structure providing a topic of active research interest for more than a century. More recently, research in this area has been stimulated by the almost routine use of various synthetic materials as replacements for bone in a variety of surgical procedures, ranging from bone grafts to total hip replacement, because there is a constant need to define precisely the mechanical properties of the natural tissue being replaced.

The mechanical behavior of a structure such as bone depends not only on the size and shape of the structure but also on the mechanical properties of the materials of which it is composed, and knowledge of the properties of bone tissue is essential to understanding the behavior of whole bones. Furthermore, apart from having some unique properties, bone is self-repairing and can alter its properties and configuration in response to changes in mechanical demand. For example, decreases in bone density are commonly observed after long periods of disuse, and increases are observed after periods of greatly increased function. Changes are also observed in bone shape during fracture healing and after certain postoperative bone procedures.[1]

This chapter is concerned with the structure and mechanical properties of cortical or compact bone and its behavior under different loading conditions. Any direct comparisons of data are often misleading, and the inclusion of all published experiments on the mechanical properties of bone in any review would generally leave anyone discouraged. This chapter, therefore, is more of a selec-

tive summary rather than a comprehensive literature review and is concerned with cortical or compact bone, which constitutes the outer, load-bearing, shell of the major support bones.

STRUCTURE OF BONE

Bone is a complex system of structure and function on the macroscopic, microscopic, and ultramicroscopic levels, with numerous and varied chemical and physiologic interrelations. Bone is a dynamically adaptable and metabolically active tissue whose form is continuously undergoing subtle remodeling to conform to its functions. It is a highly vascular tissue composed of interconnected cells in an intercellular substance, with an outstanding capacity for self-repair. Bone forms the framework or skeleton of most vertebrates and has the following functions:

- Supports the body
- Protects vital organs
- Provides kinematic links and attachment sites for muscles
- Facilitates muscle action and body movement

In biologic terms, bone can be described as a "specialized" form of connective tissue. Connective tissue connects body parts and is an aggregation of similarly specialized cells that are united to perform a particular function. Typical forms of connective tissue other than bone include hyaline cartilage, found only in a few places in the body, and dense fibrous tissue, such as tendons and ligaments. Hyaline cartilage is the avascular soft tissue that forms the supporting structures of the larynx (or voice box), attaches the ribs to the breastbone, and covers the ends of bones where they form joints. Tendons and ligaments are the soft, ropelike structures made of dense fibrous tissue; tendons attach skeletal muscle to bone, and ligaments connect bone to bone at joints.

Certain characteristics differentiate bone from these other forms of connective tissue. The most striking difference is that bone is hard—only dentin and enamel in teeth are harder. This hardness is the result of the deposition within a soft organic matrix (collagen) of a complex mineral substance known as *calcium hydroxyapatite,* which is composed of calcium, phosphorus, sodium, magnesium, fluoride, and other ions in trace amounts. Bone, therefore, not only forms the framework or skeleton of most vertebrates, providing support and protection to the body, but also acts as a mineral reservoir, playing a vital role in the maintenance of steady-state levels of ions in the body. Apart from collagen and mineral, bone also contains small amounts of mucopolysaccharides (also known as *ground substance*) and water (Table 3–1).

To understand the properties and behavior of bone, it is necessary to consider the various levels of structural organization in bone, namely the ultrastructural, microstructural, and macrostructural levels, which interact in providing bone with its characteristic properties.

ULTRASTRUCTURE

At the ultrastructural level, bone is unique in the body in that it contains both the mineral component, hydroxyapatite, and the organic component, collagen. The mineral is dispersed in microcrystalline form throughout the collagen matrix, and despite numerous investigations into the nature of bonding between these two phases, their relationship still remains to be fully elucidated.

Collagen is the most abundant protein found in the body and can be found in places such as the skin, cartilage, tendons, and blood vessels. In cartilage, collagen opposes the swelling pressure of proteoglycans to yield a shock-absorbing material; in skin and blood vessels, it is mixed with elastin to combine strength and elasticity; and in tendons, where only tensile strength is of primary importance, it is almost the only component. The

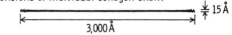

A Amino acid sequence

gly—x—y—gly—pro—hypro—gly—x—y

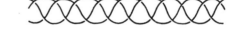

B Dimensions of individual collagen chain

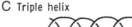

15 Å

3,000 Å

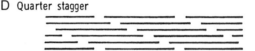

C Triple helix

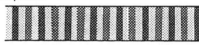

D Quarter stagger

E Banded pattern

FIGURE 3–1   Collagen structure. *A,* Amino acid sequence—repeating tripeptide. *B,* Molecular dimensions. *C,* Triple helix—three alpha chains. *D,* Quarter stagger of collagen molecules. *E,* Banded pattern resulting from alternating overlap and hole zones. (From Owen R, Goodfellow J, Bullough P: Scientific Foundations of Orthopaedics and Traumatology. Philadelphia, WB Saunders, 1980, sec 1, p 30.)

primary building unit of collagen is the tropocollagen molecule (Fig. 3–1), which is a long, rigid molecule (300×1.5 nm) and is composed of three spiral chains of peptides (monomers of proteins, i.e., amino acids), known as α chains, bound together in a triple helix. Different types of collagen for the function in question can be obtained depending on the amounts and sequence of the amino acids on the chain. Type I collagen is typically found in bone and skin, type II in cartilage, and type III in blood vessels.

The tropocollagen molecules are aligned in a quarter-stagger array (Fig. 3–2), with an overlap

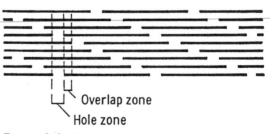

Overlap zone

Hole zone

FIGURE 3–2   Two-dimensional quarter stagger of collagen molecules with alternating overlap and hole zones. (From Owen R, Goodfellow J, Bullough P: Scientific Foundations of Orthopaedics and Traumatology. Philadelphia, WB Saunders, 1980, sec 1, p 31.)

TABLE 3–1   **Composition of Adult Cortical Bone**

COMPONENT	DRY WEIGHT (%)	WET WEIGHT (%)
Collagen	18.5	15.5
Mineral	70.0	59.9
Ground substance	3–3	2.8
Water	8.2	22.7

zone of 26.5 nm and a hole zone of 37.5 nm between subsequent molecules. A collection of tropocollagen molecules forms a collagen fibril, and bundles of fibrils form fibers that have diameters ranging from 0.2 to 12 μm. Under an electron microscope, the fibrils appear to have a banded pattern, which repeats every 64 nm as a direct consequence of the quarter-stagger array.

As previously stated, the most important mechanical properties of collagen are its tensile stiffness and strength. The only information available about collagen's mechanics as a tensile material is that about the properties of vertebrate tendon and ligament (collagen is the major component of tendon, making up 70% to 80% of the dry weight). Tendon is the structure that provides the rigid attachment of muscle to bone, and as such, it must transmit the muscle force with a minimum of loss. This is achieved through the parallel arrangement of the collagen fibers to form ropelike structures with a high modulus of elasticity and high tensile strength. Table 3–2 compares some of the properties of collagen with other materials.

Figure 3–3 illustrates the stress–strain behavior of collagen and shows that collagen can be extended reversibly to strains of about 4%, but strains above this level result in irreversible changes (under normal working conditions, collagen is strained within the limits of 0% to 3%). The collagen fibers fracture at strains of about 8% to 10%, which on examination reveal that it is a consequence from the pulling apart of adjacent molecules rather than from the fracture of the rodlike molecules. It also indicates that intermolecular cross-linking is an important factor in mechanical properties.

In the case of Young's modulus, this increases gradually over the first few percent of extension and then reaches a value of about 1 giga-pascal (GPa). Experiments with polarized light have shown that collagen fibers, particularly in tendon, are crimped and that on extension, the fibers straighten and become parallel. The initial rounded portion of the stress–strain curve reflects the straightening of these crimps, and the linear

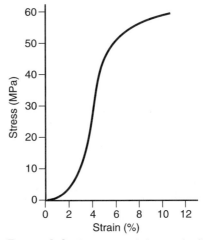

FIGURE 3–3   Stress–strain behavior of collagen.

portion of the curve indicates that the force is being applied directly to extended collagen fibers.

Surrounding the collagen fibrils in a highly organized geometric arrangement are small crystallites of hydroxyapatite ($Ca_{10}[PO_4]_6OH_2$), the major inorganic phase of bone, which are 20 to 40 nm long and about 5 nm thick. It is not known with any certainty how the crystals and the collagen are bound together, although some form of bonding is certainly present. The mineral is apparently initially deposited in the holes between the "heads" and "tails" of the tropocollagen molecules (Fig. 3–4). More mineral is later deposited all over and within the collagen fibrils, with the long axis of the mineral plates being fairly well aligned with the collagen fibrils.

As a material on its own, hydroxyapatite is quite stiff compared with collagen (Table 3–3). Its Young's modulus (E = 130 GPa) is well over half that of steel (E = 210 GPa) and is greater than that of aluminium (70 GPa), but it fractures easily and consequently possesses a low fracture toughness. This superimposition of two quite diverse materials with significantly different mechanical properties results in an ultrastructural composite.

MICROSTRUCTURE

On the microscopic level, above the level of the collagen fibril and its associated mineral (and dependent on the manner in which the fibers are laid down), bone exists in two forms: woven bone and lamellar bone. Woven bone is characterized by an isotropic nonlamellar pattern of collagen fibers, which are usually laid down very quickly. This type of bone is most characteristically found in the fetus and is also the first type of bone to form

TABLE 3–2   Comparison Between Some of the Properties of Collagen and Other Engineering Materials

MATERIAL	YOUNG'S MODULUS (GPa)	TENSILE STRENGTH (MPa)
Collagen	1–2	50–1000
Aluminum	70	150
Steel	220	700

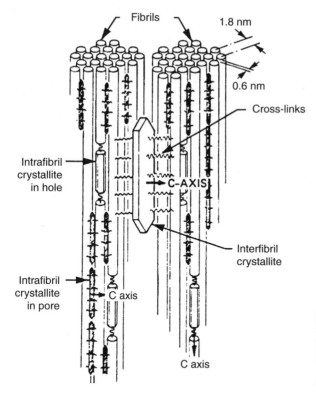

Fibrils

1.8 nm

0.6 nm

Cross-links

Intrafibril crystallite in hole

C-AXIS

Interfibril crystallite

Intrafibril crystallite in pore

C axis

C axis

FIGURE 3–4   Distribution of apatite crystallites in collagen matrix showing orientation of the C axis. (From Lees S, Davidson CL: The role of collagen in the elastic properties of calcified tissues. J Biomechanics 10:473–486, 1977. Copyright 1977, reprinted with permission from Elsevier Science.)

during healing from a fracture. The collagen in woven bone is fine fibered, 0.1 μm in diameter, and randomly oriented. It contains cells (osteocytes) and blood vessels, and the spaces surrounding the blood vessels are extensive.

In contrast to woven bone, lamellar bone is laid down more slowly and has a preferred orientation. The collagen and associated mineral are arranged in sheets about 5 μm thick. It has been suggested that the collagen fibrils in a lamella are all oriented in the same direction, but this is probably not the case. In many lamellae, the fibrils are in small domains; within a domain, the fibril orientation is constant, but it changes from one domain to the next and from one lamella to another. The collagen in lamellar bone is thicker than in woven bone (about 2 to 3 μm). The division between one lamella and the next is abrupt, and there appears to be a sheet of interlamellar bone about 0.1 μm

thick with a high mineral content and little collagen between the pairs of lamellae. Lamellar bone can extend for many millimeters and has three major patterns: osteonal, circumferential, and interstitial.

In the case of osteonal lamellar bone, lamellae can be seen formed into densely packed concentric lamellar structures, which combine concentrically around vascular or haversian canals to build up the next hierarchical structure (i.e., the haversian canal, or osteon). This is essentially a cylindrical structure (Fig. 3–5) whose long axis courses somewhat irregularly along the long axis of the bone. It contains thick walls and a narrow lumen or haversian canal about 22 to 110 μm in diameter surrounded by 4 to 20 concentrically arranged lamellae, with each lamella being 3 to 7 μm thick and having its collagen fibers oriented parallel to each other. Each adjacent lamellar layer has a different orientation of collagen fibers, and as a result, the successive lamellations appear as alternating bright and dark layers. Circumscribing the outermost concentric lamella of the haversian system is a narrow zone known as the *cement line*, which contains calcified mucopolysaccharides and is devoid of collagen. It is 1 to 2 μm thick and is the weakest constituent of bone. These concentric lamellar structures bonded to one another by means of these cement lines form a fiber-rein-

TABLE 3–3   Comparison of the Individual Components of Bone

PROPERTY	COLLAGEN	MINERAL	BONE
E (GPa)	1	130	8–30
UTS (MPa)	50	100	120

E, Young's modulus; UTS, ultimate tensile strength.

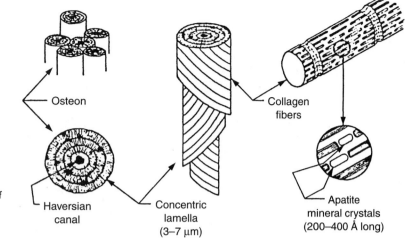

FIGURE 3–5 Detailed structure of an osteon. (Adapted from Park JB: Biomaterials. New York, Plenum Press, 1979, p 105.)

Osteon

Haversian canal

Concentric lamella (3–7 μm)

Collagen fibers

Apatite mineral crystals (200–400 Å long)

forced composite on the microstructural level. Developmentally, two distinct types of osteons exist, namely primary and secondary. Primary osteons are formed by the deposition of lamellae around a previously existing vascular canal and are different morphologically and mechanically from secondary osteons. Primary osteons do not have cement lines because they are not the product of bone remodeling, and they have smaller vascular canals and fewer lamellae than secondary osteons.

In circumferential bone, lamellae can be seen uninterrupted around the circumference of the shaft, located on the external surfaces of cortical bone immediately beneath the periosteum and on the internal surface adjacent to the endosteum (Fig. 3–6).

In interstitial lamellae, fragments of previous concentric and circumferential lamellae fill the gaps between haversian systems. They are continuous with the osteons, and their makeup is identical to that of the osteons, apart from their geometric form. As in the case of osteons, no point in the interstitial lamellae is farther than 100 μm from its blood supply.

Associated within or on the matrix can be found three characteristic cell types: the osteocyte, the osteoblast, and the osteoclast, each of which is associated with specific functions. Osteocytes are contained in small disk-shaped cavities, known as *lacunae* (Fig. 3–7), that lie along the boundaries of each layer, or lamella. A number of theories exist as to the function of osteocytes, but it is generally believed that they assist in the exchange of materials between tissue fluids and bone matrix. The lacunae interconnect with each other and with the haversian canal through a matrix of tiny channels, called *canaliculi,* that are about 0.35 μm in diameter. According to calculations of Martin,[2] 1

mm³ of bone can contain as many as 26,000 lacunae and 10 canaliculi, which indicates that they occupy a major proportion of the bone matrix. Osteoblasts lie at the end farthest from the bone surface and are actively engaged in the manufacture and secretion of components of bone matrix. They are mononucleated cells, vary considerably in size (15 to 80 μm), and can take different shapes, from ovoid to columnar to cuboidal. During bone formation, osteoblasts become trapped within the calcified tissue and differentiate into osteocytes.[3] Osteoclasts are large, 20- to 100-μm, multinucleated cells (2 to 100 cells) found on or near bone surfaces and are associated with bone resorption. They are particularly abundant in areas of active bone resorption.

MACROSTRUCTURE

At the macroscopic level, bone is composed of two types: cortical, or compact, bone and cancellous, or trabecular, bone (see Fig. 3–7). Compact bone appears solid; the only microscopic spaces present are haversian and Volkmann's canals, lacunae, canaliculi, and resorption sites, and these are invisible to the naked eye. Cancellous bone, on the contrary, is a porous material and is composed of trabeculae that join to form a network. It is generally accepted that cortical and cancellous bone are similar in their material and morphologic characteristics,[4, 5] and the main distinction between the two types of bone lies in their porosity. Cortical bone has a porosity of 5% to 30%; porosity of cancellous bone is 30% to 90%.

A typical long bone such as the tibia or femur is composed of (1) the diaphysis, which is the main central cylindrical shaft and contains walls of dense compact bone; (2) the epiphyses, the

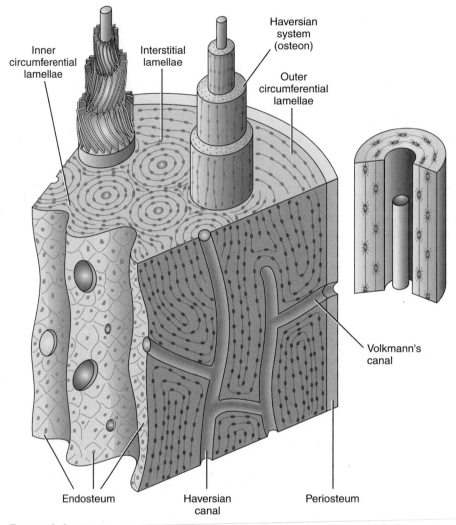

Inner circumferential lamellae

Interstitial lamellae

Haversian system (osteon)

Outer circumferential lamellae

Volkmann's canal

Endosteum

Haversian canal

Periosteum

FIGURE 3–6   Microstructural features of cortical bone. (Redrawn from Junqueira LC, Carneiro J, Kelley RO: Basic Histology, 9th ed. Norwalk, CT, Appleton & Lange, 1999, p 136.)

extreme ends of the bone that are composed of cancellous bone, covered at the surface by a thin layer of compact bone; and (3) the metaphyses, the two intermediate conelike regions connecting the shaft and articular ends (see Fig. 3–7). The articular regions and the metaphyses are spongy in form, consisting of weblike trabeculae that divide the interior volume of the metaphyses and epiphyses into intercommunicating pores filled with marrow. The sizes of the pores vary considerably throughout the bone interior and thus present a structure of variable porosity. The arrangement of the trabeculae is functional. Their orientation closely parallels the trajectories of maximum stress (Fig. 3–8) and thus gives the skeleton maximum rigidity and resistance to mechanical stresses and strains. The compact bone of the diaphysis

region encloses the medullary or marrow-filled cavity, which is lined with a fibrous membrane known as the *endosteum*. This cavity contains yellow bone marrow and communicates freely with that of the trabecular bone.

The exterior bone surface is enclosed by the periosteum, a membranous tissue whose vascular network directly communicates with the underlying bone, except at the joints, where articular cartilage forms the covering.

BIOMECHANICAL CONSIDERATIONS

From the description given previously, it is clear that bone may be regarded as a two-phase hierar-

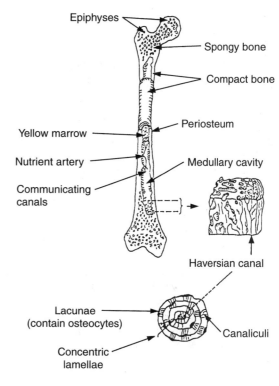

Epiphyses

Spongy bone

Compact bone

Periosteum

Yellow marrow

Nutrient artery

Medullary cavity

Communicating canals

Haversian canal

Lacunae (contain osteocytes)

Canaliculi

Concentric lamellae

FIGURE 3–7   Structure of a long bone.

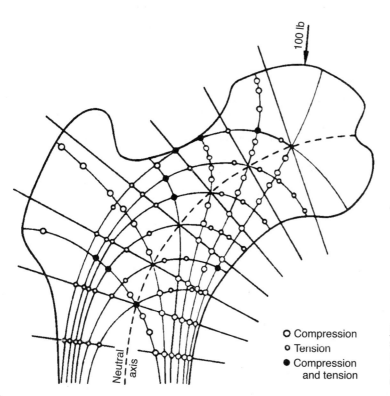

100 lb

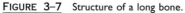

Neutral axis

○ Compression
○ Tension
● Compression and tension

FIGURE 3–8   Diagram of the lines of stress in the upper femur. (From Margel-Robertson DR: Studies of Fracture in Bone. PhD Thesis. Stanford, CA, Stanford University, 1973.)

chical composite. As a result of the way it is built and the functional requirements placed on it, bone can exhibit a variety of mechanical properties. Furthermore, it can adapt in vivo to suit the loading environment.

The present state of knowledge of the mechanical properties of bone has been well documented.[1, 6-10] Two of the most important mechanical properties of bone are its strength and stiffness. At the ultrastructural level, these and other properties are dominated by the contribution of collagen fibers and hydroxyapatite crystals and the bonding between them. When compared with conventional engineering composites, bone has its fibrous structure, collagen, as the matrix, as opposed to the strong, reinforcing element of the composite. At the microstructural level, bone again exhibits a composite nature consisting of lamina of tissue arranged in a number of organized patterns, previously described and separated by weak interfaces. Even at the macrostructural level, bone can be considered as a composite, consisting of dense cortical bone to form the shafts and peripheries and trabecular bone at the extremities to provide a means of distributing applied loads. The stresses produced in bone are complex. They comprise both normal and shear stresses that vary topographically in magnitude and direction. To determine the behavior of materials, they must be examined under simple stress conditions initially and the results then applied in more complex conditions. Standard mechanical tests, such as simple tension, compression, shear, torsion, impact, and fatigue tests, can supply mechanical constants and information that can in turn be used to determine the behavior of a material under conditions of normal use. This section reviews some of the major findings with respect to the properties that describe the mechanical behavior of bone.

STRESS–STRAIN BEHAVIOR

Influence of Orientation

A typical stress–strain curve for bone in tension is shown in Figure 3–9 and illustrates that bone behaves in a manner similar to that of engineering materials in that it consists of an initial elastic region followed by yielding, namely the onset of nonelastic deformation, before failure. The nonelastic portion of the curve, often referred to as the *plastic region,* represents irreversible microdamage in the bone, whereas the linear slope of the curve provides a direct measure of Young's modulus (E) of bone. Because the structure of bone is dissimilar in the transverse and longitudinal directions, it exhibits different mechanical properties when loaded along different axes, a characteristic known as *anisotropy.* For example, Young's modulus does not have a unique value but varies with orientation, with a maximum value parallel to the long axis of the bone and a minimum value (a factor of about 2 smaller) perpendicular to the long axis.[11] The absolute values measured for E depend on the precise nature of the bone specimen and its microstructure but normally range between 7 and 30 GPa.

Some of the most comprehensive examinations of the effects of orientation on the ultimate properties of human cortical bone can be found in the work of Reilly and colleagues[12, 13] and Bonfield and O'Connor,[14] who investigated the tensile and compressive behavior of cortical bone at different orientations. Reilly and Burstein[13] reported elastic modulus values of 17.4 GPa for bone loaded in the longitudinal direction compared with 12.7 GPa in the transverse direction. A similar story holds in the case of ultimate tensile and compressive strength, for which it was found that bone loaded

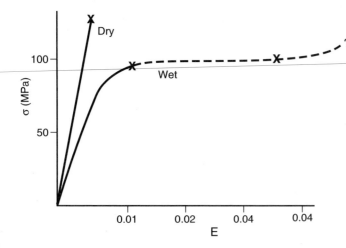

FIGURE 3–9   Stress–strain curves for wet and dry cortical bone. (From Black J: Orthopaedic Biomaterials in Research and Practice. New York, Churchill Livingstone, 1988, p 116.)

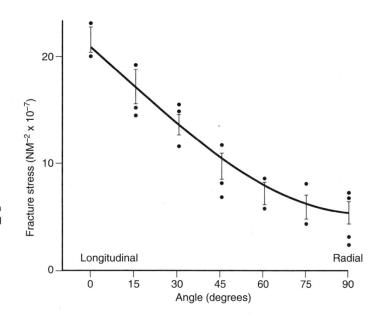

FIGURE 3–10   Variation of fracture strength as a function of angle between the longitudinal and radial axes. (From Pope MH, Outwater JO: Mechanical properties of bone as a function of position and orientation. J Biomechanics 7:61–66, 1974. Copyright 1974, reprinted with permission from Elsevier Science.)

in the transverse direction was significantly weaker in both tension (53 MPa) and compression (133 MPa) compared with bone loaded in the longitudinal direction, for which values of 135 MPa and 193 MPa have been reported.[13] Pope and Outwater[15] considered the variation in the mechanical properties of long bones as a function of position and orientation, with respect to the longitudinal axis of the bone. Their results indicated there was a distinct change of strength and elasticity of bone as a function of distance from the epiphysis, which was directly related to the manner in which the osteons were oriented. At the mid-diaphysis, the osteons are mostly oriented parallel to the longitudinal axis, and the bone is relatively much stronger, as shown in Figure 3–10. At the epiphysis, the orientation of the osteons changes, and the bone becomes better equipped for its role as a bearing surface rather than a column.

The contribution of collagen and mineral to the elastic-plastic properties was examined by Burstein and associates,[16] who found that progressive surface decalcification of bone specimens with dilute hydrochloric acid produced progressive decrease in the tensile yield stress and ultimate stress but caused no change in the yield strain or ultimate strain unless decalcification was completed (Fig. 3–11). They suggested that the mineral contributes the major portion of the tensile yield strength of bone, whereas the magnitude of the plastic modulus is a function only of the properties of collagen and is not a major contributor to the tensile yield strength of bone.

Viscoelasticity

As a consequence of bone's viscoelastic nature (mainly due to the significant amount of fibrous proteins present), the stress–strain curves depicted in Figures 3–7 and 3–8 are influenced by the rate at which bone is loaded. This effect was originally demonstrated in a convincing manner by McElhaney[17] and is shown in Figure 3–12. Young's modulus, ultimate compressive strength, and yield strength increased with increasing rate of loading; however, the failure strain and the fracture toughness of the bone reached a maximum and then decreased, implying that there is a critical rate of loading. Strain rate effects have since been confirmed by other workers, including Bonfield and Clark[18] and Currey.[19] A more recent and comprehensive study was performed by Wright and Hayes,[20] in which an increase in Young's modulus, by a factor of 2 (about 17 to 40 GPa), was reported with increases in strain rate from $5 \times 10^{-4}\text{s}^{-1}$ to $2.4 \times 10^{2}\text{s}^{-1}$. An increase of E with strain rate of this magnitude appears to represent most of the data gathered in various investigations either as a function of strain rate or at particular strain rates. The loading rate is clinically significant because it influences the fracture pattern and the amount of soft tissue damage at fracture. Depending on how rapidly the load is applied, the crack may remain a single crack or may bifurcate. The more rapidly the load is applied, the more the crack bifurcates and the greater the number of resulting bone fragments. When a bone fractures, the stored energy is released. At low rates of loading, the energy is dissipated through the formation of a

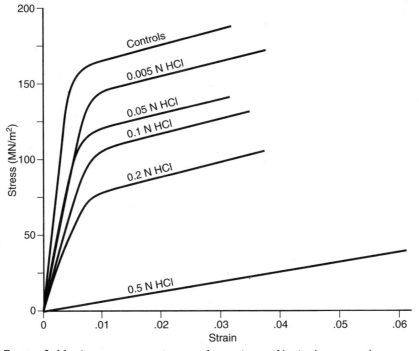

FIGURE 3–11 Average stress–strain curves for specimens of bovine bone treated to create increasing degrees of decalcification. (From Burstein AH, Zika JM, Heiple KG, Klein L : Contribution of collagen and mineral to the elastic-plastic properties of bone. J Bone Joint Surg 57A:958, 1975.)

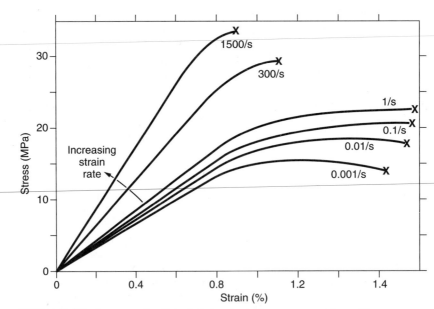

FIGURE 3–12 Stress as a function of strain rate for human compact bone. (From McElhaney JH: Dynamic response of bone and muscle tissue. J Appl Physiol 21:1231–1236, 1966.)

single crack. Under rapid loading, bone dissipates the large amount of energy through the creation of additional free bone surfaces and the creation of a large number of cracks. The number of bone fragments can therefore be directly related to the velocity of the impact.

Influence of Density

Although density has received limited attention in the literature, its importance has been recognized, with experimental studies showing that the elastic modulus correlates well with the cube of the density and that the ultimate fracture strength correlates well with the square of the density of bone tissue[21] (Fig. 3–13). Wall and coauthors[22] carried out tensile strength and density measurements on small samples of cortical bone taken from the femoral diaphysis and showed increases in ultimate tensile strength from 58 to 88 MNm^{-2} for density increases ranging between 1.8 and 2 Mgm^{-3}. Abendschein and Hyatt,[21] investigating

Young's modulus in normal and pathologic human cortical bone in relation to bone mass and density, showed increases in Young's modulus from 7 to 21 GPa for similar density ranges.

Influence of Age

Aging is associated with significant changes in the morphology, composition, and density of cortical bone, resulting in changes in the mechanical properties. Previous investigations[23, 24] have shown that both Young's modulus and yield strength increase to maximum values in the third and fourth decades of life (Fig. 3–14) and then slowly decrease with increasing age, whereas the elongation to failure decreases throughout life. Possible improvements may result from physical activity, whereas possible negative effects may result from hormonal changes (e.g., due to menopause) or from sedentary lifestyle. In a more recent investigation,[25] average deterioration rates of 5% per decade for ultimate stress, 9% per decade for ultimate strain,

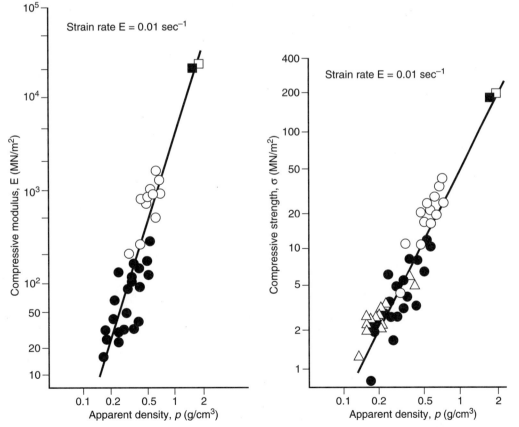

FIGURE 3–13 Influence of density on the compressive properties of compact and trabecular bone. Shown are human (triangles, filled circles, filled squares) and bovine (open circles, open squares) bone tissue. (Modified from Carter DR, Hayes WC: Bone compressive strength: The influence of density and strain rate. Science 194:1174–1176, 1976. Copyright 1976 American Association for the Advancement of Science; Galante J, Rostoker W, Ray RD: Physical properties of trabecular bone. Calcif Tissue Res 5:236–246, 1970; and McElhaney JH, Byars EF: ASME Publ. 65-WA/HUF09, 1965.)

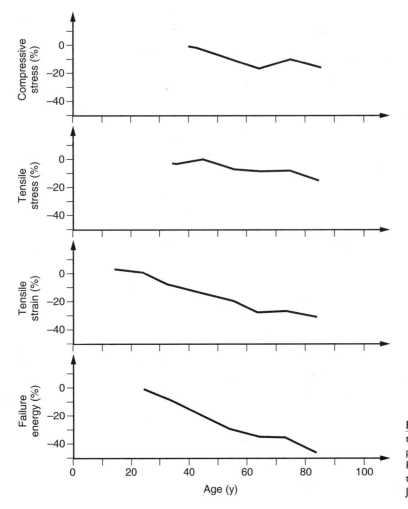

FIGURE 3-14 Summarized results of the effect of age on mechanical properties of bone. (From Burstein AH, Reilly DT, Martens M: Ageing of bone tissue: Mechanical properties. J Bone Joint Surg 58A:82–86, 1976.)

and 12% per decade for energy absorption were reported based on 235 subjects ranging in age from 20 to 102 years.

FRACTURE MECHANICS OF BONE

The fracture of bone is a complex process that has received considerable attention over the years. One of the difficulties in characterizing bone fracture is the variability in the associated microstructure among bones, and indeed for different locations in the same bone, as well as the differences related to age and sex. Moreover, because the microstructure in the major support bones is anisotropic, the resultant fracture properties also depend on the orientation.

The pioneering work of Evans[1, 6] was of considerable value in distinguishing the relative effects of microstructural parameters, strain rate, and temperature on bone fracture from measurements of the ultimate tensile and compressive strength. Given that cortical bone is a brittle solid that exhibits only a small total elongation to fracture (0.5% to 3.5%) with limited nonelastic deformation, an inevitable consequence of specimen preparation is the presence of random surface flaws. This effect was well appreciated by Evans,[6] whose careful surveys of ultimate tensile strength involved tests on many specimens to produce statistically significant results.

Because the energy to fracture a brittle solid is significantly affected by the presence of cracks, however, an alternative approach to define bone fracture is by testing precracked specimens with a single characterized crack or notch from which fracture will propagate. Bonfield and Li[26] first demonstrated that an introduced surface crack significantly reduced the energy absorbed during fracture of bovine cortical bone specimens in both the longitudinal and transverse directions. A series of significant investigations followed in which the fracture energy of precracked or notched cortical bone was determined for transverse and longitudinal directions in various bones.[15, 27, 28] Piekarski's study[27] showed that at low strain rates, a crack follows the weak interfaces of bone (i.e., the cement lines), whereas at high rates of strain, a crack propagates in a brittle manner without regard to the microstructure. The cement lines have also been shown to be a weakness by Evans and Bang,[29] Dempster and Coleman,[30] and Behiri and Bonfield.[31]

For a given bone, the considerable scatter (variability) in values in the work (energy) required to cause fracture, illustrated that the relationship between the geometry of the introduced crack and the energy or stress associated with fracture required determination if an absolute measure of bone fracture was to be established. The recognition of the dependence of fracture stress on the nature of introduced cracks provided the basis for a more precise evaluation of the fracture of bone in terms of its *fracture toughness,* defined as a measure of the resistance of a material to crack propagation. This approach utilized the concepts of linear elastic fracture mechanics,[32] developed for engineering materials, to determine values of the critical stress intensity factor (K_C, or fracture toughness) and the critical strain energy release rate (G_C) of bone. Such an approach to the failure of bone was adopted by Wright and Hayes[32] and Behiri and Bonfield.[31, 33, 34] Wright and Hayes[32] demonstrated the significant effect of an increase in bone density in producing an increase in both K_C and G_C and established the important link between fracture mechanics and microstructure.

In an independent approach, Behiri and Bonfield[31] conducted a comprehensive study of longitudinal fracture in bone and found that crack velocity increases from $1.75 \times 10^{-5} \text{ms}^{-1}$ to $23.6 \times 10^{-5} \text{ms}^{-1}$ produced increases in K_C and G_C from 4.46 to 5.38 Mnm$^{-3/2}$ and 1736 to 2796 Jm^{-2}, respectively. At higher crack velocities, fracture became catastrophic. Hence, the concept of a critical crack velocity associated with a maximum in the fracture toughness of bone was established and shown to represent a transition from controlled to catastrophic crack propagation. In later work, which embraced the effects of density and crack velocity, this transition between microstructure-dependent fracture and catastrophic crack propagation associated with a maximum in fracture toughness is shown in Figure 3–15. For controlled, slow crack velocities, the investigators correlated fracture with crack-intersecting osteon interactions, with osteon pullout similar to that noted by Piekarski.[27] The dependence of fracture on microstructure was not significant at higher crack velocities. The fracture characteristics at a range of orientations under controlled slow crack propagation were also investigated[34] (Fig. 3–16),

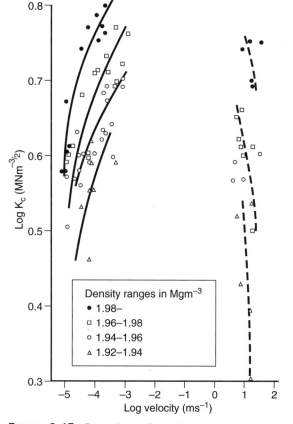

FIGURE 3–15 Dependence of critical stress intensity factor (K_c) of bovine tibia cortical bone for different density groups within the normal range. (From Behiri JC, Bonfield W: Fracture mechanics of bone: The effects of density, specimen thickness and crack velocity on longitudinal fracture J. Biomechanics 17:25–34, 1984. Copyright 1984, reprinted with permission of Elsevier Science.)

and fracture toughness values were shown to increase from 3.2 MNm$^{-3/2}$ for fracture in the longitudinal direction to 6.3 MNm$^{-3/2}$ for fracture in the transverse direction, again clearly illustrating the anisotropic nature of bone. Age was also demonstrated to have a significant effect on the fracture toughness of bone,[35] with decreases in toughness from 4.5 Mnm$^{-3/2}$ at 25 years to 2.5 Mnm$^{-3/2}$ at 90 years (Fig. 3–17).

The application of fracture mechanics techniques for an evaluation of the fracture of bone has developed to the stage at which meaningful results can be achieved that are consistent with the protocol followed for engineering materials. This approach has two advantages: first, tests can be performed on a relatively small number of specimens, which is helpful when the supply of bone is limited, as in the case of human bone; and second, a more systematic approach to prosthesis

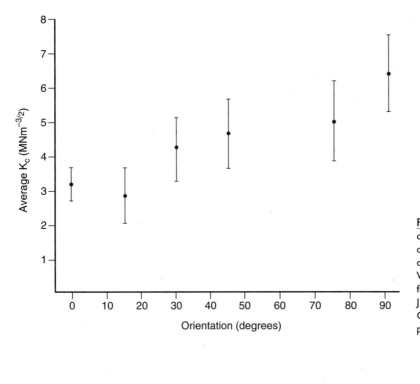

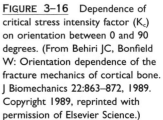

FIGURE 3–16 Dependence of critical stress intensity factor (K_c) on orientation between 0 and 90 degrees. (From Behiri JC, Bonfield W: Orientation dependence of the fracture mechanics of cortical bone. J Biomechanics 22:863–872, 1989. Copyright 1989, reprinted with permission of Elsevier Science.)

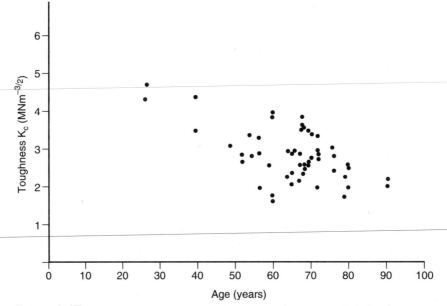

FIGURE 3–17   Critical stress intensity factor (K_c) associated with controlled, slow fracture of human tibia cortical bone specimens as a function of age (both male and female, clinically normal). (From Bonfield W, Behiri JC, Charalembides B: Orientation and age-related dependence of the fracture toughness of cortical bone. In Perren SM, Schneider E [eds]: Biomechanics: Current Interdisciplinary Research. Dordrecht, The Netherlands, Martinus Nijhoff Publishing, 1985, pp 185–189. Reprinted with kind permission from Kluwer Academic Publishers.)

design can be made with a precise knowledge of the limiting fracture toughness of the natural tissues as well as of the engineering materials considered.

FATIGUE FRACTURE

In addition to bone fractures produced by a single monotonic load at stresses that exceed the ultimate strength, fractures in bone may also occur by the repeated or cyclic application of a lower load. These types of fractures, known as *fatigue fractures* and sometimes referred to clinically as *stress fractures,* are usually sustained during continuous strenuous physical activity. Such fractures occur in bones of the lower limb, including metatarsals, calcaneus, tibia, fibula, femur, and pelvis, and occurrence of such fractures in a particular bone varies with the activities of the individual. For example, fatigue fractures of tibiae and metatarsals are more common among athletes, ballet dancers, and military recruits.

Fatigue of any material, including bone, is defined as the progressive loss of strength or stiffness under cyclic loads resulting in complete failure of the material at stresses below the static failure levels. Tests to determine fatigue characteristics are conducted by subjecting standardized subjects to a constant amplitude loading and determining the total number of cycles to failure. Tests are performed at various stress levels, and the results are used to plot stress against the number of cycles to failure (S-N curve). Figure 3–18 is a compilation of fatigue data obtained from a variety of bone studies. In the case of bone tested in vivo, the fatigue curve is asymptotic, indicating

that if the stress levels are kept below a certain level, theoretically, the material will remain intact regardless of the number of cycles of loading and unloading. Seireg and Kempke[36] conducted this in vivo fatigue test and found that the S-N curve did not exhibit a constant decline at lower loads but had a distinct knee region at 42% of the static failure load after 5×10^3 cycles. This was interpreted as the "endurance limit" of the bone beyond which it did not fatigue. This is not the case for bone when tested in vitro. Initial investigations by Swanson and colleagues[37] and later studies by other investigators did not detect any endurance limit during in vitro fatigue testing. Carter and coauthors, in a series of studies,[38–41] carried out a comprehensive investigation of the influence of stress amplitude, temperature, bone density, and microstructure on the fatigue life of compact bone. They found that (1) decreasing the stress amplitude from 108 to 65 MPa caused a four-fold increase in the fatigue life, (2) decreasing the temperature from 45° to 21°C caused a three-fold increase in the fatigue life, and (3) a 5% increase in density doubled the fatigue life.

In general, investigations into the cyclic load behavior of bone in vitro have established that cyclic loading produces microstructural damage that accumulates with each loading cycle and that damage accumulates faster at higher intensities of cyclic loading.[38] Furthermore, continued fatigue loading of bone results in loss of strength and stiffness, which has been suggested as being due to the accumulation of small microcracks. Because living bone is a dynamic and self-repairing material, a fatigue fracture occurs only when the remodeling processes outpace the fatigue processes,

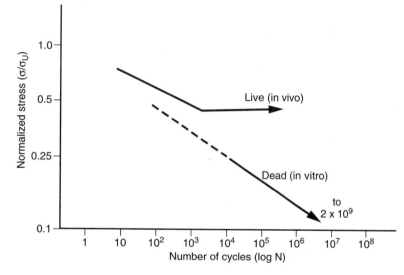

FIGURE 3–18   S-N (fatigue) curves for live and dead bone. (From Black J: Orthopaedic Biomaterials in Research and Practice. New York, Churchill Livingstone, 1988, p 116.)

and consequently, any comparisons between in vivo and in vitro fatigue data should be viewed with some caution.

References

1. Evans FG: Stress and Strain in Bones. Springfield, IL, Charles C Thomas, 1957.
2. Martin RB: Porosity and specific surface of bone. Crit Rev Biomed Eng 10:179–222, 1984.
3. Pritchard JJ: The osteoblast. *In* Bourne GH (ed): The Biochemistry and Physiology of Bone, vol. 1. New York, Academic Press, 1972, pp 21–43.
4. Carter DR, Spengler DM: Mechanical properties and composition of cortical bone. Clin Orthop 135:192–217, 1978.
5. Schaffler MB, Burr DB: Stiffness of compact bone: Effect of porosity and density. J Biomech 21:13–16, 1988.
6. Evans FG: Mechancial Properties of Bone. Springfield, IL, Charles C Thomas, 1973.
7. Kraus H: On the mechanical properties and behaviour of human compact bone. *In* Levine SN (ed): Advances in Biomedical Engineering and Medical Physics, vol 2. New York, Interscience, 1968, pp 169–204.
8. Swanson SAV: Biomechanical characteristics of bone. *In* Kenedi RM (ed): Advances in Biomedical Engineering, vol 1. New York, Academic Press, 1971, pp 137–187.
9. Currey JD: The mechanical properties of bone. Clin Orthop 73:210–231, 1970.
10. Herrmann G, Liebowitz H: Mechanics of bone fracture. *In* Liebowitz H (ed): Fracture: An Advanced Treatise, vol 7. New York, Academic Press, 1972, pp 771–840.
11. Dempster WT, Liddicoat RT: Compact bone as a non isotropic material. Am J Anat 91:331–62, 1952.
12. Reilly DT, Burstein AH, Frankel VH: The elastic modulus for bone. J Biomech 7:271, 1974.
13. Reilly DT, Burstein AH: The elastic and ultimate properties of compact bone tissue. J Biomech 8:393, 1975.
14. Bonfield W, O'Connor P: Anelastic deformation and friction stress of bone. J Mater Sci 13:202–207, 1978.
15. Pope MH, Outwater JO: The fracture characteristics of bone substance. J Biomech 5:457–465, 1972.
16. Burstein AH, Zika JM, Heiple KG, Klein L: Contribution of collagen and mineral to the elastic-plastic properties of bone. J Bone Joint Surg 57a:956, 1975.
17. McElhaney JH: Dynamic response of bone and muscle tissue. J Appl Physiol 21:1231–1236, 1966.
18. Bonfield W, Clark EA: Elastic deformation of compact bone. J Mater Sci 8:1590–1594, 1973.
19. Currey JD: The effects of strain rate, reconstruction and mineral content on some mechanical properties of bovine bone. J Biomech 8:81–86, 1975.
20. Wright TM, Hayes WC: Tensile testing of bone over a wide range of strain rates: Effects of strain rate, microstructure and density. Med Biol Eng 14:671–679, 1976.
21. Abendschein W, Hyatt GW: Ultrasonics and selected physical properties of bone. Clin Orthop 69:294–301, 1970.
22. Wall JC, Jatterji SK, Jeffery JW: Age related changes in the density and tensile strength of human femoral cortical bone. Calc Tissue Int 27:105–108, 1979.
23. McCalden RW, McGeough JA, Barker MB, Court-Brown CM: Age-related changes in the tensile properties of cortical bone. J Bone Joint Surg 75(A–8):1193–1199, 1993.
24. Burstein AH, Reilly DT, Martens M. Ageing of bone tissue: Mechanical properties. J Bone Joint Surg 58A:82–86, 1976.
25. Carter DR, Hayes WC: The compressive behaviour of bone as a two phase porous structure. J Bone Joint Surg 59A:954–962, 1977.
26. Bonfield W, Li CH: Deformation and fracture of bone. J Appl Physiol 37:869–875, 1996.
27. Piekarski K: Fracture of bone. J Appl Physiol 41:215–233, 1970.
28. Moyle DD, Welborn JW, Cooke FW: Work to fracture of canine femoral bone. J Biomech 11:435–440, 1978.
29. Evans FG, Bang S: Physical and histological differences between human fibular and femoral compact bone. *In* Evans FG (ed): Studies on the Anatomy and Function of Bone and Joints. Heidelberg, Germany, Springer-Verlag, 1966, p 142.
30. Dempster WT, Coleman RF: Tensile strength of bone along and across the grain. J Appl Physiol 16:355, 1961.
31. Behiri JC, Bonfield W: Crack velocity dependence of longitudinal fracture in bone. J Mater Sci 15:1841, 1980.
32. Wright TM, Hayes WC: Fracture mechanics parameters for compact bone: Effects of density and specimen thickness. J Biomech 10:419–430, 1977.
33. Brown W, Srawley J: Plain strain crack testing of high strength metallic materials. ASTM-STP-410. Philadelphia, ASTM, 1966.
34. Behiri JC, Bonfield W. Fracture mechanics of bone: The effects of density, specimen thickness and crack velocity on longitudinal fracture. J Biomech 17:25–34, 1984.
35. Bonfield W, Behiri JC, Charalambides B. Orientation and age-related dependence of the fracture toughness of cortical bone. *In* Perren SM, Schneider E (eds): Biomechanics: Current Interdisciplinary Research. Dordrecht, The Netherlands, Martinus Nijhoff Publishers, 1985, pp 185–189.

36. Seireg A, Kempke W: Behaviour of in vivo bone under cyclic loading. J Biomech 2:455–462, 1969.
37. Swanson SAV, Freeman MAR, Day WH: The fatigue properties of human cortical bone. Med Biol Eng 9:23–32, 1971.
38. Carter DR, Hayes WC: Compact bone fatigue damage. I. Residual strength and stiffness. J Biomech 10:325–337, 1977.
39. Carter DR, Hayes WC: Compact bone fatigue damage: A microscopic examination. Clin Orthop 127:265–274, 1977.
40. Carter DR, Hayes WC: Fatigue life of compact bone. I. Effects of stress amplitude, temperature and density. J Biomech 9:27–34, 1976.
41. Carter DR, Hayes WC, Schurman DJ: Fatigue life of compact bone. II. Effects of microstructure and density. J Biomech 9:211–218, 1976.

CHAPTER 4

BIOMECHANICS OF MUSCLE

Zeevi Dvir

Motion is perhaps the most conspicuous sign of life—so much so that someone described as lying completely motionless is presumed to be either unconscious or dead. In the latter case, however, examination of other movement-related parameters, such as pulse, would be required. These special manifestations, in particular the full spectrum of normal or pathologic biomotion, from simple reflexes to stereotyped activities to the most complex intentional movements, are the exclusive result of the capacity of muscles to generate tension.

From a control systems point of view, skeletal muscle presents a unique feature in that it operates as both an effector and a sensor. In other words, it possesses the dual abilities of producing tension, on one hand, and detecting and transmitting signals relevant to its functioning, on the other. Moreover, as discussed in Chapter 5, some muscles may be intended for positional sensing more than for the actual sharing in supporting the load. The dual abilities of skeletal muscle are without comparison among the other sense organs. Consider, for instance, production and sensing of sound; the former is the responsibility of the vocal cords, whereas the latter is that of the ear; neither organ can fulfill both roles.

This distinguishing quality is but one of many that have rendered skeletal muscle one of the most researched organ tissues in the body. Among the various fields of muscle research, biomechanics naturally occupies a special niche. Consequently, survey of all related aspects would be beyond the scope of this chapter; instead, focus is given to a number of pertinent aspects, including the following:

- Muscle structure and architecture
- Mechanism of tension generation and transmission
- Force–length (F-L) relationship
- Force–velocity (F-V) relationship
- Muscle action vector and moment arm
- Muscle moment and its relationship to joint angular position
- Statically determinate systems
- Statically indeterminate systems and common methods of solution

MUSCLE STRUCTURE AND ARCHITECTURE

Both of these general aspects of skeletal muscle are now fairly well documented. In this text, *structure* refers to the arrangement of the morphologic units that consist, in order of decreasing size, of the muscle as an integral unit, the compartment (where applicable), the fascicle, the muscle fiber, the myofibril, and the sarcomere, which contains the basic contractile proteins myosin and actin. *Muscle architecture* refers to the pennation type, fiber length, and physiologic cross-sectional area (PCSA).

STRUCTURE

The subdivisions of skeletal muscle are depicted in Figure 4–1. Within the muscle proper, an intricate latticework of connective tissue enables partitioning of the contractile machinery into the previously mentioned units. This tissue is made up predominantly of collagen fibers enmeshed with a relatively much smaller number of elastin fibers. As seen in Figure 4–2, the epimysium covers the integral unit and invades the inside of the muscle, connecting with the perimysium, which subdivides the muscle into fascicles. Lining the fibers is the endomysium, a dense mesh of delicate collagen fibers that may provide a physical continuation between the perimysium on one side and the outer (basement) membrane of the fiber on the other.[1]

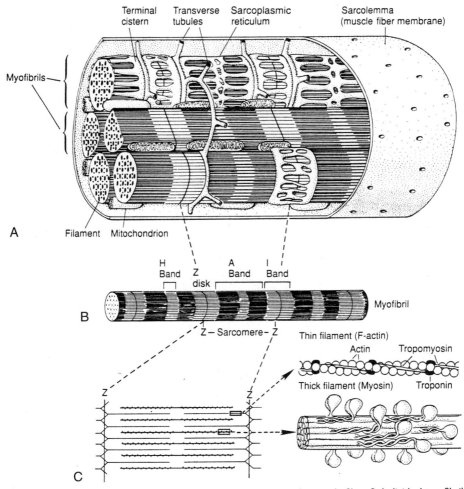

FIGURE 4–1 A, Three-dimensional reconstruction of a sector of a muscle fiber. B, Individual myofibril showing the dark bands that correspond to the regions of actin–myosin overlap. C, Schematic cross-section of an individual sarcomere. Note the stem and globular double-head configuration of the myosin molecule. (From Kandell EC, Schwartz JH, Jessel TM: Principles of Neural Science. Englewood Cliffs, NJ, Prentice Hall, 1991. Reproduced with permission of The McGraw-Hill Companies.)

In the context of gross structure, some muscles may consist of several compartments divided by transverse fibrous bands. This means that bundles of short fibers may be arranged *in series*,[2] so that the overall shortening capacity and, hence, variety of contraction may be considerably enhanced. Each compartment has its own nerve supply and is centrally represented. In humans, the sartorius has four compartments, whereas the gracilis has two.[3] To what extent this layout depends on the complexity of function or on the sheer size of the muscle is not absolutely clear. As suggested by Windhorst and colleagues,[4] however, the control of some muscles as single units poses significant problems that could be solved more effectively using compartmentalization.

The basic functional unit of the muscle is the sarcomere, which consists of parallel actin and myosin filaments. Under the electron microscope, a finer subdivision of each sarcomere into several bands is visible (see Fig. 4–1). The centrally located dark A band corresponds to the presence of myosin. Two less refractory I bands correspond to the presence of actin and insert into the thin Z disks, which also serve as the borders of the sarcomere. In a noncontracting muscle, the H zone, which occupies the middle portion of the A band, corresponds with the nonoverlapping region of the filaments. This region also contains a thin central M region, a latticework of filaments supporting the myosin filaments while maintaining an inter-filament distance. This support system, which consists of a number of proteins,[1] is essential for structural integrity as well as for the proper func-

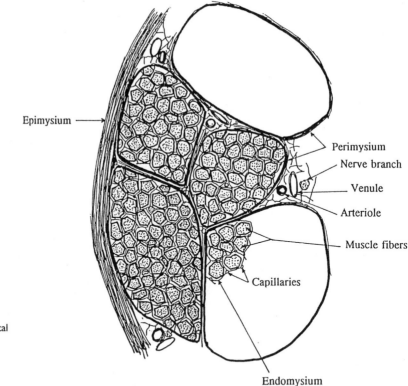

Epimysium

Perimysium
Nerve branch
Venule
Arteriole
Muscle fibers
Capillaries
Endomysium

FIGURE 4–2 Schematic cross-section of a muscle showing the three types of connective tissue sheath. (From McComas AJ: Skeletal Muscle Form and Function. Champaign, IL, Human Kinetics, 1996. Courtesy of Dr. John Maguire.)

tioning of the sliding mechanism. In addition, because of their intimate relationship with the contractile filaments, these noncontractile proteins contribute to the stiffness properties of the muscle.

The arrangement of the actin and myosin filament is revealed by the electron microscope. In principle, each myosin filament is surrounded by a hexagonal array of six actin filaments (Fig. 4–3). About 250 myosin molecules make up 1 myosin filament whose length is about 1.6 nm. These molecules are distinguished by a Z-disk–oriented head and M-region–oriented tail portions, known as heavy and light meromyosin, respectively. Along the major axis of the myosin filament, the heads of the myosin molecules, which act as the binding site during the cross-bridge formation, are arranged in pattern. The basic block is of six heads, configured as three opposing heads lying at an offset angle of 60 degrees to each other. The distance between each pair is 14.3 nm.[5] Thin filaments are made up of braided polymerized actin monomers and have a length of 1.27 nm.[6] Intertwined between them are actin-binding tropomyosin and troponin molecules.

ARCHITECTURE

Among the architectural parameters, fiber length and PCSA are the most essential because they determine, to a considerable extent, the force and velocity profile of the individual muscle. However, the individual architectural profile of a given muscle should not be confused with the motion profile of the segment it acts on. As in most instances, motion depends on the activity of a number of muscles. For instance, the soleus and gastrocnemius form the core of the plantar-flexor group, yet architecturally, they are quite different.[7]

In humans, skeletal muscle fibers may reach a length of up to 160 mm (the semitendinosus), but in most limb muscles, fiber length ranges typically between 40 and 100 mm.[8-10] The distribution of fiber length, together with several other architectural parameters in selected lower extremity muscles, is outlined in Table 4–1. Data for most muscles are based on three cadavers and are presented in terms of the range (in parentheses) and average values.[8]

Assuming that all sarcomeres have the same length and length variation (shortening, lengthening), longer fibers, which by definition have a larger number of sarcomeres, also possess a larger absolute range of excursion. It also follows that because the maximum contraction velocity of a muscle depends on the number of sarcomeres, longer fibers can produce higher velocity. On the other hand, shorter fibers are characterized by a

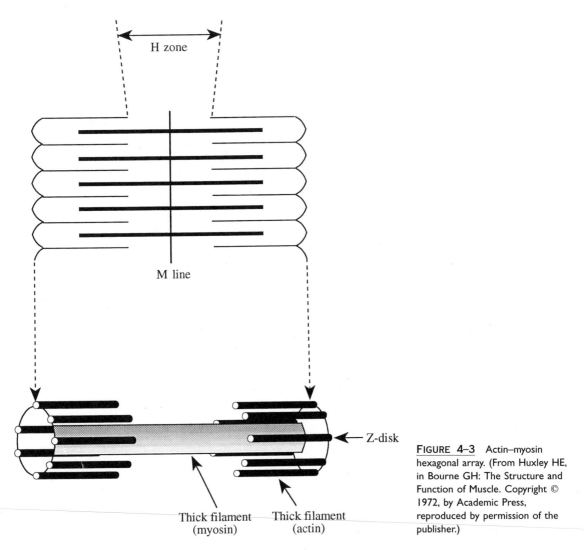

FIGURE 4–3 Actin–myosin hexagonal array. (From Huxley HE, in Bourne GH: The Structure and Function of Muscle. Copyright © 1972, by Academic Press, reproduced by permission of the publisher.)

more dominant ability to produce force. In a study of the specific mechanical nature of long and short fibers in an animal model, Woittiez and associates[11] have proposed the use of a ratio termed *index of architecture* (i_a), which is equal to the fiber length divided by the muscle belly length. Figure 4–4 depicts the major trends based on modeling and experimental findings that reveal that the i_a is positively and linearly related to the maximal velocity of contraction but negatively related to the maximal force produced. In principle, the situation with human muscles may be similar. The value of i_a for the tibialis anterior muscle is 0.26, compared with 0.14 for the medial gastrocnemius, whereas that of the semimembranosus is 0.24, compared with 0.17 in the vastus lateralis. These variations are reflected in what is perceived as the more dominant functional feature of these muscles, namely, that the knee extensors

and ankle plantar-flexors are primarily designed for the generation of high forces, whereas the knee flexors and ankle dorsiflexors are more suitable for greater excursions.[7]

Another essential architectural parameter is the PCSA of the muscle. The importance of the PCSA lies in the fact that it is linearly related to the maximal force output of the muscle under isometric conditions and at optimal length. Illuminating findings come from a study of human cadaveric material in which a number of architectural parameters were measured in muscles that compose the lower limb.[8] Figure 4–5 depicts some of these findings, which clearly support the general dichotomy into predominantly "force" or "velocity" muscles. By way of example, the gracilis and sartorius have the lowest PCSA-to-muscle weight ratio but the highest i_a. Although a geometric property, estimation of the PCSA factors in the

TABLE 4–1   **Architectural Features of Selected Lower Extremity Muscles**

MUSCLE	MUSCLE LENGTH (cm)	FIBER LENGTH (cm)	FEMUR LENGTH–TO–MUSCLE LENGTH RATIO (%)	PENNATION ANGLE (degrees)	PCSA (cm²)
Rectus femoris	31.6 (30.5–32.4)	6.6 (6.3–6.8)	21 (21–21)	5 (5–5)	12.7 (8.9–15.2)
Vastus lateralis	32.5 (30.8–35.3)	6.6 (6.4–6.7)	20 (19–22)	5 (5–5)	30.6 (21–42.9)
Vastus medialis	33.5 (31.4–36.3)	7.3 (6.4–7.5)	21 (20–22)	5 (5–5)	21.1 (13.3–28.0)
Semimembranosus	26.2 (26.0–26.5)	6.3 (5.4–7.0)	24 (21–26)	15 (10–20)	16.9 (13.9–18.6)
Biceps femoris*	34.2 (32.8–36.9)	8.5 (7.8–9.5)	25 (21–29)	0 (0–0)	12.8 (7.4–16.4)
Semitendinosus	31.7 (31.3–32.1)	15.8 (15.6–16.0)	50 (50–50)	5 (5–5)	5.4 (4.4–6.3)
Sartorius	50.3 (45.8–55.2)	45.5 (41.9–48.2)	90.6 (87–93)	0 (0–0)	1.7 (1.1–2.1)
Adductor magnus	30.5 (28.8–32.7)	11.5 (10.6–13.1)	38 (36–40)	0 (0–0)	18.2 (13.6–20.8)
Adductor longus	22.9 (21.0–25.2)	10.8 (10.5–11.2)	48 (43–50)	6 (5–8)	6.8 (4.0–10.5)
M. gastrocnemius	24.8 (23.7–26.8)	3.5 (3.2–3.9)	14.3 (13–16)	16.6 (15–25)	32.4 (29.3–38.7)
L. gastrocnemius	21.7 (19.5–22.9)	5.1 (4.0–5.9)	23.3 (21–26)	8.3 (5–10)	—
Soleus	30.9 (30.8–31.1)	1.95 (1.9–2.0)	6 (6–6)	25 (20–30)	58.0†
Tibialis anterior	29.8 (28.4–32.2)	7.7 (6.9–9.3)	25.6 (24–29)	5 (5–5)	9.7 (7.9–12.7)
Peroneus brevis	23 (20.8–25.2)	3.9 (3.4–4.6)	17 (16–18)	5 (5–5)	5.7 (4.5–7.7)
Peroneus longus	28.6 (25.8–31.8)	3.9 (3.3–4.4)	13.7 (12–16)	10 (10–10)	12.3 (7.4–17.3)

*Long (ischial) head.
†Single measurement.
PCSA, physiologic cross-sectional area.

mass of the muscle belly and its density, as follows:

$$PCSA = (m\cos\alpha) \,/\, (\text{fiber length} \times \text{muscle density})$$

where m is the mass of muscle belly, α is the angle of pennation, and the muscle density is 1.056 kg^{-3}.[12] There is some controversy regarding the representative value of the slope of the above linear relationship. Generally speaking, it has been estimated to range from 20 to 35 N/cm².[13] but factors such as fiber type distribution and its associated biochemical variations may have resulted in quotation of different values. For instance, whereas Gregor[14] quotes 22.5 N/cm² as the value, Pierrynowski[15] suggests 35 N/cm² as more reasonable.

The third architectural factor, pennation, relates to the arrangement and direction of the fibers in terms of the insertion regions. In humans, most muscles have their fibers oriented along the longitudinal axis, resulting in the so-called fusiform type. In this context, note that the "longitudinal axis" does not necessarily imply a straight line between the insertions, because, as discussed later in this chapter, muscles may more accurately be modeled as piecewise linear actuators.[15] The other way fibers may be configured is feather-like. Thus, in pennated muscles, fibers are essentially at an angle to the major axis. Variants of this include the unipennate, bipennate, and multipennate muscles. Clearly, the higher the index of architecture, the lower the pennation angle. To gain insight into the effect of pennation angle on the force transmitted by the muscle to the tendon, consider Figure 4–6, in which α is the angle of pennation. In this configuration, the force developed in the tendon (F^T) and the force developed in the muscle (F^M) are related as follows:

$$F^T = F^M\cos\alpha$$

Also note that the total length of the musculotendinous unit (L_{MT}) is computed as follows:

$$L_{MT} = L_T + L_{M\alpha}$$

where $M\alpha$ is the "co-linear" muscle length. Assuming that w, the width of the unit, remains constant, α is 30 degrees, and maximal fiber shortening is 50%, a situation may be reached in which the fibers are orthogonal to the tendon and therefore cannot transmit any force. However, both conditions may not be realized in the human body. Pennation angles rarely exceed 25 degrees,[8] whereas full shortening of the fibers is hampered by external constraints, such as the joint range of motion.

MECHANISM OF TENSION GENERATION AND TRANSMISSION

The prevailing model for muscular tension generation is based on a series of studies by Andrew Huxley and Hugh Huxley, begun almost half a

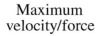

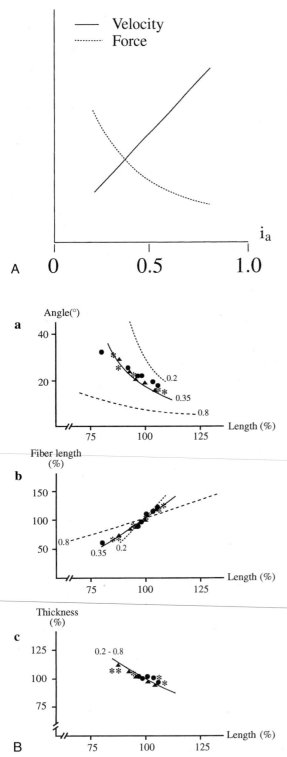

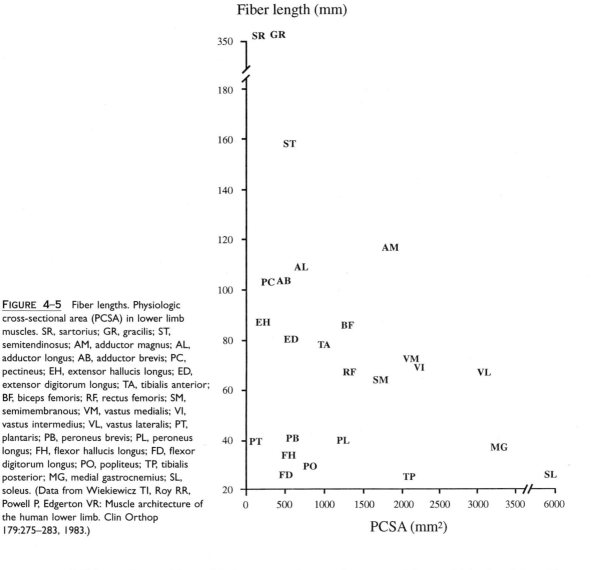

Fiber length (mm)

FIGURE 4-5 Fiber lengths. Physiologic cross-sectional area (PCSA) in lower limb muscles. SR, sartorius; GR, gracilis; ST, semitendinosus; AM, adductor magnus; AL, adductor longus; AB, adductor brevis; PC, pectineus; EH, extensor hallucis longus; ED, extensor digitorum longus; TA, tibialis anterior; BF, biceps femoris; RF, rectus femoris; SM, semimembranous; VM, vastus medialis; VI, vastus intermedius; VL, vastus lateralis; PT, plantaris; PB, peroneus brevis; PL, peroneus longus; FH, flexor hallucis longus; FD, flexor digitorum longus; PO, popliteus; TP, tibialis posterior; MG, medial gastrocnemius; SL, soleus. (Data from Wiekiewicz TI, Roy RR, Powell P, Edgerton VR: Muscle architecture of the human lower limb. Clin Orthop 179:275–283, 1983.)

century ago.[16–18] According to this model, the production of force is effected by a sequential formation of cross-bridges between the respective active sites of actin and myosin filaments. This process translates into the relative sliding of the filaments;

hence, the name of the model is the *sliding filament theory*. The model predicts that because each cross-bridge acts as an independent force generator, the sliding, which introduces a linearly growing number of cross-bridges, would, within a certain excursion, be reflected in a corresponding increase in the total force produced by the fiber. This hypothesis was indeed validated by Gordon and colleagues[19] in an experiment whose major results are depicted in Figure 4–7. It was indicated that with sarcomere length exceeding 3.65 μm, filament overlapping could not be reached, and hence no tension was produced. As the fiber ends were allowed to approximate, tension increased linearly, reaching a peak at a sarcomere length between 2 and 2.25 μm. The length (L_0) at which peak force (P_0) was reached corresponded to optimal filament overlapping. Further approximation

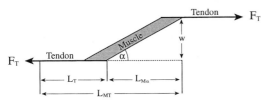

FIGURE 4-6 Geometric relation between the pennation angle and other linear length parameters in muscle. F_T, force developed in tendon; L_T, tendon's length; L_{MT}, total length of musculotendinous unit; $L_{M\alpha}$, colinear muscle length, w, tendon-to-tendon vectorial distance.

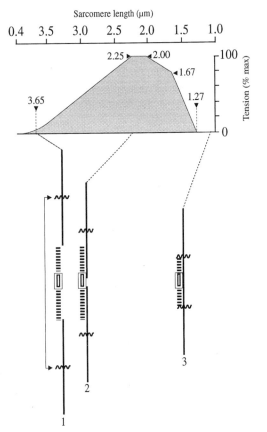

Sarcomere length (μm)

FIGURE 4–7 Relationship between sarcomere length and the relative tension it develops. (Data from Gordon AM, Huxley AF, Julian FJ: The variation in isometric tension with sarcomere length in vertebrate muscle fibers. J Physiol 184:170–192, 1966.)

pertinent points should be highlighted, however. First, actin and myosin filaments have a strong chemical affinity that, in the absence of adenosine triphosphate (ATP), results in their binding together.[22] The actin–myosin complex can therefore be described as a physiologic "default" situation, characteristic of such phenomena as rigor mortis. As soon as ATP is available on site, however, it enters a specific segment of the myosin molecule, where it causes weakening of the actin–myosin complex. Second, immediately after, the ATP entrenches within this segment, enabling a detachment of the complex, a relative movement of 5 N m, and reattachment. Third, after a series of chemical reactions, the myosin, through its head, performs the power stroke and advances another 5 N m. Fourth, after other reactions, the cycle is concluded by freeing the ATP site and reformation of the actin–myosin complex. Experiments have shown that the total unresisted excursion covered within one such cycle, which lasts about 50 ms, is on average 11 N m.[23] The actual binding time, however, is 2 ms. This, of course, must be interpreted in terms of whole muscle, as should the force generated by a single myosin head: 3 to 4 $\times\ 10^{-12}$N.

Once generated within its fibers, muscle tension is transmitted to the bones. This is normally done through tendons, and owing to the passive properties of the latter, consideration is given to the combined musculotendinous unit. When muscle exerts force on tendons, a deformation results that reflects two independent properties: one that is structural and another that is purely mechanical. Structurally, tendons are made up of a woven mesh of collagen fibers, which under no tension have a wavy appearance. Mechanically, tendons are viscoelastic materials, but the elastic component is by far the more dominant.[24] Thus, when force acts on the tendon, the initial effect is that of straightening out the waviness (slackness). Sufficiently high force further results in elongation of the fibers (deformation). This elongation is linearly proportional to the stress (force/unit area of tendon material); that is, the stiffness of the tendon is kept almost constant with a tangent modulus of 1.2 giga-pascal (GPa).[25] From the functional point of view, tendon elasticity may serve a protective role: momentary loads exerted by the muscle are not transmitted directly to the bone. Even more important, however, is the fact that energy dissipation in the tendons, as indicated by the area inside the hysteresis loop, is small.[26] This means that tendons manifest a high degree of elastic recoil, that is, that energy injected into the system may in part be recovered.

resulted in a reduction of force, probably owing to electrostatic repulsion between adjacent and opposing actin filaments. In vivo studies indicate that the length–tension behavior of whole muscle is similar, provided that the involved muscle's lever arm does not change during movement of the mobile relative to the stationary segment. A good approximation of the in vitro findings may be found in a study by Sale and associates,[20] in which isometric movement records of calf muscles under various stimulation conditions were employed. These relationships may also be derived from an isokinetic strength curve by dividing the resulting moment by the corresponding length of the lever arm.[21] Further discussion of the length–tension relationship is provided later in this chapter.

A detailed description of the activation and deactivation of myosin–actin cross-bridges is beyond the scope of this chapter, and interested readers are referred to the work by McComas.[1] Some

FORCE–LENGTH RELATIONSHIP

The F-L relationship is one of the most discussed in muscle mechanics. As the term implies, the main issue is the way in which muscle force varies with its length under zero-velocity (isometric) conditions. A general Hill-type model is commonly used to explain the major mechanical inter-actions. In this model, which precludes the tendon, the active contractile element (CE) operates in a series with the series elastic element (SEE), which represents stiffness residing in the cross-bridges and in parallel with the passive element (PE). However, other than in muscles operating through short tendons, or unless contrary to the accepted theory,[17, 27] positive indications for Z-disk extensi-bility exist, and the energy stored in SEE is con-sidered to be negligible compared with that stored by the tendon; hence, the SEE may be ignored.

As previously indicated, muscle fibers reach their maximal force when the sarcomere length is 2 to 2.25 μm. Moreover, the fiber-specific F-L

relationship takes the form of an inverted U shape (see Fig. 4–7). When a whole muscle specimen is considered, it is predominantly the effect of the passively resisting viscoelastic elements that con-tributes to the change in the total force recorded and the way it varies with the muscle's length (Fig. 4–8). In vivo analysis of the F-L relationship in humans is, of course, a rarity. Measurements carried out on some arm muscles in volunteer cineplastic amputees, however, have shown that muscles behave in quite the same way.

Passive muscles whose length is equal to or below the resting length offer little resistance to pull. Once past its resting length, unstimulated muscle records increasing resistance to deforma-tion whose main source could be myofibrillar elas-ticity.[28] This passive resistance does not vary with the level of muscular activation, as may be seen in Figure 4–8. On the other hand, a lower activa-tion level leads to lower total tension and, conse-quently, to lower net (active) force. Because the active force cannot physically be divorced from

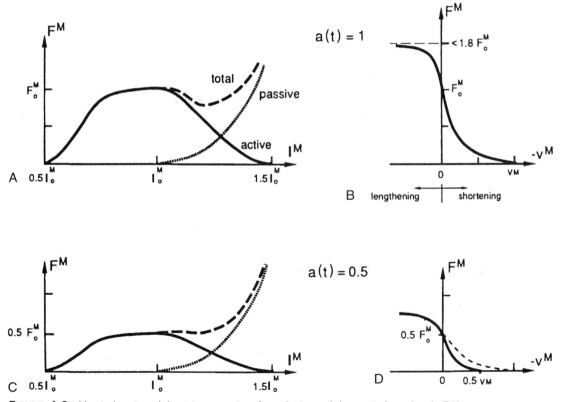

FIGURE 4–8 Nominal static and dynamic properties of muscle tissue. A, Isometric force–length (F-L) relationship with passive (dotted) and active (dashed) components. F^M, muscle force; F_o, peak force; l_o, optimal length. B, Less than fully activated muscle develops less force, but the passive component is unaffected. a(t), level of activation C, Force–velocity (F-V) relationship in fully activated tissue when measured at l_o. VM, maximal shortening velocity. D, When activated at a level lower than its maximum, muscle may contract at a lower rate. $-v^M$, maximal velocity.

the passive force, biomechanical calculations of joint forces equilibrium refer to the total (active plus passive force) as the *muscle force*.

The shape of the F-L relationship depends on the architectural properties of fiber length and pennation. Two variants of the F-L curve, which are based on an animal study,[11] are shown in Figure 4–9, where the semimembranosus (SM, i_a = 0.7) is compared with the gastrocnemius (GM, i_a = 0.3). The active tension of both muscles is of the inverted U shape form, where the maximal value is reached at the normalized length of 100%. Likewise, in both, the passive resistance can be closely approximated by an exponential curve. On the other hand, the falloff toward both ends is much sharper in the gastrocnemius owing to its greater pennation and hence significantly more limited range of excursion. This difference affects the normalized length at which active muscle force can be produced, which is greater in the gastrocnemius. It is also apparent with regard to other interconnected parameters: the active slack

length, meaning the shortest length at which the muscle exerts resistance, 83% for the gastrocnemius and 71% for the semimembranosus, and the passive stiffness in relation to the muscle optimum length, which in the gastrocnemius is almost twice that in the semimembranosus.

The above parameters may vary as a result of length changes imposed on skeletal muscle. Using an animal model, Williams and Goldspink[29] were able to shift the F-L curve, this shift being dependent on the age of the animal. Compared with the typical control curve, the F-L relationship, after imposed lengthening, shifted to the right in adult animals and to the left in young people (Fig. 4–10A and B, respectively). As evident from the adults' curves, although the L_0-based active force was higher in the lengthened position than in the control group, at an original muscle length of 95% L_0 and below, it was lower than that measured in the control group. Gossman and associates[30] speculated that this finding, if allowed to be applied in live human muscle, would explain the

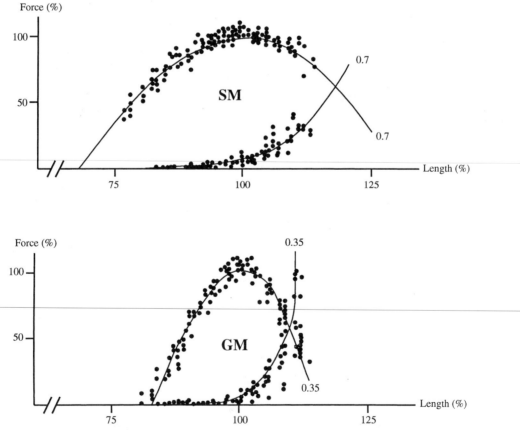

FIGURE 4–9   Force–length relationship in semimembranosus (SM) and medial gastrocnemius (GM). Numbers on the curves refer to the index of architecture. (From Woittiez RD, Huijing PA, Boom H, Rozendal RH: A three dimensional muscle model: A quantified relation between form and function of skeletal muscles. J Morphol 182:95–113, 1984. Copyright © 1984. Reprinted by permission of Wiley-Liss, Inc., a subsidiary of John Wiley & Sons, Inc.)

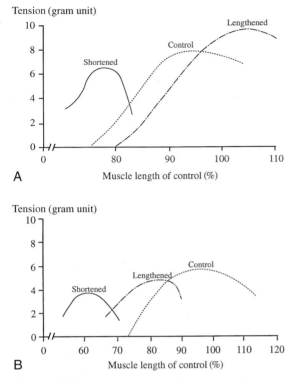

Tension (gram unit)

A Muscle length of control (%)

Tension (gram unit)

B Muscle length of control (%)

FIGURE 4–10 A, Length-associated changes in *adult* animal muscles following immobilization in lengthened and shortened positions relative to control. B, Length-associated changes in *young* animal muscles following immobilization in lengthened and shortened positions relative to control. (A and B, Adapted from Williams PE, Goldspink G: Changes in sarcomere length and physiological properties in immobilised muscle. J Anat 127:459–468, 1978. Reprinted with the permission of Cambridge University Press.)

phenomenon of stretch weakness, namely, the tendency of muscles that are stretched because of postural malalignment to test stronger at the new L_0 but weaker at the natural length. However tempting this theory is, because of the variation in the muscle's lever arm and because of inherent methodologic problems, conclusive proof of this speculation with respect to active muscle contraction may not be possible. In young people, lengthening of muscle results in its actual weakening. The difference may be due to the different mechanism operating: in adults, there is an increase in the sarcomere number, whereas in children, it is the tendon that grows disproportionately in length, placing the muscle belly in a shortened position, which in turn leads to a reduction in the sarcomere length and total force.[29, 31, 32] When shortening is imposed in animals, the result in both adult and young animals is a reduction in the number of sarcomeres and the force produced.

The clinical significance of the F-L relationship

is highlighted in some pathologic states amenable to intervention.[30] In the present context, special reference is made to the treatment of children with cerebral palsy using tone-reducing casts. The aim of using the cast is to elongate hypoextensible muscles to improve function. This intervention is effected by imposing a neutral foot position where equinus exists and then firmly casting for a period of several weeks. Assessment of improvement may be conducted using a force or movement measurement instrument applied at the same ankle joint positions before and after casting. Tardieu and associates[32] indicated that patients whose muscles could adapt well to the new imposed length obtained better compliance (passive torque) after cast removal.

FORCE–VELOCITY RELATIONSHIP

The F-V relationship is the second mechanical function of skeletal muscle that has been the focus of numerous studies over the years. Similar to the studies concentrating on the F-L relationship, research has been directed at the muscle fiber level, at a whole muscle under stimulation, or at muscle in the live body. In the last case, the measured quantity in in vivo studies is the torque rather than the actual force developed by the muscle.

The general description of the F-V relationship was intensively explored by Hill in the late 1930s. The experiments were based on maximal stimulation of a muscle that was allowed to shorten or lengthen against a series of discrete loads, rendering the situation truly isotonic. The graphical presentation of the findings (see Fig. 4–8) clearly evidences two branches: the concentric and the eccentric. During the concentric contractions, F and V were inversely related according to the following equations:

$$v = b(F - F_0)/F + a$$

where v is muscle velocity, F_0 is maximal muscle force at isometric conditions and optimal sarcomere length, F is muscle force, and a and b are constants derived experimentally. By rearranging, this hyperbolic relationship could be solved for F as follows:

$$F = (F_0 b - av)/(b + v)$$

Likewise, one may obtain the maximal velocity (v_0) by setting F = 0, which leads to the following equation:

$$v_0 = bF_0/a$$

Power, the rate at which work is done by muscle (dW/dt), may also be derived from the previous equations because W = Fds and therefore dW/dt = Fds/dt = Fv. In Figure 4–11, the power curve is obtained by multiplying the velocity by the respective force value. Power reaches its peak at about $0.3v_0$, and its value there is equal to about $0.1F_0v_0$.[5]

These relationships do not apply in the eccentric branch of the curve. In vitro findings demonstrate that the force produced is generally independent of the velocity at which the muscle lengthens and that theoretically its maximum may not be higher than $1.8F_0$. The former observation is amply supported by in vivo (isokinetic) studies of eccentric contractions.

Similar to the passive resistance to elongation, characteristic of the F-L curve, in the F-V relationship there is a velocity-dependent response that reflects the inherent viscoelastic makeup of muscles and is therefore not related to a reflexive component. Furthermore, of definite clinical significance is the question of whether velocity sensitivity varies in patients with chronic spasticity. A recent study[33] compared the nonreflexive resistive torque (NRT) of the plantar-flexors in spinal cord injury patients and in control subjects using isokinetic dynamometry. It was revealed that in both groups, NRT increased positively with the velocity, which was varied over a range of 5 to 180 degrees/s. Moreover, although the NRT was generally larger in patients than in control subjects, it tended to plateau in the former group at 60 degrees/s, whereas a proportional linear trend was maintained in the control group throughout the tested velocity spectrum. It was suggested that spasticity and disuse could alter the tensile properties of muscle and that this change should be accounted for, namely, by avoiding rapid vigorous and intensive stretching techniques.

MUSCLE ACTION VECTOR AND MOMENT ARM

Analysis of muscle action in terms of the forces it generates and the reactions produced in the joints and associated structures necessitates further information that cannot be obtained from the previously described physiologic and mechanical parameters: muscle and fiber length, muscle belly versus tendon, angle of pennation, and PCSA. Specifically, because the dominant expression of muscle activity is rotational motion in the joints it spans, knowledge of factors such as the instantaneous direction of the force vector and the moment arm vector is essential. To determine these factors, the human body must be represented spatially as a system of rigid links (segments) whose positions relative to each other are known. Once link position is known, a process of scaling is undertaken in which fitting of the so-called normative databases to the patient's anthropometric parameters (height, weight, skin-fold thickness, somatotype, and segmental length and girth) is performed. The location of the insertion regions of the muscles (and other structures) relative to the links can then be calculated.

Although ostensibly a straightforward procedure, scaling is not without some severe limitations.[15] For example, cadaveric material may not be sufficiently representative because of the actual preservation method, and because cadavers are normally older, their dimensions may not be directly applicable to the younger population. Because no better approach is available, the largely accepted theory of elastic similarity deems that scaling is basically a linear process, measuring increase or decrease proportionately in all dimensions.[34, 35]

There are two major issues concerning the di-

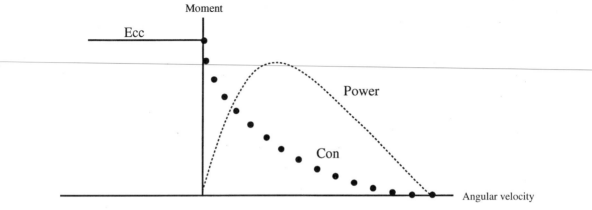

FIGURE 4–11   Schematic strength and power relationships. Con, in concentric contraction; Ecc, in eccentric contraction.

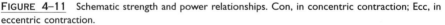

rection of the muscle action vector. One is associated with the fact that in many cases, muscles connect insertion areas rather than insertion points. The other, which is more difficult to tackle, relates to the curvature, or pulley design, of muscles, that is, that some of them cannot be treated as straight lines and hence their action vector does not simply point from the origin to the insertion (or vice versa). As for the former issue, the common method is to represent the insertion area by its centroid, which is basically the geometric average of the area, for example, the center of a circle or an ellipse. With regard to the latter, a few approaches have been adopted for representing the action vector. In the simplest case, muscle may be represented as a straight line using the scaled coordinates of the origin ($X°$, $Y°$, $Z°$) and insertion (X^I, Y^I, Z^I) to obtain the direction cosines of the vector, its length, and its describing equation. The equation may then be employed to solve for the instantaneous length of the moment arm given the coordinates of the instantaneous center or axis of rotation of the relevant joints.

In a detailed analysis of 47 human lower extremity muscles, more than half were represented by nonjointed straight lines.[15] Prominent among these were various components of the gluteus minimus and medius. On the other hand, a more complex course indicated by a pronounced change of direction, at least once, required three anchor points (two sections). One such example is the superficial part of the gluteus minimus. Highly deflected muscles such as those acting on the toes (the extensor and flexor digitorum longus and the extensor and flexor hallucis longus) required no less than six anchor points and hence five linear segments for their representation.

If the muscle has a truly curved trajectory, curve fitting better serves the purpose. This may be done using parametric cubic polynomials, namely, of the form $F(m) = am + bm^2 + cm^3 + d$, where m is the parameter and the values of a, b, c, and d are related to two points and their corresponding tangent vectors through which the muscle passes.[15] In vivo estimation of action vectors currently employs imaging techniques and is based on sequential sections of the specific territory.[36] For example, the magnetic resonance imaging–based approximated muscle moment arms of the lumbar musculature with respect to the disk centroid were calculated by McGill and colleagues[37] using the following matrix:

$$MA = \begin{bmatrix} ri & rj & rk \\ Fi & Fj & Fk \\ Ui & Uj & Uk \end{bmatrix}$$

where MA is the corrected moment arm, r(ijk) is the distance from the disk centroid, F(ijk) is the unit vector of the fiber's line of action, and U(ijk) is the unit vector of the orthopedic axis. However, although magnetic resonance imaging provides an accurate platform for measuring both the disks and muscles, this method depends on the position assumed by the subject during imaging. Moreover, as pointed out by McGill and colleagues,[37] lumbar muscle boundaries are not easy to delineate, neither with respect to other soft tissues nor with respect to adjacent muscles.

On a different level and with respect to these muscles, it would be erroneous to assume that the force contributed by individual muscles can be determined using a single section (lumbar level) because the PCSA of some muscles can change dramatically from one vertebral level to another. These and other factors render the derivation of an exact moment an almost impossible task in some cases. In cases in which the geometry of the muscles and joints concerned is less complex, however, reasonable accuracy may be established, leading to improved prediction of the force and load-sharing mechanisms operating in a specific joint territory.

MUSCLE MOMENT AND ITS RELATIONSHIP TO JOINT ANGULAR POSITION

Muscle moment, which is obtained by the vector product of the muscle force and its moment arm, is the mechanical equivalent of the physiologic *strength*. This is a typical in vivo entity as it relates to the turning effect of the muscle when it operates on the joints it spans. Both the force and the moment arm vary with the change in the angular position of the joint. Although variation in the former is largely dictated by the F-L relationship, the latter is a function of the degree of sliding, spinning, and rolling taking place in the joint. These distinct types of motion are in turn a result of a number of elements, such as the ligamentous-capsular configuration and its laxity, congruence of the articular surfaces, and the joint-loading profile, all of which manifest intimate angle dependency. Consequently, the moment generated by the muscle must be angle dependent.

The determination of the in vivo L_0 is to a large extent arbitrary. On the other hand, it is reasonable that for most uniarticular muscles, the ends of the range of motion are likely to coincide with the shortest or longest muscle belly length. Because the F-L relationship is a monotonically decreasing function from L_0 toward the shortest possible length, and muscles may generally exceed L_0 by more than 10%, it is reasonable to expect that the muscle moment–joint angular position relationship will basically reflect variations in the moment arm. The moment–joint angular position relationship obtained in maximal contractions may be derived by either static (isometric) or dynamic (low-velocity isokinetic) testing.

STATICALLY DETERMINATE SYSTEMS

Up to this point, several parameters associated with the structure and basic mechanical descriptors of the skeletal muscle have been presented. It is now time to consider the variable force that may be generated in the course of purposeful contraction. This information is essential in clinical instances involving the effect of the force on the relevant joints, ligaments, capsule, disks, or muscle itself. For example, the magnitude of bone-to-bone forces depends intimately on the level of muscular forces. Thus, after joint replacement or resurfacing, close monitoring of the level of permissible forces is crucial. For example, quadriceps force is the dominant factor in the tension generated within the anterior cruciate ligament. Consequently, in rehabilitation of the conservatively treated or surgically reconstructed anterior cruciate ligament, extreme care should be taken in designing clinically adequate exercises. Additionally, for the muscle's own sake, it is crucial to know the magnitude of contraction (relative to the maximal tension) that a given muscle may be allowed to exert after, for example, partial tear of its tendon.

Had the situation been that each distinct muscle was responsible for only one motion (e.g., in the case of the elbow joint: brachialis for flexion, triceps for extension, supinator for supination, and pronator for pronation), simple mathematical models of the kind described below would have sufficed to find the force exerted by the muscles for a specific activity. Biomotion, however, is distinguished by a significant extent of redundancy; that is, there are normally more muscles than what is strictly necessary, although in some pathologies, the opposite could be true.[38] This creates a cardinal and fundamental biomechanical problem whose essence is the determination of the exact contribution each muscle is making to the total joint load system.

An attempt to solve it using direct (in vivo) measurements of muscle force proves to be a formidable task. Although it is possible to implant a force transducer and measure the force exerted by the muscle, this intervention is obviously lim-

ited to animal models[39] and even then may prove to be a partial solution only. For example, instrumentation of the patellar tendon can yield information about the level of tension transmitted by the heads of the quadriceps but may hardly solve the problem of intervasti force distribution. Implanting a number of transducers might enhance our understanding but at the same time would introduce serious technical problems. For many reasons, employment of electromyography (EMG) is still not a viable solution for assessing muscle forces. Although much less invasive than sensor implantation, this technology, notwithstanding some major developments, has not yet been perfected for purposes of dynamic contraction analysis as much as it is effective for static analysis. On the other hand, it should be conceded that EMG may be used effectively for either endorsing analytic solutions or guiding the selection of a more appropriate solution set. At any rate, the governing approach in modern biomechanical analysis of musculoskeletal problems is by mathematical modeling. Such analysis extends from the simplistic methods discussed in this section to the advanced methods reviewed in the next section.

Both methods model a "force-movement unit," which consists of the interaction of two basic components: the *biologic component,* comprising the joint, its associated passive structures, and the muscles; and the *external force system,* which is the *resistance* the body has to overcome (or restrain) (that is, objects lifted). Among the main tenets of the model are the following:

1. Muscles generate only those tensile forces whose location with respect to an arbitrary coordinate system can be determined.
2. Ligaments (and capsule) exert tensile forces only.
3. Joints are frictionless and transmit compressive forces.
4. Joints have a well-defined axis of rotation with respect to which the moment arms of all forces may be calculated.

According to the simpler approach, biomechanical force systems have a unique solution that can be arrived at by reducing the number of unknowns, mostly muscle forces, to the number of equipollence equations. This can be done by lumping several muscles into one "working group,"[40-42] by ascribing specific force proportions between muscles,[43] or by ignoring certain muscles whose contribution to the moment is considered negligible.[44] These procedures result in a *statically determinate system* in which the number of unknowns equals the number of equations.

The most basic statically determinate system

requires no reduction. Consider the simple planar situation in which segment 2 is to be held at a certain position relative to segment 1 with which it shares a common joint (Fig. 4–12). In principle, *one* muscle (m) would suffice to support the counter (resisting) moment provided it can generate enough tension. Assuming that the magnitude of the resisting moment (M_{ext}) can be calculated, the force generated by the muscle (F_m) can readily be derived using the following equilibrium equation:

$$\Sigma \overrightarrow{M} = r_m \times F_m + M_{ext} = 0$$

where r_m is the vector representing the muscle's moment arm. In this hypothetical example, suppose that m has a moment arm of 40 mm, and the external moment is 30 newton-meters (N m). The force (F_m) is therefore equal to 30 divided by 0.04, or 750 N. If another muscle, q, is operating along with m, and it is assumed (e.g., owing to their respective PCSAs) that $F_m = 2F_q$, the following equation can readily be solved for F_m and then F_q:

$$\Sigma \overrightarrow{M} = r_m \times F_m + r_q \times F_q + M_{ext} =$$
$$r_m \times F_m + 0.5r_q \times F_m + M_{ext} = 0$$

To solve for the reactive forces, the force equilibrium equation is used, as follows:

$$\Sigma \overrightarrow{F} = 0$$

The forces acting on the joint are then commonly resolved along the compression and shear axes of the joint. Clearly, the compressive component does not require additional balancing because

it is operating against a "solid" plate of articular cartilage (with or without disk or bursae, when relevant). Depending on the geometry of the joint, however, passive tension of a ligamentous or a capsular nature would be required to offset the shear component, which invariably tends to sublux or dislocate the joint.

Problems involving motion of the segment are solved likewise. For instance, consider the case in which segment 2 moves radially relative to segment 1. Providing that its moment of inertia and its kinematics are known, the following equations are equally applicable and yield a unique solution:

$$\Sigma \overrightarrow{F} = 0$$
$$\Sigma \overrightarrow{M} = 0$$

where the relevant components of $I\alpha$ are added. If, on the other hand, owing to the inertia imparted by muscle m, segment 2 approaches the end of range too quickly and antagonistic activity is initiated in muscle n (see Fig. 4–12) in such a way that m and n do not co-contract, F_n can be derived in a similar fashion.

Inherent in these simple models is the assumption that neither synergism (m and q) nor antagonistic coactivation (m and n or m, q, and n) takes place. This assumption is obviously erroneous and therefore may be used only when there is good grounds for its existence. On the other hand, reduction methods can sometimes yield a reasonable approximation to the real situation, hence their applicability.

STATICALLY INDETERMINATE SYSTEMS AND COMMON METHODS OF SOLUTION

From a purely mathematical viewpoint, the situation changes dramatically when the assumptions given previously are no longer valid, that is, when the number of muscles (or other load-transmitting elements) is larger than the number of equations. This results in *redundancy* or the so-called distribution problem,[45] both of which relate to the determination of the force magnitude developed by P muscles based on R equations, where P is greater than R. Because in principle there is an infinite number of solutions to such a system, it is not possible to determine a unique solution, and thus the system becomes *statically indeterminate*.

Such systems are the rule in musculoskeletal biomechanics, and their solution poses one of the main challenges in modern studies. For example,

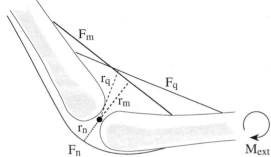
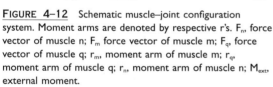

FIGURE 4–12 Schematic muscle–joint configuration system. Moment arms are denoted by respective r's. F_n, force vector of muscle n; F_m force vector of muscle m; F_q, force vector of muscle q; r_m, moment arm of muscle m; r_q, moment arm of muscle q; r_n, moment arm of muscle n; M_{ext}, external moment.

in the foregoing problem, suppose that m, q, and n are simultaneously contracting, that is, that there is an agonist–antagonist coactivation in addition to synergy. The equation to be solved thus would be as follows:

$$\Sigma \vec{M} = r_m \times F_m + r_q \times F_q + r_n \times F_n + M_{ext} = 0$$

If the method of simple reduction is ruled out, this equation must be supplemented by other conditions or equations to be solved. To that aim, there are two general approaches. One approach that has attracted considerable attention, *optimization*, is based on the arbitrary yet physiologically reasonable assumption that activation of muscles is done according to some criterion. Furthermore, this criterion, which is known by the terms *cost, objective,* or *penalty function,* is to be minimized or maximized—for instance, muscular stresses or muscular endurance, respectively. The other approach is based on testing all possible combinations within a solution space and selecting those that are physiologically viable or meet certain accepted criteria.[46] Methodologically, the second approach is reminiscent of the reduction technique, although it is by far more sophisticated. In this chapter, a more detailed presentation is given to the first (optimization) method, although it should by no means be construed as the better of the two.

One of the first formulations of a cost function in this kind of problem was by MacConaill,[47] who proposed the minimal total muscular force principle according to which "no more total force than is both necessary and sufficient to maintain a body posture or perform a motion is used."[45] Other cost functions (see later) have been tested during the past 20 years, and some have proved highly successful in predicting temporal activity patterns when compared with EMG traces. The magnitude of the forces, however, could not be validated. The fact that temporal patterns are predictable proves, at least partially, that the body works according to some optimization principle. On the other hand, because the nature of the optimization is yet unknown, it may well be that more than one principle is operating. Furthermore, cost functions that reasonably operate in intact and normal musculoskeletal systems may not necessarily apply in other instances. In this context, one could speculate about the significance of specific cost functions in movements provoking joint-related pain or the need to exercise or when a need arises for extremely delicate movements. It is therefore not surprising that the specific selection of the optimization technique is paramount in deciding the sort of solutions at which one arrives.[48] The evolution of optimization methods in musculoskeletal biomechanics started with the use of linear models.[49] This approach enjoys the relative ease of linear programming, but its results are not always consistent physiologically. The nonlinear approach pioneered by Pedotti and associates[50] and Crownshield and Brand[45] is more complicated mathematically but yields physiologically interpretable solutions.

To demonstrate the elegance of the optimization technique as well as its drawbacks, the following relatively simple example, taken from a study by Dul and coworkers,[44] was selected. The problem to be solved was that of finding the load distribution among the muscles performing planar quasistatic knee flexion in the seated position (Fig. 4–13) while the force exerted by subjects in-

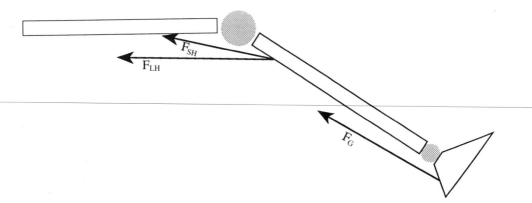

FIGURE 4–13 Schematic muscle–joint configuration for solving the optimization problem. F_{LH}, long hamstring; F_{SH}, short hamstring; F_G, gastrocnemius. (Adapted from Dul J, Townsend MA, Shiavi R, Johnson GE: Muscular synergism. I. On criteria for load sharing between synergistic muscles. J Biomechanics 17:663–673, 1984, with permission from Elsevier Science.)

creased from 30 to 275 N. The problem was first reduced to three muscle groups by the following lumping procedure:

Long hamstrings comprising the long biceps femoris, semimembranosus, and semitendinosus

Short hamstrings comprising the short biceps femoris

Gastrocnemius comprising the lateral and medial heads

The small popliteus and plantaris muscles were ignored owing to a small motion arm and small PCSA, respectively. Also, no consideration was given to ligamentous (e.g., posterior longitudinal) forces. There were three joint equipollence equations: two relating to the planar forces and one to the moment. On the other hand, the system included five unknown forces (three muscle forces and two joint reactions), hence the optimization.

In the second stage, the design variables and constraint functions were determined. The design variables are those elements that are included in the cost function and that are systematically varied (normally by an iterative process) until the cost function is minimized. In the present context, they are invariably the magnitudes of the muscular forces.[51] The constraint functions are those mathematical relationships aimed at restricting the solution to certain boundary conditions.

In formulating the optimization problem, the following equations were applied:

$$\text{Minimize: } \Sigma_i x_i^p \ (i = 1\text{–}3)$$

where x_i is a decision variable that stands for either the i-th muscle force (N) or stress (N/cm^2), the latter being defined as F/PCSA of the individual muscle; p is the power of the decision variable to be minimized. The equation $p = 1$ renders the system linear; otherwise, it is nonlinear, subject to the following:

$$x_i \geq 0 \ (i = 1\text{–}3)$$

where x_i is the force or stress.

$$\Sigma C_i x_i = M$$

where c_i (in cm or cm^3) is a constant derived from the moment equation and M is the resultant moment (in Ncm).

$$x_i \leq x_{max}$$

where x_{max} refers to the maximal force or stress of the i-th muscle; in the present case, 30 N/cm^2 was selected as the constraint.

$$x_i = Kx_j \ (i \neq j)$$

where K is a force ratio that dictates that when muscle x_i is contracting, so does muscle x_j; that is, there is a synergistic pattern. However, the force (stress) in i is K times greater than that in j.

The results of this problem subject to several different cost functions are presented next. For the sake of simplicity, the joint reactions were not included in the figures.

In the simplest situation, the design variables are muscle forces, $p = 1$; that is, optimization is done using the Simplex method, and the cost function is the *sum of forces* (ΣF_i). No upper force limit is imposed, and synergy is not assumed. The solution takes the form depicted in Figure 4–14A, which shows that the only muscle operating is the long hamstring because it has the longest motion arm and hence is the least expensive (minimal force) to use. As pointed out before, this may not be a realistic solution because coactivation takes place. Another linear optimization is illustrated in Figure 4–14B, in which the cost function is the same as in the former example, but this time, the previous two equations are imposed, so that the long and short heads of the hamstrings are contracting simultaneously. Moreover, the stress developed in each of these muscles is equal (K = 1); that is, $F_{LH} = 4.9F_{SH}$. As a consequence, F_{LH} and F_{SH} depart together from the x axis, but the slope is different, reflecting the force proportion.

Nonlinear optimization of the sum of cubed forces (ΣF_i^3; $p = 3$) imposing the same constraints as in the second example is shown in Figure 4–14C. Note that in this case, the F_{LH}-F_{SH} force pattern is strikingly similar, but F_G follows a different recruitment pattern; that is, instead of being delayed until the external force reaches about 130 N, it is contracting parallel to the hamstrings. Finally, another cost function, the *sum of the cubed stresses* ($\Sigma [F_i/PCSA_i^3]$), is used under the same constraints, and the results are depicted in Figure 4–14D. Note the significant change in the order of strength occurring between F_{LH} and F_G.

These examples emphasize that the solution to the distribution problem is dependent on the choice of the cost function and on the decision and constraint variables; that is, the solution is arbitrary. Nevertheless, such selection can be rendered physiologically sound and therefore can yield a reasonable solution.

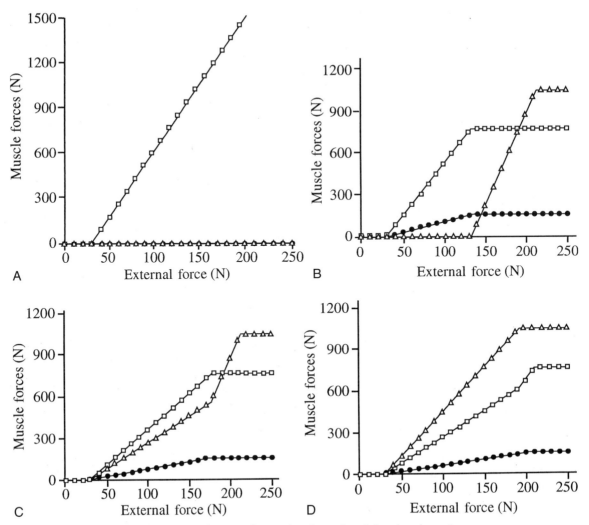

FIGURE 4–14 Solutions to different cost functions. Squares, long hamstring; circles, short hamstring; triangles, gastrocnemius.

References

1. McComas AJ: Skeletal Muscle Form and Function. Champaign, IL, Human Kinetics, 1996.
2. Coers C, Woolf AL: The Innervation of Muscle. Oxford, UK, Blackwell Scientific Publications, 1959.
3. Barrett B: The length and mode of termination of individual muscle fibers in the human sartorius and posterior femoral muscles. Acta Anat 48:242–251, 1962.
4. Windhorst U, Hamm TM, Stuart DG: On the function of muscle and reflex partitioning. Behav Brain Res 12:629–681, 1989.
5. Herzog W: Muscle. *In* Nigg BM, Herzog W (eds): Biomechanics of the Musculoskeletal System. New York, John Wiley & Sons, 1994.
6. Walker SM, Schrodt GR: I-segment lengths and thin filaments periods in skeletal muscle fibers of the rhesus monkey. Anat Rec 178:63–82, 1973.
7. Lieber RL, Bodine-Fowler SC: Skeletal muscle mechanics: Implications for rehabilitation. Phys Ther 73:844–856, 1993.
8. Wiekiewicz TI, Roy RR, Powell PL, Edgerton VR: Muscle architecture of the human lower limb. Clin Orthop 179:275–283, 1983.
9. Lieber RL, Fazeli BM, Botte MJ: Architecture of selected wrist flexor and extensor muscles. J Hand Surg (Am) 14:244–250, 1990.
10. Lieber RL, Jacobson MD, Fazeli BM: Architecture of selected muscles of the arm and forearm: Anatomy and implications for tendon transfer. J Hand Surg (Am) 17:787–798, 1992.
11. Woittiez RD, Huijing PA, Boom H, Rozendal RH: A three dimensional muscle model: A quantified

relation between form and function of skeletal muscles. J Morphol 182:95–113, 1984.

12. Lieber RL, Blevins FL: Skeletal muscle architecture of the rabbit hindlimb: Functional implications of muscle design. J Morphol 199:93–101, 1989.

13. Alexander RMcN, Vernon A: The dimensions of knee and ankle muscles and the forces they exert. J Hum Movement Studies 1:115–123, 1975.

14. Gregor RJ: Skeletal muscle mechanics and movement. *In* Grabiner MD: Current Issues in Biomechanics. Champaign, IL, Human Kinetics, 1993.

15. Pierrynowski MR: Analytic representation of muscle line of action and geometry. *In* Allard P, Stokes IAF, Blanchi J-P (eds): Three Dimensional Analysis of Human Movement. Champaign, IL, Human Kinetics, 1995.

16. Huxley AF, Niedergerke R: Structural changes in muscle during contraction: Interference microscopy of living muscle fibers. Nature 173:971–973, 1954.

17. Huxley AF, Simmons RM: Proposed mechanism of force generation in striated muscle. Nature 233:533–536, 1971.

18. Huxley HE, Hanson J: Changes in the cross striations of muscle during contraction and stretch and structural interpretations. Nature 173:973–976, 1954.

19. Gordon AM, Huxley AF, Julian FJ: The variation in isometric tension with sarcomere length in vertebrate muscle fibers. J Physiol 184:170–192, 1966.

20. Sale DG, Quinlan J, Marsh E, et al: Influence of joint position on ankle plantarflexion in humans. J Appl Physiol 52:1636–1642, 1982.

21. Dvir Z: Isokinetics: Muscle Testing, Interpretation and Clinical Applications. Edinburgh, Churchill Livingstone, 1995.

22. Rayment, I, Holden HM, Whittaker M, et al: Structure of actin-myosin complex and its implications for muscle contractions. Science 261:58–65, 1993.

23. Finner JT, Simmons RM, Spudich JA: Single myosin molecule mechanics: PicoNewton forces and nanometre steps. Nature 368:113–119, 1994.

24. Latash ML, Zatiorsky VM: Joint stiffness: Myth or reality? Hum Movement Sci 12:653–692, 1993.

25. Zajac EF: Muscle and tendon: Properties, models, scaling and application to biomechanics and motor control. Crit Rev Biomed Eng 17:359–411, 1989.

26. Alexander RMcN: Elastic mechanisms in animal movement. Cambridge, Cambridge University Press, 1988.

27. Ford LE, Huxley AF, Simmons RM: Tension responses in sudden length change in stimulated frog muscle fibers near slack length. J Physiol (Lond) 269:441–449, 1977.

28. Magid A, Law DG: Myofibrils bear most of the resting tension in frog skeletal muscle. Science 230:1280–1282, 1985.

29. Williams PE, Goldspink G: Changes in sarcomere length and physiological properties in immobilized muscle. J Anat 127:459–468, 1978.

30. Gossman MR, Sahrmann SA, Rose SJ: Review of length-associated changes in muscle. Phys Ther 62:1799–1808, 1982.

31. Tabray JC, Tabray C, Tardieu C: Physiological and structural changes in the cat's soleus muscle due to immobilization at different lengths by plaster casts. J Physiol (Lond) 224:231–244, 1972.

32. Tardieu C, Tabray JC, Tabray C: Comparison of the sarcomere number adaptation in young and adult animals: Influence of tendon adaptation. J Physiol (Paris) 73:1045–1055, 1977.

33. Lamontagne A, Malouin F, Richards C, Dumas F: Impaired viscoelastic behavior of spastic plantarflexors during passive stretch at different velocities. Clin Biomech 12:508–515, 1997.

34. Gunther B: Dimensional analysis and theory of biological similarity. Physiol Rev 55:659–699, 1975.

35. McMahon TA: Muscles, Reflexes and Locomotion. Princeton, NJ, Princeton University Press, 1984.

36. Koolstra JH, van Eijden TMGJ, Weijs WA: An iterative procedure to estimate muscle lines of action in vivo. J Biomech 22:911–920, 1989.

37. McGill SM, Santaguida L, Stevens J: Measurement of the trunk musculature from T_4 to L_5 using MRI scans of 15 young males corrected for muscle fiber orientation. Clin Biomech 8:171–178, 1993.

38. Dul J: The biomechanical prediction of muscle forces. Clin Biomech 1:27–30, 1986.

39. Whiting QC, Gregor RJ, Roy RR, Edgerton VR: A technique for estimating mechanical work of individual muscles in the cat during treadmill locomotion. J Biomech 17:685–691, 1984.

40. Paul JP: Bioengineering studies of the forces transmitted by joints. *In* Kenedi RM (ed): Engineering Analysis, Biomechanics and Related Bioengineering Topics. Oxford, UK, Pergamon Press, 1965, pp 369–380.

41. Morrison JB: The mechanics of the knee joint in relation to normal walking. J Biomech 3:51–71, 1970.

42. Procter P: Ankle Joint Biomechanics. Unpublished PhD thesis, Strathclyde University, Glasgow, UK, 1980.

43. Nicol A: Biomechanics of the Elbow Joints. Unpublished PhD thesis, Strathclyde University, Glasgow, UK, 1977.

44. Dul J, Townsend MA, Shiavi R, Johnson GE: Muscular synergism. I. On criteria for load sharing between synergistic muscles. J Biomech 17:663–673, 1984.

45. Crownshield RD, Brand RA: The prediction of forces in joint structures: distribution of intersegmental resultants. Exer Sport Sci Rev 9:159–181, 1981.

46. Collins JJ: The redundant nature of locomotor optimization laws. J Biomech 28:251–268, 1995.

47. MacConnail MA: The ergonomic aspect of articular mechanics. *In* Evans FG (ed): Studies on the Anatomy and Function of Bones and Joints. Berlin, Springer, 1967.
48. An K-N, Kaufman K, Chao EYS: Estimation of joint and muscle forces. *In* Allard P, Stokes IAF, Blanchi J-P (eds): Three Dimensional Analysis of Human Movement. Champaign, IL, Human Kinetics, 1995.
49. Seireg A, Arkivar RJ: A mathematical model for evaluation of forces in lower extremities of the musculoskeletal systems. J Biomech 6:313–326, 1973.
50. Pedotti A, Krishnan VV, Starke L: Optimization of muscle-force sequencing in human locomotion. Math Biosci 38:57–76, 1978.
51. Herzog W, Binding P: Mathematically indeterminate systems. *In* Nigg BM, Herzog W (eds): Biomechanics of the Musculoskeletal System. New York, John Wiley & Sons, 1994.

CHAPTER 5

BIOMECHANICS OF THE THORACOLUMBAR SPINE

Stuart M. McGill

Most clinicians reading this chapter will already have studied basic biomechanics and anatomy. The study of biomechanics becomes an exercise in basic science if the clinical relevance is ignored. The intent of this chapter is to describe some normal biomechanics of the thoracolumbar spine, then to describe the injury process, and finally to revisit some anatomic-biomechanical features, possibly in a way not previously considered, and to relate these to function, the reduction of the risk of low-back injury or reinjury, and the design of optimal rehabilitation programs. The professional challenge is to make wise decisions from the blending of laboratory and empirical evidence with clinical experience.

NORMAL BIOMECHANICS OF THE THORACOLUMBAR SPINE

ANATOMIC FEATURES AND THEIR CLINICAL RELEVANCE

Vertebrae

The Body

It is assumed that the reader knows there are 12 thoracic and 5 lumbar vertebrae. The construction of the vertebral bodies themselves may be likened to a barrel whereby the round walls are formed with relatively stiff cortical bone (Fig. 5–1). The top and bottom of the barrel are formed with a more deformable cartilage plate (end plate) that is about 0.6 mm thick but is thinnest in the central region.[1] The end plate is porous for passage of nutrients such as oxygen and glucose, whereas the inside of the barrel is filled with cancellous bone.

The trabecular arrangement within the cancellous bone is aligned with the trajectories of stress to which it is exposed. Three orientations dominate—one vertical and two oblique[2] (Fig. 5–2). This is a special architecture in terms of how the vertebral bodies bear compressive loading and how they fail under excessive loading. Although the walls of the vertebrae appear to be rigid on compression, the nucleus of the disk pressurizes (see the classic works by Nachemson[3, 4]) and causes the cartilaginous end plates of the vertebrae to bulge inward, seemingly to compress the cancellous bone.[5] In fact, under compression, it is the cancellous bone that fails first,[6] making it the determinant of failure tolerance of the spine (at least when the spine is not positioned at the end range of motion). It is difficult to injure the disk anulus this way (anular failure is discussed later).

Although this notion is contrary to the concept that the vertebral bodies are rigid, the functional interpretation of this anatomy suggests the presence of a clever shock-absorbing and load-bearing system. Farfan[7] proposed that the vertebral bodies act as shock absorbers of the spine, although he based this on vertebral body fluid flow and not end-plate bulging. Because the nucleus is incompressible, bulging end plates suggest fluid expulsion from the vertebral bodies, specifically blood through the perivertebral sinuses.[8] This would suggest protective dissipation on quasistatic and dynamic compressive loading of the spine. The question is: how do the end plates bulge inward into seemingly rigid cancellous bone? The answer appears to be in the architecture of the cancellous bone, which is dominated by the system of columns of bone (shown in Fig. 5–2) with much smaller transverse bony ties. On axial compres-

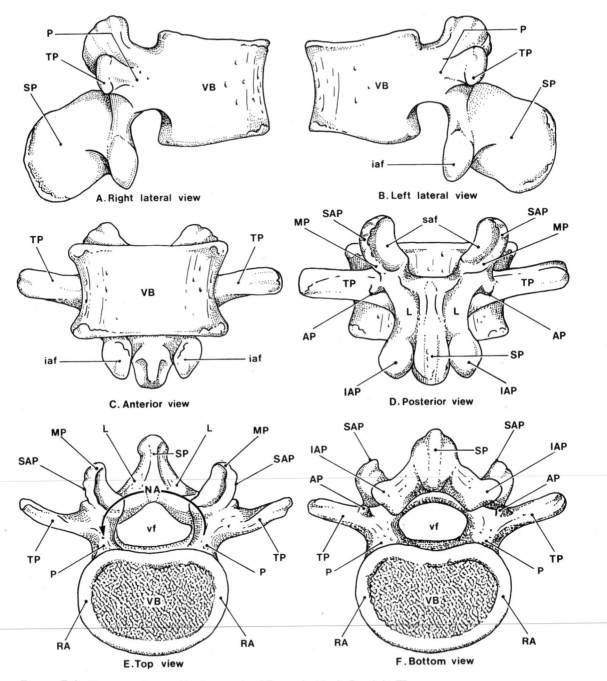

FIGURE 5–1   The parts of a typical lumbar vertebra. VB, vertebral body; P, pedicle; TP, transverse process; SP, spinous process; L, lamina; SAP, superior articular process; LAP, inferior articular process; saf, superior articular facet; iaf, inferior articular facet; MP, mamillary process; AP, accessory process; vf, vertebral foramen; RA, ring apophysis; NA, neural arch. (From Bogduk N, Twomey LT: Clinical Anatomy of the Lumbar Spine. New York, Churchill Livingstone, 1987.)

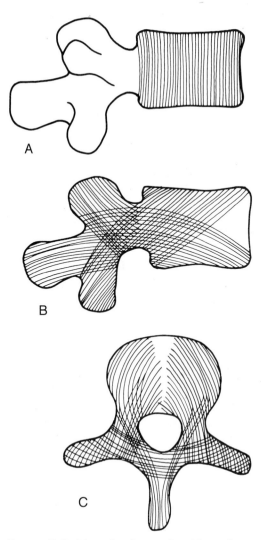

FIGURE 5-2 The trabeculae are aligned (according to Gallois and Japoit, 1925[2]) with the dominant trajectories of stress. *A*, Vertical trabecular system. *B*, Inferior and superior oblique systems. *C*, Oblique systems viewed from above. (From Dupuis PR, Kirkaldy-Willis WM: The spine: Integrated function and pathophysiology. *In* Cruess RL, Rennie WRJ [eds]: Adult Orthopaedics, vol 2. New York, Churchill Livingstone, 1984, p 683.)

its original structure and function. It would appear that cancellous fracture could heal quickly when damaged given the small amount of osteophyte activity needed, at least compared with the length of time needed for repair of collagenous tissues.

Both the disk and the vertebrae deform while supporting spinal loads. Under excessive compressive loading, the bulging of the end plates into the vertebral bodies also causes radial stresses in the end plate sufficient to cause fracture in a stellate pattern. These fractures, or cracks, in the end plate are sometimes sufficiently large to allow the nucleus of the disk to squirt through into the vertebral body,[10] resulting in the formation of the classic Schmorl's node (Fig. 5–4). This type of injury is associated with compression of the spine when the spine is not at the end range of motion (i.e., not flexed, bent, or twisted). I believe that this type of common compressive injury is often misdiagnosed as a herniated disk owing to the flattened interdiscal space seen on planar radiographs. The anulus of the disk, however, does remain intact. It is simply a case of the nucleus' leaving the disk and progressing through the end plate into the cancellous core of the vertebrae.

The Posterior Elements

The posterior elements of the vertebrae (pedicles, laminae, spinous processes, and facet joints) have a shell of cortical bone but contain a cancellous bony core in the thicker parts. The transverse processes project laterally together with a superior pair and inferior pair of facet joints (see Fig. 5–1). On the lateral surface of the bone that forms the superior facets are the accessory and mamillary processes, which, together with the transverse process, are major attachment sites of the longissimus and iliocostalis extensor muscle groups (described later). The facet joints are typical synovial joints in that the articulating surfaces are covered with hyaline cartilage and are contained in a capsule. Fibroadipose enlargements or miniscoids are found around the rim of the facet, although mostly at the proximal and distal poles,[11] which have been implicated as a possible structure that could "bind" and lock the facet joint (Fig. 5–5).

The neural arch in general (pedicles and laminae) appears to be somewhat flexible. In fact, Bedzinski[12] demonstrated flexibility of the pars during flexion and extension of cadaveric spines, whereas Dickey and associates[13] documented up to 3-degree changes of the right pedicle with respect to the left pedicle during mild daily activities using pedicle screws in vivo. Failure of these elements, together with facet damage, leading to spondylolisthesis, is often blamed exclusively on

sion, as the end plates bulge into the vertebral bodies, these columns experience compression and appear to bend in a buckling mode; under excessive load, they buckle as the smaller bony transverse ties fracture, as documented by Fyhrie and Schaffler[9] (Fig. 5–3). In this way, the cancellous bone can rebound to its original shape (at least 95% of the original unloaded shape) when the load is removed, even after suffering fracture and delamination of the transverse ties. This architecture appears to afford superior elastic deformation, even after marked damage, and then heal to regain

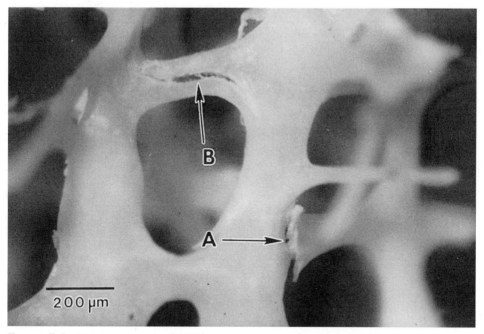

FIGURE 5–3 Under compressive loading, bulging of the end plate causes buckling stresses in the vertical trabeculae (A) that, when excessive, cause damage in the transverse trabeculae (B). (From Fyhrie DP, Schaffler MB: Failure mechanisms in human vertebral cancellous bone. Bone 15[1]: 105–109, 1994, with permission from Elsevier Science.)

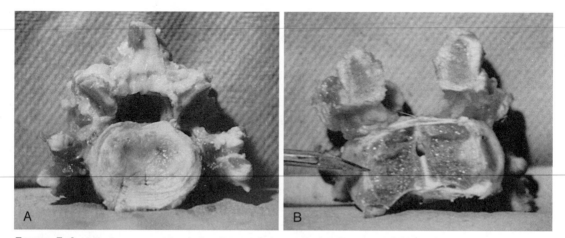

FIGURE 5–4 A, Stellate-patterned end-plate fracture. B, Intrusion of nuclear material (shown at the tip of the scalpel) into the vertebral body from compressive loading of a spine in a neutral posture. These are porcine specimens.

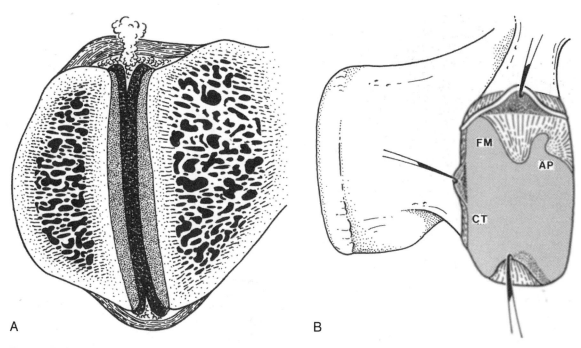

FIGURE 5–5 Lateral view of the facet face revealing the fibroadipose meniscoids (FM) and the adipose tissue pad (AP), which have been implicated in joint binding. CT, connective tissue rim. (From Bogduk N, Twomey LT: Clinical Anatomy of the Lumbar Spine. New York, Churchill Livingstone, 1987, p 31.)

anteroposterior shear forces. A case could be made from epidemiologic evidence, however, that the damage to these posterior elements may also be associated with full range of motion in athletes such as gymnasts and Australian cricket bowlers.[14]

It would appear that injury to the posterior bony elements in these sorts of activities is a fatigue injury caused by cyclic full flexion and extension, fatiguing the arch with repeated bending. On the other hand, there is no doubt that excessive shear forces also cause injury to these elements. Posterior shear of the superior vertebrae can lead to ligamentous damage but also failure in the vertebrae itself as the end plate avulses from the rest of the vertebral body (Fig. 5–6). Anterior shear of the superior vertebrae has been documented to cause pars and facet fracture, leading to spondylolisthesis with a typical tolerance of an adult lumbar spine of about 2000 N.[15] Although similar injury mechanisms and tolerance values were observed in young porcine spine specimens,[6] the type of injury appeared to be modulated by loading rate. Specifically, anterior shear forces produced undefinable soft tissue injury at low load rates (100 N/s), but fractures of the pars, facet face, and vertebral body were observed at higher load rates (7000 N/s). Posterior shear forces applied at low load rates produced undefinable soft tissue failure and vertebral body fracture, whereas higher load rates produced wedge fractures and facet damage.

Intervertebral Disk

The disk comprises three major components: the nucleus pulposus, the anulus fibrosus, and the end plates. The nucleus is a gel-like substance with collagen fibrils suspended in a base of water and various mucopolysaccharides, giving it both viscosity and some elastic response when perturbed in vitro. Although there is no distinct border with the anulus, the lamellae of the anulus become more distinct, moving radially outward. The collagen fibers of each lamina are obliquely oriented; the obliquity runs in the opposite direction in each concentric lamella. The ends of the collagen fibers anchor into the vertebral body with Sharpey's fibers in the outermost lamellae, whereas the inner fibers attach to the end plate (discussed earlier). The disks in cross-section resemble a rounded triangle in the thoracic region and an ellipse in the lumbar region, suggesting anisotropic facilitation of twisting and bending.

The disk appears to be a hydrostatic structure that allows 6-degrees-of-freedom motion between vertebrae, but its ability to bear load is dependent on its shape and geometry, as determined by the adjacent vertebrae. Because of the orientation of

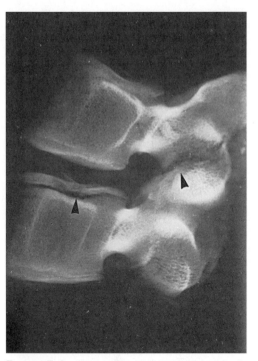

FIGURE 5-6 Shear injuries include fracture of the facet base and end-plate avulsion from the vertebrae.

support compressive load as the nucleus pressurizes, applying hydraulic forces to the end plates and to the anulus and causing the anulus collagen fibers to bulge outward, which places them under tension.

Many years ago, Markolf and Morris[16] elegantly demonstrated that a disk with the nucleus removed lost height but preserved properties of axial stiffness, creep, and relaxation rates. It would appear that the nucleus is required to preserve disk height, which has implications on facet loading, shear stiffness, ligament mechanics, and so forth. Consideration of progressive disk injury is in order here. If little hydrostatic pressure is present, perhaps the nucleus has been lost through end-plate fracture or herniation; when the disk is compressed, not only does the outer anulus bulge outward but also the inner anulus bulges inward (Fig. 5–7). This double-convex bulging causes the laminae of the anulus to separate, or delaminate, and has been hypothesized to form a pathway for nuclear material to leak through the lamellar layers and finally extrude, creating a frank herniated disk.[17]

From a review of the literature, one can make three general conclusions about anulus injury and resulting bulging or herniation. First, it appears that the disk must be bent to the full end range of motion to herniate,[18] and herniations tend to occur in younger spines[19] (those with higher water content[20] and more hydraulic behavior). Second, disk herniation is associated with extreme deviated posture, fully flexed, and the risk is higher with repeated loading of at least 20,000 or 30,000 times, highlighting the role of fatigue as a mechanism of injury.[21, 22] Third, epidemiologic data link herniation with sedentary occupations and the sit-

the collagen fibers within the concentric rings of the anulus, with half of the fibers oblique to the other half, the anulus is able to resist loads in twist; however, only half of the fibers are able to support this mode of loading, and the other half become disabled, resulting in a substantial loss of strength or ability to bear load. When the disk is subjected to bending and to compressive load, it has been argued that the anulus and the nucleus

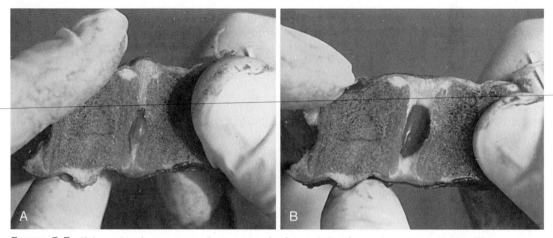

FIGURE 5-7 If the nucleus loses pressure (e.g., as a result of an end-plate fracture) upon compression (A), the anulus compresses, resulting in radial bulging both outward and inward, causing delaminating stresses. When the nucleus is contained in a healthy disk, these stresses are minimal (B).

ting posture.[23] In fact, Wilder and associates[24] documented anular tears in young calf spines from prolonged simulated sitting postures and cyclic compressive loading (i.e., simulated truck driving). Older spines appear not to exhibit the classic extrusion of nuclear material but rather are characterized by delamination of the anulus layers and by radial cracks, which appear to progress with repeated loading (see the review by Goel and colleagues[25]).

Muscles

Most textbooks present the major thoracic and lumbar musculature from a posterior view. However, many of the functionally relevant aspects are better viewed in the sagittal plane (see the synopsis of the sagittal plane lines of action presented by Bogduk and colleagues[26–28]). Furthermore, there is a tendency to obtain a mechanical appreciation of function by simply interpreting the lines of action, region of attachment, and lines of pull of the musculature, which may be misleading. Together with knowledge of muscle morphology, knowledge of activation of the musculature in a wide variety of movement and loading tasks is required to understand the function and purpose of each muscle and how the motor control system activates the musculature to support external loads. Therefore, this section provides an anatomic description of the musculature together with the results of various electromyography (EMG) studies to help interpret function.

Muscle Size

The physiologic cross-sectional area of muscle determines the force-producing potential, whereas the line of action and moment arm determine the effect of the force in moment production, stabilization, and so forth. It is erroneous to estimate force based on muscle volume without accounting for fiber architecture or from taking transverse scans to measure anatomic cross-sectional areas.[29] Muscle forces are often underestimated because a large number of muscle fibers are not "seen" in a single transverse scan of a pennated muscle, and magnetic resonance imaging (MRI) or computed tomography (CT) scans must be corrected for architecture and scan plane obliquity.[30] Transverse scans of one subject show the changing shape of the torso muscles over the thoracolumbar region (Fig. 5–8), highlighting the need to obtain fiber architecture data from dissection. In this example, the thoracic extensors seen at T9 provide extensor moment at L4 even though they are not seen in the L4 scan; only their tendons

overlying the L4 extensors are seen. Raw muscle relative physiologic cross-sectional areas and moment arms are provided in Tables 5–1 to 5–3,[30] whereas areas corrected for oblique lines of action, for some selected muscles at several levels of the thoracolumbar spine, are shown in Table 5–4. Guidelines for estimating true physiologic areas are provided by McGill and associates.[29]

Moment arms of the abdominal musculature reported in CT- and MRI-based studies have recently been shown to underestimate true values by 30% as a result of the supine posture adopted in MRI and CT scanners, which causes the abdominal contents to collapse under gravity.[31] In real life, the abdominals are pushed away from the spine with the visceral contents when a person is standing.

The Rotatores and Intertransversarii

Many anatomic textbooks describe the small rotator muscles of the spine, which attach adjacent vertebrae, as fulfilling the role of creating axial twisting torque (Fig. 5–9). Similarly, the intertransversarii are assigned the role of lateral flexion. There are several problems with these proposals. First, these small muscles are of such small physiologic cross-sectional area that they can generate only a few newtons of force, and second, they work through such a small moment arm that their total contribution to rotational axial twisting and bending torque is minimal. It would appear that they have some other function. There is evidence to suggest that these muscles are highly rich in muscle spindles (4.5 to 7.3 times more rich than multifidus[32]), such that they would be involved as length transducers or vertebral position sensors at every thoracic and lumbar joint.

In some indwelling EMG experiments performed on ourselves a couple of years ago, we placed some electrodes very close to the vertebrae. In one case, we strongly suspected that the electrode was in a rotator. Isometric twisting efforts with the spine untwisted (or in a neutral posture) were attempted in both directions, which produced no EMG activity from the rotator—only the usual activity in the abdominal obliques and so forth. When nonresisted twisting was attempted in one direction there was no response, whereas in the other direction there was major activity. It appeared that this particular rotator was not activated through torque development but rather acted in response to position change. Thus, its activity resulted as a function of twisted position; it was not consistent with the role of creating torque to twist the spine. From a clinical perspective, it is likely

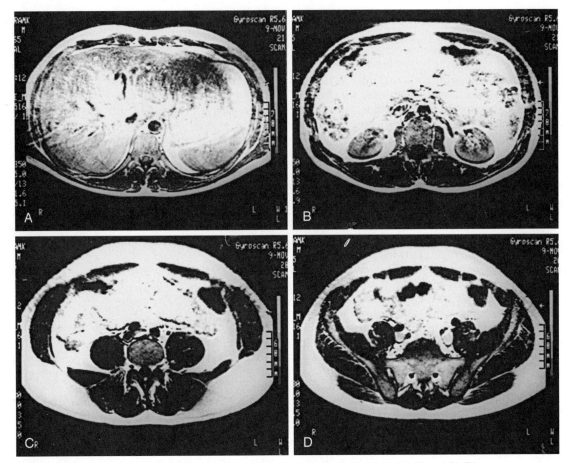

FIGURE 5–8   Transverse scans of one subject (supine) at the levels of T9 *(A)*, L1 *(B)*, L4 *(C)*, and S1 *(D)* showing the musculature in cross-section.

that these structures are effected during therapeutic manipulation with the joint at end range of motion.

The Extensors: Longissimus, Iliocostalis, and Multifidus Groups

The major extensors of the thoracolumbar spine are the longissimus, iliocostalis, and multifidus groups. The longissimus and iliocostalis groups are often separated in anatomy books, although it may be more productive to recognize the thoracic portions of both muscles separately from their lumbar portions because they are architecturally[26] and functionally different.[33] Even fiber-typing studies have noted differences between the lumbar and thoracic sections; the thoracic sections contain about 75% slow twitch, whereas the lumbar sections are generally evenly mixed.[34] Bogduk[26] partitioned the lumbar and thoracic portions of these muscles into longissimus thoracis pars lumborum

and pars thoracis, and iliocostalis lumborum pars lumborum and thoracis. These two functional groups (pars lumborum and pars thoracis) form quite a marvelous architecture for several reasons and are discussed with this distinction (i.e., lumbar versus thoracic).

The pars thoracis components of these two muscles attach to the ribs and vertebral components and have relatively short contractile fibers with long tendons that run down the spine, to their origins over the posterior surface of the sacrum and medial border of the iliac crests (Fig. 5–10). Their basic line of action is parallel to the compressive axis of the spine. Furthermore, their line of action over the lower thoracic and lumbar region is superficial, such that forces in these muscles have the greatest possible moment arm and therefore produce the greatest amount of extensor moment with a minimum of compressive penalty to the spine. When seen on a transverse MRI or CT scan at a lumbar level, their tendons have the greatest extensor moment arm, overlying the

TABLE 5–1 Raw Cross-Sectional Areas (mm²) Measured Directly From Magnetic Resonance Imaging Scans

	VERTEBRAL LEVEL*												
MUSCLE	L5	L4	L3	L2	L1	T12	T11	T10	T9	T8	T7	T6	T5
R. Rectus abdominis	787 (250)	750 (207)	670 (133)	712 (239)	576 (151)								
L. Rectus abdominis	802 (247)	746 (181)	693 (177)	748 (240)	514 (99)								
R. External oblique		915 (199)	1276 (171)	1158 (222)									
L. External oblique		992 (278)	1335 (213)	1351 (282)									
R. Internal oblique		903 (83)	1515 (317)	1055 (173)									
L. Internal oblique		900 (115)	1424 (310)	1027 (342)									
R. Trans. abdominis	119 (22)	237 (82)	356 (110)	596 (50)									
L. Trans. abdominis	175 (57)	224 (48)	376 (115)	646 (183)									
R. Abdominal wall†	1104 (393)	2412 (418)	3269 (422)	3051 (463)									
L. Abdominal wall†	1146 (377)	2420 (475)	3329 (468)	3111 (556)									
R. Longissimus thor.			747 (162)	1175 (370)	1248 (228)	1095 (222)	938 (49)						
L. Longissimus thor.			782 (129)	1089 (251)	1180 (184)	1258 (347)	938 (21)						
R. Iliocostalis lumb.			1368 (341)	1104 (181)	1181 (316)	921 (339)	556 (234)						
L. Iliocostalis lumb.			1395 (223)	1150 (198)	1158 (247)	835 (400)	551 (170)						
R. Multifidus			447 (271)	343 (178)	290 (96)	289 (66)	331 (89)	351 (90)	312 (97)				
L. Multifidus			472 (269)	366 (157)	324 (95)	312 (76)	327 (80)	353 (53)	355 (73)				
R. Latissimus dorsi			232 (192)	429 (202)	717 (260)	1014 (264)	1254 (281)	1368 (330)	1458 (269)	1581 (159)	1764 (289)	1876 (432)	2477 (246)
L. Latissimus dorsi			256 (217)	372 (161)	682 (260)	960 (310)	1102 (316)	1239 (257)	1417 (293)	1582 (281)	1697 (189)	2013 (422)	2596 (721)
R. Erector mass‡	905 (331)	2151 (539)	2831 (458)	2854 (547)	2615 (405)	2614 (584)	1832 (282)	1690 (210)	1413 (304)	1049 (201)	842 (165)	777 (189)	743 (70)
L. Erector mass‡	986 (338)	2234 (476)	2933 (382)	2833 (456)	2723 (428)	2601 (559)	2041 (285)	1722 (279)	1471 (351)	1129 (100)	879 (114)	779 (95)	675 (76)
R. Psoas	1606 (198)	1861 (347)	1594 (369)	1177 (285)	513 (329)	330 (210)							
L. Psoas	1590 (244)	1820 (272)	1593 (291)	1211 (298)	488 (250)	462 (190)							
R. Quadratus lumb.		725 (209)	701 (212)	552 (192)	392 (249)	320 (197)							
L. Quadratus lumb.		625 (249)	746 (167)	614 (189)	404 (220)	326 (5)							
Disc area	1360 (276)	1459 (270)	1415 (249)	1332 (294)	1334 (285)	1241 (166)	1133 (124)	1015 (125)	933 (112)	798 (91)	797 (104)	741 (80)	671 (82)
Total area	52912 (9123)	51813 (9845)	54286 (8702)	55834 (8112)	59091 (6899)	63287 (9153)	59249 (7272)	61051 (7570)	61732 (6960)	65794 (5254)	67782 (3982)	66410 (2372)	69337 (2233)

*Standard deviation is given in parentheses.
†Abdominal wall includes external and internal oblique and transverse abdominis.
‡Erector mass includes longissimus thoracis, iliocostalis lumborum, and multifidus.

TABLE 5–2 Raw Lateral Distances (mm) Between Muscle Centroids and Intervertebral Disk Centroid

							VERTEBRAL LEVEL*						
MUSCLE	L5	L4	L3	L2	L1	T12	T11	T10	T9	T8	T7	T6	T5
R. Rectus abdominis	32 (5)	38 (7)	43 (7)	46 (8)	37 (8)								
L. Rectus abdominis	−33 (6)	−36 (7)	−38 (8)	−43 (7)	−35 (17)								
R. External oblique		125 (13)	130 (10)	140 (5)									
L. External oblique		−120 (9)	−125 (9)	−133 (7)									
R. Internal oblique		109 (11)	116 (8)	123 (9)									
L. Internal oblique		−103 (9)	−112 (8)	−121 (11)									
R. Transverse abdominis	99 (1)	108 (11)	112 (9)	117 (9)									
L Transverse abdominis	−101 (1)	−101 (9)	−107 (7)	−109 (9)									
R. Abdominal wall†	102 (8)	113 (12)	119 (8)	123 (9)									
L. Abdominal wall†	−102 (9)	−115 (14)	−114 (7)	−120 (9)									
R. Longissimus thoracis			22 (4)	32 (2)	32 (6)	30 (2)	29 (1)						
L. Longissimus thoracis			−19 (5)	−30 (6)	−37 (12)	−34 (4)	−36 (7)						
R. Iliocostalis lumborum			52 (4)	58 (4)	68 (10)	65 (7)	61 (4)						
L. Iliocostalis lumborum			−48 (6)	−60 (10)	−65 (9)	−67 (7)	−67 (11)						
R. Multifidus			11 (1)	13 (4)	13 (3)	10 (3)	8 (2)	11 (2)	12 (2)				
L. Multifidus			−14 (7)	−12 (3)	−11 (3)	−11 (2)	−12 (2)	−12 (2)	−15 (10)				
R. Latissimus dorsi			102 (8)	108 (8)	122 (12)	129 (10)	129 (9)	140 (9)	141 (8)	145 (7)	146 (7)	153 (7)	153 (4)
L. Latissimus dorsi			−104 (15)	−107 (9)	−117 (11)	−128 (7)	−129 (10)	−137 (9)	−139 (8)	−143 (6)	−147 (10)	−153 (5)	−151 (5)
R. Erector mass‡	22 (6)	34 (7)	40 (4)	42 (4)	44 (5)	42 (3)	34 (4)	34 (4)	32 (4)	31 (7)	30 (4)	25 (5)	27 (2)
L. Erector mass‡	−21 (5)	−33 (6)	−38 (5)	−41 (6)	−41 (7)	−40 (4)	−40 (3)	−36 (3)	−35 (4)	−33 (6)	−31 (2)	−29 (3)	−27 (6)
R. Psoas	54 (4)	50 (3)	44 (3)	39 (2)	32 (3)	32 (3)							
L. Psoas	−54 (5)	−48 (4)	−42 (3)	−38 (3)	−31 (3)	−32 (2)							
R. Quadratus lumborum		81 (5)	75 (6)	63 (5)	46 (6)	46 (11)							
L. Quadratus lumborum		−78 (12)	−73 (4)	−64 (5)	−50 (6)	−47 (5)							
Total area	0 (2)	1 (3)	−2 (4)	−1 (3)	−1 (4)	0 (3)	1 (3)	0 (2)	0 (2)	2 (1)	2 (1)	1 (3)	2 (3)

*Standard deviation is given in parentheses.

†Abdominal wall includes external and internal oblique and transverse abdominis.

‡Erector mass includes longissimus thoracis, iliocostalis lumborum, and multifidus.

112

TABLE 5-3 Raw Anterior-Posterior Distances (mm) Between Muscle Centroids and Intervertebral Disk Centroid

Muscle	T5	T6	T7	T8	T9	T10	T11	T12	L1	L2	L3	L4	L5
R. Rectus abdominis									109 (8)	90 (14)	79 (13)	73 (14)	81 (16)
L. Rectus abdominis									112 (6)	92 (14)	80 (14)	73 (14)	80 (15)
R. External oblique										28 (12)	20 (14)	35 (10)	
L. External oblique										28 (11)	19 (11)	32 (18)	
R. Internal oblique										36 (17)	25 (9)	41 (12)	
L. Internal oblique										40 (16)	26 (12)	41 (17)	
R. Transverse abdominis										36 (6)	22 (11)	28 (11)	55 (0)
L. Transverse abdominis										44 (5)	23 (10)	30 (14)	50 (5)
R. Abdominal wall†										30 (15)	17 (12)	31 (12)	58 (16)
L. Abdominal wall†										31 (11)	20 (12)	32 (13)	59 (17)
R. Longissimus thoracis							−56 (4)	−60 (6)	−60 (7)	−62 (7)	−61 (6)		
L. Longissimus thoracis							−52 (4)	−59 (8)	−60 (7)	−63 (6)	−61 (5)		
R. Iliocostalis lumborum							−57 (1)	−59 (7)	−62 (5)	−61 (7)	−57 (7)		
L. Iliocostalis lumborum							−56 (2)	−58 (6)	−61 (4)	−61 (6)	−57 (7)		
R. Multifidus					−48 (2)	−49 (4)	−47 (5)	−51 (3)	−52 (6)	−55 (6)	−55 (7)		
L. Multifidus					−47 (2)	−47 (3)	−47 (5)	−50 (3)	−51 (5)	−56 (5)	−53 (7)		
R. Latissimus dorsi	−17 (5)	−12 (3)	−17 (6)	−18 (9)	−22 (7)	−24 (7)	−32 (7)	−39 (8)	−47 (10)	−47 (12)	−45 (16)		
L. Latissimus dorsi	−19 (3)	−11 (7)	−15 (8)	−17 (7)	−19 (7)	−23 (7)	−28 (9)	−37 (8)	−46 (7)	−46 (10)	−43 (17)		
R. Erector mass‡	−50 (3)	−47 (4)	−52 (4)	−52 (3)	−52 (4)	−54 (4)	−54 (4)	−56 (5)	−59 (5)	−61 (5)	−61 (5)	−61 (5)	−64 (6)
L. Erector mass‡	−50 (3)	−46 (5)	−51 (4)	−51 (3)	−51 (4)	−52 (4)	−52 (4)	−57 (5)	−60 (4)	−62 (5)	−61 (5)	−61 (5)	−63 (5)
R. Psoas								−14 (2)	−11 (6)	−9 (5)	−7 (5)	1 (5)	18 (9)
L. Psoas								−11 (1)	−11 (4)	−8 (2)	−6 (4)	2 (4)	19 (8)
R. Quadratus lumborum								−31 (6)	−35 (4)	−37 (6)	−37 (6)	−36 (9)	
L. Quadratus lumborum								−32 (8)	−34 (4)	−36 (5)	−34 (6)	−31 (5)	
Total area	34 (5)	32 (10)	37 (6)	36 (7)	32 (7)	30 (9)	29 (8)	24 (7)	18 (5)	9 (8)	1 (8)	−2 (9)	1 (10)

Vertebral Level*

*Standard deviation is given in parentheses.
†Abdominal wall includes external and internal oblique and transverse abdominis.
‡Erector mass includes longissimus thoracis, iliocostalis lumborum, and multifidus.

113

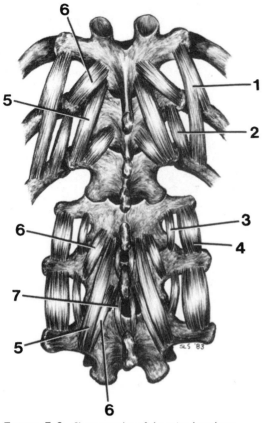

6

5

1

2

6

3

4

7

5

SLS '83

6

lumbar bulk—often by more than 10 cm[29, 30] (see Fig. 5–8).

The lumbar components of these muscles (iliocostalis lumborum pars lumborum and longissimus thoracis pars lumborum) are very different anatomically from their thoracic namesakes. They connect to the mamillary, accessory, and transverse processes of the lumbar vertebrae and originate, once again, over the posterior sacrum and medial aspect of the iliac crest. Each vertebra is connected bilaterally with separate laminae of these muscles (Fig. 5–11). Their line of action is not parallel to the compressive axis of the spine; rather, they have a posterior caudal obliquity that causes them to generate posterior shear forces together with extensor moment on the superior vertebrae. These posterior shear forces support

any anterior-reaction shear forces of the upper vertebrae produced as the upper body is flexed forward in a typical lifting type of posture (this possible injury mechanism is addressed later).

The multifidus muscles perform a different function, particularly in the lumbar region, where they attach posterior spines of adjacent vertebrae or span two or three segments. Their line of action tends to be parallel to the compressive axis or, in some cases, runs anteriorly and caudad in obliquity. The major mechanically relevant feature of multifidus, however, is that because it spans only a few joints, its forces affect only local areas of the spine. Therefore, the multifidus muscles are involved in producing extensor torque, but they provide the ability for corrections or moment support only at specific joints that may be foci of stresses. In a later section, we propose an injury mechanism involving inappropriate neural activation signals to multifidus, using an example of injury observed in the laboratory.

The Abdominal Wall

Although many classic anatomy texts consider the abdominal wall to be an important flexor of the trunk, it appears that the rectus abdominis is the major trunk flexor (and the most active during sit-ups and curl-ups[35]). It is interesting to consider why the rectus abdominis is partitioned into sections, rather than being a single long muscle, given that the sections share a common nerve supply and that a single long muscle would have the advantage of broadening the force–length relationship over a greater range of length change. Perhaps a single muscle would bulk upon shortening, compressing the viscera, or be stiff and resistant to bending. Not only does the sectioned rectus abdominis limit bulking upon shortening, but also the sections have a "bead effect," which allows bending at each tendon to facilitate torso flexion and extension or abdominal distention or contraction as the visceral contents change volume.[36]

The three layers of the abdominal wall (external oblique, internal oblique, transverse abdominis) perform several functions. They are involved in flexion and appear to have their flexor potential enhanced as a result of their attachment to the linea semilunaris (Fig. 5–12),[37] which redirects the oblique muscle forces down the rectus sheath to increase their flexor moment arm. The obliques are involved in torso twisting[38] and lateral bend[39] and appear to play some role in lumbar stabilization because they increase their activity, to a small degree, when the spine is placed under pure axial

TABLE 5–4 Examples of Corrected Cross-Sectional Areas and Anteroposterior and Lateral Moment Arms Perpendicular to the Muscle Fiber Line of Action

		VALUES*		
MUSCLE	**VERTEBRAL LEVEL**	**CROSS-SECTIONAL AREA (mm)²**	**ANTEROPOSTERIOR MOMENT ARM (mm)**	**LATERAL MOMENT ARM (mm)**
Longissimus pars lumborum†	L3–L4	644	51	17
Quadratus lumborum	L1–L2	358	31	43
	L2–L3	507	32	55
	L3–L4	582	29	59
	L4–L5	328	16	39
External oblique	L3–L4	1121	17	110
Internal oblique	L3–L4	1154	20	89

*Data are derived from the cosines listed in McGill and colleagues.[30] These are the values that should be used in biomechanical models, rather than the uncorrected values obtained directly from scan slices.

†Longissimus pars lumborum at the L4–L5 level would have been listed here by virtue of their cosines but were not because they could not be distinguished on all scan slices.

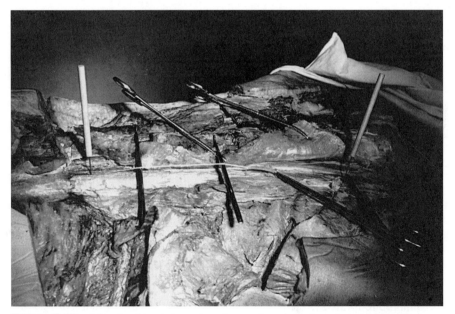

FIGURE 5–10 A bundle of longissimus thoracis pars thoracis has been isolated (inserting on the ribs at T6). Their tendons, lifted by the probes, course over the full lumbar spine to their sacral origin. They have a very large extensor moment arm.

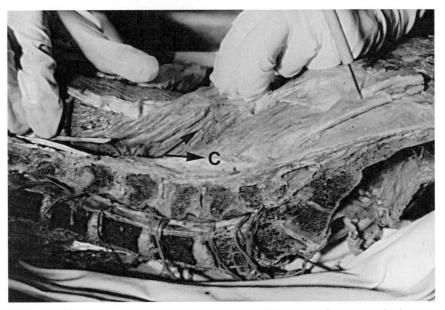

FIGURE 5–11   Iliocostalis lumborum pars lumborum and longissimus thoracis pars lumborum originate over the posterior surface of the sacrum, follow a superficial pathway, and then dive obliquely to their vertebral attachments. The compressive axis is shown (C). They create posterior shear forces and extensor moment on each successive superior vertebra.

compression[40] (this functional notion is developed later in this chapter).

The Special Case of Quadratus Lumborum and Psoas

Although the psoas has often been claimed to be a good stabilizer of the lumbar spine, I think that this is unlikely and that, rather, quadratus lumborum is the major stabilizer, particularly of the lower thoracic and lumbar regions. It is true that the psoas complex attaches to T12 and to every lumbar vertebra on its course over the pelvic ring, but its activation profile (see Juker and colleagues[35] for indwelling EMG data of psoas and McGill and associates[40] for quadratus lumborum) is not consistent with that of a spine stabilizer, instead indicating that the role of psoas is purely as a hip flexor. In contrast, it appears that quadratus lumborum is the major stabilizer of the lumbar spine, for two reasons. First, during flexion-dominant, extensor-dominant, or lateral-bending tasks, the quadratus lumborum is always active (e.g., 12% of maximum voluntary contraction (MVC) during bent-knee sit-ups, 74% during heavy lifts, 42% during standing isometric twists, 54% during side-supported isometric lateral-bending holds[40]). Second, in a task in which the subjects stood upright but held buckets in both hands, and in which load was incrementally added to each bucket, the quadratus lumborum increased its acti-

vation level with each increase in hand load more than any other muscle. After measuring the activation of the psoas, the obliques, the extensors, and the quadratus lumborum, it was clearly the quadratus lumborum that the major muscle incrementally activated to stabilize the spine in this special situation in which only compressive loading was applied to the spine in the absence of any bending moments. In addition, the architecture of the quadratus lumborum suits a stabilizing role by attaching each transverse process (therefore, bilateral vertebral buttressing) with the more rigid pelvis and rib cage.

Ligaments

The column formed by the vertebrae is joined with two ribbon-like ligaments, the anterior longitudinal and posterior longitudinal ligaments, which assist in restricting excessive flexion and extension (Fig. 5–13). Both have bony attachments to the vertebral bodies and to the anulus. Posterior to the spinal cord is the ligamentum flavum, which is characterized by a composition of about 80% elastin and 20% collagen, signifying a special function for this ligament. It has been proposed that this highly elastic structure, which is under pretension throughout all levels of flexion, appears to act as a barrier to material that would otherwise encroach on the cord in some regions of the full range of motion. Furthermore, this

Furthermore, with its oblique line of action, it protects against posterior shearing of the superior vertebrae and is implicated in an injury scenario described later on in this chapter. The supraspinous ligament, on the other hand, is aligned more or less parallel to the compressive axis of the spine, connecting the tips of the posterior spines, and it appears to provide resistance against excessive forward flexion.

The facet capsule consists of connective tissue with bands that restrict joint flexion as well as distraction of the facet surfaces resulting from axial twisting. Other ligaments in the thoracolumbar spine include the intertransverse ligaments, which span the transverse processes and have been argued by Bogduk and Twomey[42] to be sheets of connective tissue rather than true ligaments. These authors suggested that the intertransverse liga-

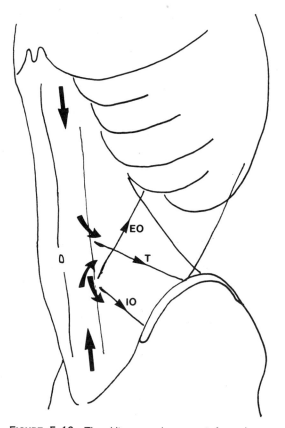

FIGURE 5–12 The oblique muscles transmit force along their fiber lengths and then redirect force along the rectus abdominis, through their attachment to the linea semilunaris, to enhance their effective flexor moment arm. EO, anterior portion of external oblique; IO, anterior portion of internal oblique; T, transverse abdominis. (From McGill SM: A revised anatomical model of the abdominal musculature for torso flexion efforts. J Biomech 29[7]:973–977, 1996, with permission from Elsevier Science.)

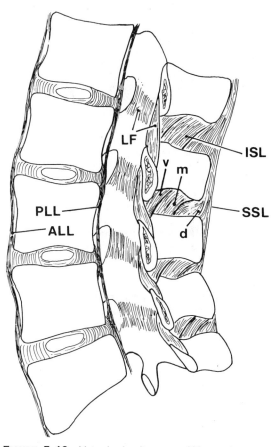

FIGURE 5–13 Major lumbar ligaments. ALL, anterior longitudinal ligament; PLL, posterior longitudinal ligament; SSL, supraspinous ligament; ISL, interspinous ligament; v, ventral part; m, middle part; d, dorsal part; LF, ligamentum flavum, viewed from within the vertebral canal, and in sagittal section at the midline. (From Bogduk N, Twomey LT: Clinical Anatomy of the Lumbar Spine. New York, Churchill Livingstone, 1987, p 34.)

prestretched elastic structure prevents any sort of buckling folds that would otherwise impinge the cord.

The interspinous and supraspinous ligaments are often classed as a single structure in most anatomy texts, although functionally they appear to have different roles. The interspinous ligaments connect adjacent posterior spines but are not oriented parallel to the compressive axis of the spine. Rather, they have a large angle of obliquity (Fig. 5–14).[41] Although many anatomy textbooks suggest that this ligament serves to protect against excessive flexion, I disagree. Heylings[41] suggested that the ligament acts like a collateral ligament similar to the knee, whereby the ligament controls the vertebral rotation to follow an arc throughout the flexion range, which in turn assists the facet joints to remain in contact, gliding with rotation.

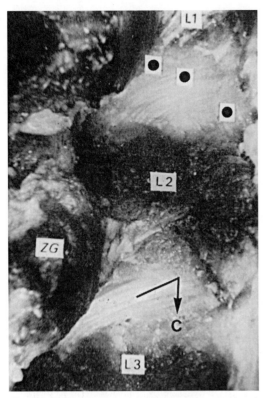

FIGURE 5-14 The interspinous ligament runs obliquely to the compressive axis and thus has limited capacity to check flexion rotation of the superior vertebrae. On the contrary, the interspinous ligament may act as a collateral ligament, controlling vertebral rotation and imposing anterior shear forces on the superior vertebrae. The compressive axis (C) is indicated, together with the zygopophyseal joint (ZG) and the posterior spines of L1, L2, and L3. (From Heylings DJ: Supraspinous and interspinous ligaments of the human lumbar spine. J Anat 125[1]:129, 1978. Reprinted with the permission of Cambridge University Press.)

ment-membrane forms a septum between the anterior and posterior musculature that is an embryologic holdover from the development of these two sections of muscle.

Determining the roles of ligaments has involved qualitative interpretation using their attachments and lines of action, together with functional tests in which successive ligaments were destroyed and the joint motion reassessed. Early studies to determine the relative contribution of each ligament to restricting flexion in particular were performed on cadaveric preparations that were not preconditioned before testing. This suggests that early data that described the relative roles of various ligaments were incorrect. For example, upon death, the disks, because they are hydrophilic, increase their water content and consequently their disk height. The "swollen" disks in cadaveric specimens resulted in an artificial preload on the liga-

ments closest to the disk, causing the earlier studies to suggest that the capsular and longitudinal ligaments may be more important in resisting flexion than is actually true in vivo. The work of Sharma and coauthors[43] has shown that the major ligaments for resisting flexion are those making up the supraspinous complex.

Mechanical failure of the ligaments is a topic worthy of consideration. King[21] noted that soft tissue injuries are much more common during high-energy traumatic events, such as automobile collisions. Our own observations on pig and human specimens loaded at slow rates in bending and shear suggests that excessive tension in the longitudinal ligaments usually results in avulsion or bony failure as the ligament pulls some bone away near its attachment. Noyes and colleagues[44] noted that slower strain rates (0.66% per second) produced more ligament avulsion injuries, whereas faster strain rates (66% per second) resulted in more ligamentous failure to the fiber bundles (in the middle region of the ligament), at least in monkey knee ligaments. It is interesting, however, to interpret the clinical report by Rissanen[45] that about 20% of cadaveric spines possessed visibly ruptured lumbar interspinous ligaments (in their middle, not at their bony attachment) and that dorsal and ventral portions of interspinous, together with supraspinous, ligaments remained intact.

Given the oblique fiber direction of the interspinous complex (see Fig. 5–6B), a likely scenario to damage this ligament would be slipping and falling and landing on one's behind, driving the pelvis forward on impact, creating a posterior shearing of the lumbar joints when the spine is fully flexed. The interspinous ligament is a major load-bearing tissue in this example of high-energy loading, in which anterior shear displacement is combined with full flexion. Given the available data, I believe that damage to the ligaments of the spine during lifting or other normal occupational activities, particularly to the interspinous complex, is more uncommon than common. Rather, it appears much more likely that ligament damage occurs during a more traumatic event, particularly landing on one's behind during a fall, which then leads to joint laxity and acceleration of subsequent arthritic changes. As has been often said in reference to the knee joint, "ligament damage marks the beginning of the end."

The Lumbodorsal Fascia

Although a functional interpretation of the lumbodorsal fascia (LDF) is provided later in this chapter, a short anatomic description is given here.

First, the transverse abdominis and internal oblique muscles obtain their posterior attachment to the fascia, as does the latissimus dorsi over the upper regions of the fascia. The fascia forms a compartment around the lumbar extensors (multifidus and pars lumborum groups of iliocostalis and longissimus) and has been implicated in compartment syndrome.[46, 47] Some have suggested that the abdominals work through their fascia attachments to create extension of the spine[48]; however, this notion is highly questionable. Perhaps the most tenable explanation for the role of the fascia is that of a large extensor retinaculum to constrain the long tendons of the thoracic and lumbar extensors throughout all levels of lordosis.

KINEMATICS AND KINETIC PROPERTIES OF THE THORACOLUMBAR SPINE

The ranges of thoracic and lumbar segmental motion around the three principal axes (Table 5–5) demonstrate the greater flexion, extension, and lateral bending capability of the lumbar region and the relatively greater twisting capability of the thoracic region. Although the segmental ranges shown in the table are population averages, there is a great amount of variability between subjects and between segments in a single person. Specifically, there are individual asymmetries in bending to the right and left, for example, and twisting clockwise and counterclockwise; these are of great importance to the clinician, who may sometimes

suspect pathology at a specific location but is simply noticing normal anatomic asymmetry.

Joint stiffness values convey the amount of translational and rotational deformation of a spine section under the application of force or moment. The average stiffness values (Table 5–6)[49] document the stiffness of the spine in a neutral posture, indicating the greater stiffness under compression loads than shear loads and the greater stiffness in axial torsion than in rotation around the other two axes of flexion and extension and lateral bend. Generally, range of motion decreases with age, but certain injuries, particularly disk injuries, can increase the range of motion in bending and shear translations,[50] a situation that has often been implicated in subsequent facet joint derangement.[51]

Loads on the Low Back During Lifting and Walking

Low-back loads during lifting result from the muscle and ligament tension required to support the posture and facilitate movement. This is why lifting technique is so important to reduce low-back moment demands and the risk of excessive loading. The following example demonstrates this concept.

The components of muscular moment generation are detailed in Table 5–7 for the period of peak loading in a sample squat lift of 27 kg, which provided a reaction moment in the low back of 450 newton-meters (N m) and a total compressive load of more than 7000 N. The individual muscle forces, subsequent joint moment, and components of compression and shear that are imposed on the joint are useful information. In this particular example, the lifter avoided full spine flexion, minimizing ligament and other passive tissue tension and relegating the moment restoration responsibility to the musculature.

Compressive and especially shear components of muscular force have been greatly neglected during assessment of injury mechanisms. The very large magnitude of force in the pars lumborum laminae results from their large individual cross-sectional area. These forces produce a large proportion of the extensor moment. Negative moments observed in Table 5–7 correspond to the flexor contributions of abdominal co-contraction. The abdominal co-contraction in this lifting example, and in most sagittal plane lifting tasks, was small at the instant of peak extensor moment.

The compression penalty from even mild abdominal activity can be observed from the individual muscle forces shown in Table 5–7. To meet the requirements of the net moment, additional extensor activity is necessary to offset the flexor

TABLE 5–5   **Range of Motion of Each Spine Level**

LEVEL	FLEXION	EXTENSION	LATERAL BENDING	AXIAL TWIST
T1–T2		4	6	9
T2–T3		4	6	8
T3–T4		4	6	8
T4–T5		4	6	8
T5–T6		4	6	8
T6–T7		5	6	8
T7–T8		6	6	8
T8–T9		6	6	7
T9–T10		6	6	4
T10–T11		9	7	2
T11–T12		12	9	2
T12–L1		12	8	2
L1–L2	8	5	6	2
L2–L3	10	3	6	2
L3–L4	12	1	8	2
L4–L5	13	2	6	2
L5–S1	9	5	3	5

All data are from White and Panjabi,[108] except for flexion and extension lumbar data, which are from Pearcy and colleagues[109] and Pearcy and Tibrewal.[110]

TABLE 5-6   **Average Stiffness Values for the Adult Human Spine*

SPINE LEVEL	COMPRESSION	SHEAR		BENDING		AXIAL TORSION
		ANTERIOR/POSTERIOR	LATERAL	FLEXION/EXTENSION	LATERAL	
T1–T12	1250	86/87	101	155/189	172	149
L1–L5	667	145/143	132	80/166	92	395
L5–S1	1000	78/72	97	120/172	206	264

*Shear values are given in Newtons per millimeter and bending and axial torsion in newton-meters per radian.
Data on T1–T2 are from White and Panjabi[108]; data on L1–L5 are from Schultz and colleagues[111] and Berkson and associates[112]; data on L5–S1 are from McGlashen and colleagues.[113]

moment produced by the abdominals. However, this creates a double contribution to joint compression: compression from abdominal activity and compression from the additional extensor forces. Even so, when all of the component forces are summed, the total predicted joint compression is less than what would have been predicted by a simple analysis using a single equivalent muscle model (5-cm extensor moment arm has been used in the past). Obviously, abdominal activity would result in a shorter equivalent moment arm. The ability of an individual to reduce compression appears to be determined by the degree of abdominal activity. As is often observed in elite lifters, however, the abdominals are not completely uninvolved, exhibiting varying degrees of activity. This suggests that they are sacrificing minimum compression for some other benefit. Interviews with some elite lifters about why co-contraction is

observed often reveal that the lifters feel that it stiffens the trunk to prevent buckling of the spine. This idea has been tested by Cholewicki and McGill[52] and is discussed in a later section of this chapter.

Negative shear forces from the muscles (shown in Table 5–7) correspond to L4 shearing posteriorly on L5. Hence, a powerful anti-anterior shear mechanism is observed, in the tabulated forces, owing to the obliquity of the pars lumborum extensors. These muscles help to offset the anterior reaction shear force from lifting a load when they are activated presumably to contribute extensor moment.[33] The implication of these forces is a reduced load on the facet joints. Some subjects whom we have tested have offset the reaction shear force almost completely, depending on the forward inclination of the disk (and trunk) and on the magnitude of force in these obliquely orien-

TABLE 5-7   **Musculature Components for Moment Generation of 450 N m During Peak Loading for a Squat Lift of 27 kg**

MUSCLE	FORCE (N)	MOMENT (N m)*	COMPRESSION (N)	SHEAR (N)*
Rectus abdominis	25	−2	24	5
External oblique 1	45	1	39	24
External oblique 2	43	−2	30	31
Internal oblique 1	14	1	14	−2
Internal oblique 2	23	−1	17	−16
Longissimus thoracis pars lumborum (L4)	862	35	744	−436
Longissimus thoracis pars lumborum (L3)	1514	93	1422	−518
Longissimus thoracis pars lumborum (L2)	1342	121	1342	0
Longissimus thoracis pars lumborum (L1)	1302	110	1302	0
Iliocostalis lumborum pars thoracis	369	31	369	0
Longissimus thoracis pars thoracis	295	25	295	0
Quadratus lumborum	393	16	386	74
Latissimus dorsi (L5)	112	6	79	−2
Multifidus 1	136	8	134	18
Multifidus 2	226	8	189	124
Psoas (L1)	26	0	23	12
Psoas (L2)	28	0	27	8
Psoas (L3)	28	1	27	6
Psoas (L4)	28	1	27	5

*Negative moments correspond to flexion, whereas negative shear corresponds to L4 shearing posteriorly on L5.

tated pars lumborum fibers.[53] The clinical implications of these shear forces are discussed in a subsequent section of this chapter.

During walking every day, thousands of low-level loading cycles are endured by the spine. Although the small loads in the low back during walking suggest a noninjurious activity, walking has been found to provide relief to some persons but is painful to others—particularly fast walking as opposed to strolling. The compressive loads of about 2.5 times body weight and the shear forces are well below any known in vitro failure load. Strolling, however, reduces spine motion and produces static loading of tissues, whereas faster walking with arm swinging causes cyclic loading of tissues,[54] which may begin to explain the relief experienced by some patients who undertake this activity.

ANATOMIC CONSISTENCY IN EXAMINING THE ROLE OF INTRAABDOMINAL PRESSURE

It has been claimed for many years that intraabdominal pressure (IAP) plays an important role in support of the lumbar spine, especially during strenuous lifting. Anatomic accuracy has been influential in this debate. This issue has been considered in lifting mechanics for years and, for some, has formed a cornerstone for prescription of abdominal belts to industrial workers and has motivated various abdominal strengthening programs. Some research reports suggest that IAP may be a mechanism to reduce lumbar spine compression directly.[55, 56] Some, however, have indicated that they believe the role of IAP in reducing spinal loads has been overemphasized.[57–59] In fact, some experimental evidence suggests that somehow, in the process of building up IAP, the net compressive load on the spine is increased! Increased low-back EMG activity with higher IAP was noted by Krag and coauthors[60] during voluntary Valsalva maneuvers. Nachemson and colleagues[61, 62] showed an increase in intradiscal pressure during a Valsalva maneuver, indicating a net increase in spine compression with an increase in IAP, presumably a result of abdominal wall musculature activity.

In our own investigations, which used an anatomically detailed modeling approach, an evaluation of the net spine compression benefit and penalty to build up IAP and produce concomitant abdominal activity was performed. The size of the cross-sectional area of the diaphragm and the moment arm used to estimate force and moment produced by IAP have a major effect on conclusions reached about the role of IAP.[63] The diaphragm surface area was 243 cm², and the centroid

of this area was 3.8 cm anterior to the center of the T12 disk (compare with a 511-cm² pelvic floor and 465-cm² diaphragm, together with moment arm distances up to 11.4 cm, which were outside of the chest in most subjects used in other studies). During squat lifts, it appears that the net effect of the involvement of the abdominal musculature and IAP is to increase compression rather than alleviate joint load. (A detailed description and analysis of the forces can be found in McGill and Norman[63]). This predicted finding agrees with experimental evidence of Krag and colleagues,[60] who used EMG, and with Nachemson and associates,[62] who documented increased intradiscal pressure with an increase in IAP.

The generation of appreciable IAP during load-handling tasks is well documented, but the role of IAP is not. Farfan[7] has suggested that IAP creates a pressurized visceral cavity to maintain the hoop-like geometry of the abdominals. Recent work measuring the distance of the abdominals to the spine (their moment arms) was unable to confirm substantial changes in abdominal geometry when activated in a standing posture.[31] The compression penalty of abdominal activity, however, cannot be discounted. It appears that the spine prefers to sustain increased compression loads if intrinsic stability is increased. An unstabilized spine buckles under extremely low compressive load (e.g., about 20 N).[64] The geometry of the musculature suggests that individual components exert lateral and anteroposterior forces on the spine that perhaps can be thought of as guy wires on a mast to prevent bending and compressive buckling.[52] In addition, activated abdominals create a rigid cylinder of the trunk, resulting in a stiffer structure. Thus, it appears that increased IAP, commonly observed during many activities, including lifting, as well as in patients with back pain, does not have a direct role in reducing spinal compression but rather is an agent used to stiffen the trunk and prevent tissue strain or failure from buckling.

WHAT IS THE ROLE OF THE LUMBODORSAL FASCIA?

Recent studies have attributed various mechanical roles to the LDF. In fact, there have been some attempts to recommend lifting postures based on LDF hypotheses. Suggestions were originally made that lateral forces generated by internal oblique and transverse abdominis are transmitted to the LDF through their attachments to the lateral border, claiming that the fascia could support substantial extensor moments.[48] This lateral tension was hypothesized to increase longitudinal tension, from Poisson's effect, pulling in the direction of the posterior midline of the lumbar spine and causing the posterior spinous processes to move together, resulting in lumbar extension. This proposed sequence of events formed an attractive proposition because the LDF has the largest moment arm of all the extensor tissues. As a result, any extensor forces within the LDF would impose the smallest compressive penalty to vertebral components of the spine.

This hypothesis was examined by three studies, all published about the same time, which collectively questioned its viability: Tesh and colleagues,[65] who performed mechanical tests on cadaveric material; Macintosh and associates,[66] who recognized the anatomic inconsistencies with the abdominal activation; and McGill and Norman,[67] who tested the viability of LDF involvement with latissimus dorsi as well as with the abdominals. Regardless of the choice of LDF activation strategy, the LDF contribution to the restorative extension moment was negligible compared with the much larger low-back reaction moment required to support the load in the hands.

Although the LDF does not appear itself to be a significant active extensor of the spine, it is a strong tissue with a well-developed lattice of collagen fibers. Its function may be that of an extensor muscle retinaculum.[68] The tendons of longissimus thoracis and iliocostalis lumborum pass under the LDF to their sacral and ilium attachments. Perhaps the LDF provides a form of "strapping" for the low-back musculature. Hukins and coauthors,[69] on theoretical grounds only at this time, have proposed that the LDF acts to increase by up to 30% the force per unit cross-sectional area that muscle can produce. They suggest that it does this by constraining bulging of the muscles when they shorten. This contention remains to be proved. Tesh and colleagues[65] have suggested that the LDF may be more important for supporting lateral bending. No doubt, this notion will be pursued in the future. Given the confused state of knowledge about the role, if any, of the LDF, the promotion of movement strategies based on intentional LDF involvement, for either low-back pain patients or healthy people, cannot be justified at this time.

BIOMECHANICS OF LOW-BACK INJURY

Reducing the risk of low-back injury, as perceived by many clinicians, engineers, and ergonomists, is thought to involve the reduction of applied loads to the various anatomic components at risk of injury. This is an overly simplistic view—optimal tissue health requires an envelope of loading, not too much or too little. Although some occupations require lower loads to reduce the risk, in other sedentary occupations, the risk can be better reduced with more loading and with varying the nature of the loading. To decide which is best, the clinician must understand the biomechanics of injury.

MECHANICAL LOADING AND THE PROCESS OF INJURY

A generic scenario for injury is presented first, and references for injury from repeated and prolonged loading to specific tissues are provided in the following section. The purposes of this section are to motivate consideration of the many factors that modulate the risk of tissue failure and to generate hypotheses to probe the causes of injury.

Injury, or failure of a tissue, occurs when the applied load exceeds the failure tolerance or strength of the tissue. For the purposes of this chapter, *injury* is defined as the full continuum from the most minor of tissue irritations (but microtrauma nonetheless) to the grossest of tissue failures, for example, vertebral fracture or ligament avulsion. I proceed on the premise that such damage generates pain. Obviously, a load that exceeds the failure tolerance of the tissue, applied once, produces injury (e.g., the snowmobiler, airborne and about to experience an axial impact with the spine fully flexed, is at risk of posterior disk herniation on landing). This injury process is depicted in Figure 5–15, in which a margin of safety is observed in the first cycle of subfailure load. In the second loading cycle, the applied load increases in magnitude, simultaneously decreasing the margin of safety to zero, and injury occurs. Although this description of low-back injury is common, particularly among medical community members who are required to identify an event when completing injury reporting forms or workers' compensation reports, I believe that relatively few low-back injuries occur in this manner. (More detail on the types of loads which create injury is provided in the next section.)

Some more likely scenarios that result in injury, when considering occupational and athletic endeavors, involve cumulative trauma from subfailure magnitude loads. In such cases, injury is the result of accumulated trauma produced by either the repeated application of a relatively low load or the application of a sustained load for a long duration (as in sitting). Figure 5–16 shows a person loading boxes on a pallet, repeatedly loading the tissues of the low back (several tissues could be at risk) to a subfailure level and causing a slow degradation of their failure tolerance (e.g., vertebrae[5, 19]). As the margin of safety approaches

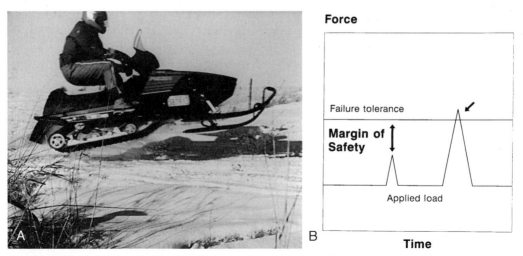

FIGURE 5-15 *A,* The snowmobile driver is about to experience an axial compressive impact load to a fully flexed spine. One-time application of load can reduce the margin of safety to zero as the applied load exceeds the strength or failure tolerance of the supporting tissues *(small arrow in B).* (From McGill SM: Biomechanics of low back injury: Implications on current practice and the clinic. J Biomech 30[5]:465–475, 1997.)

zero, this person experiences low-back injury. Obviously, the accumulation of trauma is more rapid with higher loads[70]; however, at least with bone, fatigue failure occurs with fewer repetitions when the applied load is closer to the yield strength.

Yet another way to produce injury with a subfailure load is to induce stresses over a sustained period of time. For example, rodmen (Fig. 5–17), with their spines fully flexed for a prolonged period of time, are loading the posterior passive tissues and initiating changes in disk mechanics. The sustained load causes a progressive reduction in the margin of safety, whereby injury is associated with the nth percentage of tissue strain. Analysis of injury is further complicated by the interaction between the various tissues in the low back. For example, a prolonged, stooped posture loads the posterior ligaments of the spine and posterior

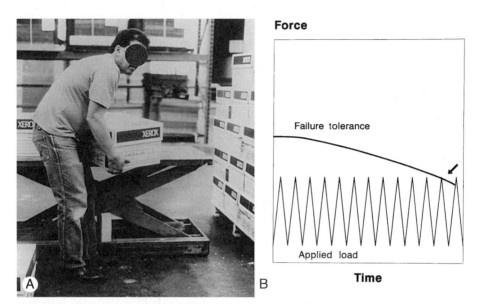

FIGURE 5-16 Repeated subfailure loads lead to tissue fatigue *(A),* reducing the failure tolerance and resulting in failure on the nth repetition of load *(B)* (or box lift in this example). (From McGill SM: Biomechanics of low back injury: Implications on current practice and the clinic. J Biomech 30[5]:465–475, 1997.)

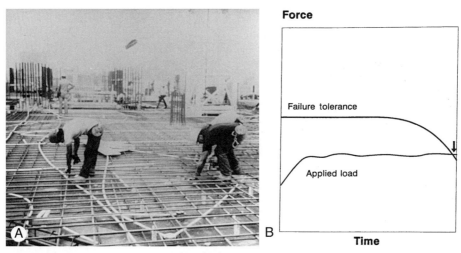

FIGURE 5–17 A, These "rodmen" are loading posterior passive tissues for a long duration, reducing the failure tolerance leading to failure at the nth percentage of tissue strain (*arrow* in B indicates where the margin of safety has reduced to zero and the injury occurs). (From McGill SM: Biomechanics of low back injury: Implications on current practice and the clinic. J Biomech 30[5]:465–475, 1997.)

fibers of the intervertebral disk, causing creep deformation, possibly to the point of microfailure.[71, 72] This could initiate another chain of events: "stretched" ligaments increase joint laxity, increasing the risk of hyperflexion injury (to the disk) as well as the risk of local instability, leading to injury of unisegmental structures and to ever-increasing shearing and bending loads on the neural arch. It would appear that the most appropriate injury intervention strategies must appreciate the complexities of tissue overload.

The objective of injury avoidance strategies is to ensure that tissue adaptation, stimulated by exposure to load, keeps pace with, and ideally exceeds, the accumulated tissue damage. Thus, exposure to load is necessary, but in the process of accumulating microtrauma, the applied loads must be removed to allow the healing and adaptation process to increase the failure tolerance gradually to the necessary level. Tissue loading and the risk of injury form an optimum U-shaped relationship, whereby the determination of the safety optimum for individual tissue loading encompasses both the art and science of medicine and biomechanics.

In summary, the injury process need be associated not only with very high loads but also with relatively low loads that are repeated or sustained, justifying the need for consideration of injury and tissue loading experienced by an individual for substantial periods of time before the culminating injury event. Simply focusing on a single variable, such as one-time load magnitude, may not result in a successful index of risk of injury, particularly across a wide variety of activities.

AN EXAMPLE OF INJURY

The work that many have reported over recent years has demonstrated the extraordinary magnitudes of forces within the various components of the trunk musculature, even during nonstrenuous tasks. Although these forces have been interpreted for their mechanical role, clinicians have expressed interest in their potential to cause injury. Damage to bony attachments remains a possibility that may be wrongfully attributed to alternative mechanisms. One such example follows.

Pain in the sacroiliac region is common and often attributed to disorders of the sacroiliac joint or to the iliolumbar ligament.[73, 74] For this reason, the role of the musculature may have been neglected. A large proportion of the extensor musculature has its origin in the sacroiliac and posterior superior iliac spine region.[26] The area of tendon–periosteum attachment and extensor aponeurosis is relatively small in relation to the volume of muscle in series with the tendon complex. From this, a hypothesis evolved that the seeming mismatch of large muscle tissue to small attachment area for connective tissue places the connective tissue at high risk of sustaining microfailure, resulting in pain.[75] Knowledge of the collective muscle force–time histories enables speculation about one-time failure loads and cumulative trauma. For example, if the forces of muscles that originate in the sacroiliac region are tallied for the trial illustrated in Table 5–7, the total force transmitted to the sacroiliac region during peak load exceeds 5.6 kiloNewtons (kN). Such a load would lift a small car off the ground!

The failure tolerance of these connective tissues is not known, which makes speculation about the potential for microfailure difficult. No doubt, the risk of damage must increase with the extremely large loads observed in the extensor musculature and with the frequency of application. Task analysis of many industrial tasks has documented that lifting three containers in excess of 18 kg per minute during an 8-hour day is not an unusual task, suggesting there is significant potential for cumulative trauma.

This mechanical explanation may account for local tenderness on palpation associated with most cases of sacroiliac syndrome. In addition, muscle strain and spasm often accompany sacroiliac pain. Nonetheless, treatment is often directed toward the articular joint despite the extreme difficulty in diagnosing the joint as the primary source of pain. Although reduction of spasm through conventional techniques would reduce the sustained load on the damaged connective fibers, patients should be counseled on techniques to reduce internal muscle loads through effective lifting mechanics. This example of sacroiliac syndrome, just one of many, of which there may be several, illustrated how knowledge of individual muscle force–time histories suggested a mechanism for injury for which a specific treatment modality would be prescribed.

USING BIOMECHANICS FOR BETTER PREVENTION OF LOW-BACK INJURY

LUMBAR POSTURE: A GENERAL CONSIDERATION FOR INJURY AVOIDANCE

A generalization that appears to have justification based on knowledge of how injury occurs is that a neutral spine (at least avoiding end range of motion) reduces the risk of many of the injuries listed previously. Many injuries are associated with the spine at end range of motion.

The following example demonstrates the shifts in tissue loading, predicted from our modeling approach, which has dramatic effects on shear loading of the intervertebral column and the resultant injury risk. First, the dominant direction of the pars lumborum fibers of longissimus thoracis and iliocostalis lumborum have been noted earlier (see Figs. 5–10 and 5–11), producing a posterior shear force on the superior vertebra. In contrast, the interspinous ligament complex generates forces with the opposite obliquity to impose an anterior shear force on the superior vertebra (see Fig. 5–14). This is one example of how spine posture determines the interplay between passive tissues and muscles that ultimately modulates the risk of several types of injury. For example, if a subject holds a load in the hands with the spine flexed enough to achieve myoelectric silence in the extensors (reducing their tension), and with all joints held still so that the low-back moment remains the same, the recruited ligaments appear to add to the anterior shear to levels well over 1000 N, which is of great concern from an injury risk viewpoint (Fig. 5–18). However, a more neutral lordotic posture is adopted, and the extensor musculature is responsible for creating the extensor moment and at the same time will support the anterior shearing action of gravity on the upper body and hand-held load. Disabling the ligaments greatly reduces shear loading (Table 5–8). In this example the spine is at much greater risk of sustaining shear injury (>1000 N) than compressive injury (3000 N), simply because the spine was flexed, or in a position at the end range of motion (for a more comprehensive discussion see Potvin and colleagues,[53] McGill and Norman,[76] and McGill and Kippers[77]). This example also illustrates the need to consider more loading modes than simple compression—in this case the real risk was anteroposterior shear load.

CHANGES IN THE FUNCTION OF THE SPINE THROUGHOUT THE DAY

The task of reducing injury becomes more involved as the biomechanical function of the spine changes throughout the day depending on the previous tasks and the time since rising from bed. The diurnal variation in spine length together with the ability to flex forward has been well documented. Losses in sitting height over a day have been measured at up to 19 mm by Reilly and coworkers,[78] who also noted that approximately 54% of this loss occurred in the first 30 minutes after rising. Over the course of a day, and depending on the task history, hydrostatic pressures cause a net outflow of fluid from the disk, resulting in narrowing of the space between the vertebrae, which in turn reduces tension in the ligaments. When a person lies down at night, osmotic pressures in the disk nucleus exceed the hydrostatic pressure, causing the disk to expand (and the spine to lengthen). Adams and colleagues[79] noted that the range of lumbar flexion increased by 5 degrees throughout the day. The increased fluid content after a person rises from bed causes the lumbar spine to be more resistant to bending, while the musculature does not appear to compensate by restricting the bending range. Adams and colleagues estimated that disk bending stresses increased by 300% and ligament stresses

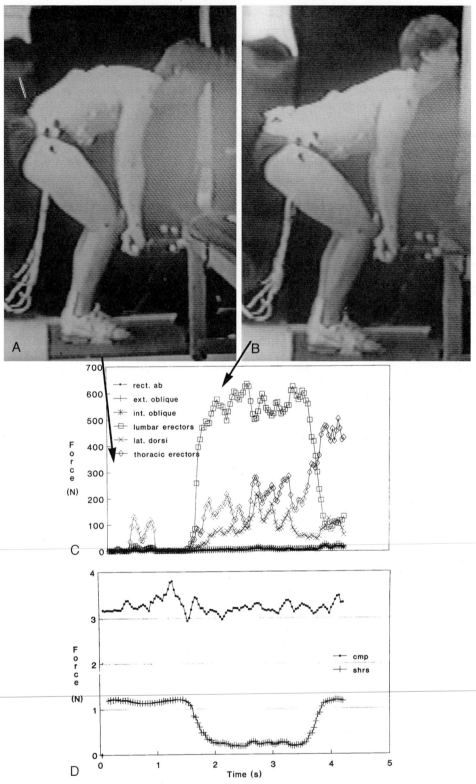

FIGURE 5–18 The fully flexed spine (A) is associated with myoelectric silence in the back extensors and strained posterior passive tissues and high shearing forces on the lumbar spine (from both reaction shear on the upper body and interspinous ligament strain; see Fig. 5–14). A more neutral spine posture (B) recruits the pars lumborum muscle groups (large activity shown in C) to support the reaction shear (see Fig. 5–11), thus reducing total joint shear (to about 200 N in this example) shown in D. (From McGill SM: Biomechanics of low back injury: Implications on current practice and the clinic. J Biomech 30[5]:465–475, 1997.)

TABLE 5–8 Individual Muscle and Passive Tissue Forces and the Associated Lumbar Moments, Compression, and Shear Forces*

| | | FULLY FLEXED LUMBAR SPINE | | | | | | NEUTRAL LUMBAR SPINE |
| | FORCE (N) | MOMENT (N m) | | | COMPRESSION (N) | SHEAR (N) | | FORCE (N) |
		Flexion	Lateral	Twist		Anteroposterior	Lateral	
Muscle								
R. Rectus abdominis	16	−2	1	1	15	5	−4	39
L. Rectus abdominis	16	−2	−1	−1	15	5	4	62
R. External oblique 1	10	−1	1	1	8	7	−3	68
L. External oblique 1	10	−1	−1	−1	8	7	3	40
R. External oblique 2	7	−1	1	0	6	2	−3	62
L. External oblique 2	7	−1	−1	0	6	2	3	31
R. Internal oblique 1	35	0	3	−2	21	−19	20	130
L. Internal oblique 1	35	0	−3	2	21	−19	−20	102
R. Internal oblique 2	29	−2	2	−3	8	−17	21	116
L. Internal oblique 2	29	−2	−2	3	8	−17	−21	88
R. Pars lumborum (L1)	21	2	1	0	21	6	2	253
L. Pars lumborum (L1)	21	2	−1	0	21	6	−2	285
R. Pars lumborum (L2)	27	2	1	0	26	8	2	281
L. Pars lumborum (L2)	27	2	−1	0	26	8	−2	317
R. Pars lumborum (L3)	31	1	1	0	29	−4	6	327
L. Pars lumborum (L3)	31	1	−1	0	29	−4	−6	333
R. Pars lumborum (L4)	32	1	1	0	30	−7	6	402
L. Pars lumborum (L4)	32	1	−1	0	30	−7	−6	355
R. Iliocostalis lumborum	58	5	4	1	57	14	−1	100
L. Iliocostalis lumborum	58	5	−4	−1	57	14	1	137
R. Longissimus thoracis	93	7	4	0	91	23	−6	135
L. Longissimus thoracis	93	7	−4	0	91	23	6	179
R. Quadratus lumborum	25	1	2	0	25	−1	1	155
L. Quadratus lumborum	25	1	−2	0	25	−1	−1	194
R. Latissimus dorsi (L5)	15	1	1	0	14	−1	−6	101
L. Latissimus dorsi (L5)	15	1	−1	0	14	−1	6	115
R. Multifidus 1	28	1	1	1	26	6	9	80
L. Multifidus 1	28	1	−1	−1	26	6	−9	102
R. Multifidus 2	28	1	1	0	28	6	0	87
L. Multifidus 2	28	1	−1	0	28	6	0	90
R. Psoas (L1)	25	1	2	0	24	0	6	61
L. Psoas (L1)	25	−1	−2	0	24	0	−6	69
R. Psoas (L2)	25	−1	2	0	24	0	6	62
L. Psoas (L2)	25	0	−2	0	24	0	−6	69
R. Psoas (L3)	25	0	1	0	24	0	7	62
L. Psoas (L3)	25	0	−1	0	24	0	−7	69
R. Psoas (L4)	25	0	1	1	24	0	8	61
L. Psoas (L4)	25	0	−1	−1	24	0	−8	69
Ligament								
Anterior longitudinal	0	0	0	0	0	0	—	0
Posterior longitudinal	86	2	0	0	261	44	—	0
Ligamentum flavum	21	1	0	0	21	2	—	3
R. Intertransverse	14	0	0	0	13	3	—	0
L. Intertransverse	14	0	0	0	13	3	—	0
R. Articular	74	2	1	1	65	40	—	0
L. Articular	74	2	−1	−1	65	40	—	0
R. Articular 2	103	3	2	2	84	−3	—	0
L. Articular 2	103	3	−2	−2	84	−3	—	0
Interspinous 1	301	18	0	0	273	142	—	0
Interspinous 2	345	14	0	0	233	268	—	0
Interspinous 3	298	10	0	0	194	238	—	0
Supraspinous	592	41	0	0	591	79	—	0
R. Lumbodorsal fascia	122	8	1	0	109	−1	—	0
L. Lumbodorsal fascia	122		−1	0	109	−1	—	0
Passive tissue								
Disk	—	9	0	0	—	—	—	1
Gut, etc.	—	11	0	0	—	—	—	2

*During full flexion, with just the forces in a more neutral lumbar posture demonstrating the shift from muscle to passive tissue and the resultant effects on joint compression and shear. The extensor moment with full lumbar flexion was 171 N m, producing 3145 N of compression and 954 N of anterior shear; in the more neutral posture of 170 N m, the forces produced 3490 N of compression and 269 N of shear.

increased by 80% (owing to the swollen disks and longer spine) and concluded that there is an increased risk of injury to these tissues when one bends forward when first arising. This risk is a variable that is modulated with disk hydration level, which is directly linked to the activity history and the time since rising from bed.

MEMORY OF THE SPINE

The function of the spine is modulated by a patient's activity history in terms of disk hydration (explained in the previous paragraph) as well as viscoelastic creep in the disk and ligaments. In effect, the loading of any activity determines disk hydration (and therefore the size of the disk space and disk geometry), which, in turn, modulates ligament rest length, joint mobility, stiffness, and load distribution. It has been proposed that the nucleus within the anulus "migrates" anteriorly during spinal extension and posteriorly during flexion.[80] McKenzie's program of passive extension of the lumbar spine (which is presently popular in physical therapy) was based on the supposition that an anterior movement of the nucleus pulposus would decrease pressure on the posterior portions of the anulus fibrosus, the most problematic site of herniation. Because of the viscous properties of the nuclear material, such repositioning of the nucleus does not occur immediately upon postural change but rather takes time.

Krag and colleagues[81] demonstrated anterior movement, albeit minute, from an elaborate experiment that placed radiopaque markers in the nucleus of cadaveric lumbar motion segments. Whether this observation reflects simply the redistribution of the centroid of the wedge-shaped nuclear cavity moving forward with flexion or migration of the whole nucleus remains to be seen. Nonetheless, hydraulic theory would suggest lower bulging forces on the posterior anulus if the nuclear centroid moved anteriorly during extension. If compressive forces were applied to a disk in which the nuclear material was still posterior (as in lifting immediately after a prolonged period of flexion), a concentration of stress would occur on the posterior anulus, modulating the risk of injury.

Although this specific area of research needs more development, there does appear to be a time constant (indicating viscosity) associated with this redistribution of nuclear material, suggesting that it would be unwise to lift an object immediately after prolonged flexion—such as when sitting, or stooping, as would a stooped gardener who may stand erect and lift a heavy object. Furthermore, it was suggested by Adams and coauthors[79] that prolonged full flexion may cause the posterior ligaments to creep, which may allow damaging flexion postures to go unchecked if lordosis is not controlled during subsequent lifts. The data of McGill and Brown,[82] in a study of posterior passive tissue creep while sitting in a slouched posture, showed that during the 2 minutes after 20 minutes of full flexion, subjects regained only half of their intervertebral joint stiffness, and even after 30 minutes of rest, some residual joint laxity remained. Thus, the spine has a memory. This is of particular importance for those people whose work is characterized by cyclic bouts of full end range-of-motion postures followed by exertion. Before lifting exertions after a stooped posture, or after prolonged sitting, a case could be made for standing or even consciously extending the spine for a short period. Allowing the nuclear material to "equilibrate" or move anteriorly to a position associated with normal lordosis may decrease forces on the posterior nucleus. Ligaments will regain some protective stiffness.

In conclusion, the anatomy and geometry of the spine is not static. Much remains to be accomplished before we will understand the importance of tissue loading history on subsequent biomechanics, rehabilitation therapies, and injury mechanics.

THE ANATOMIC FLEXIBLE BEAM AND TRUSS: MUSCLE CO-CONTRACTION AND SPINE STABILITY

The ability of the joints of the lumbar spine to bend in any direction is accomplished with large amounts of muscle coactivation. These coactivation patterns are counterproductive to generating the torque necessary to support the applied load in a way that minimizes the load penalty imposed on the spine from muscle contraction. Several ideas have been postulated to explain muscular coactivation: the abdominals are involved in the generation of intraabdominal pressure[83] or in providing support forces to the lumbar spine through the LDF.[48] These ideas, however, have not been without opposition.[63]

It appears that another explanation for muscular coactivation is tenable. A ligamentous spine will fail under compressive loading in a buckling mode, at about 20 N[64]; in other words, a bare spine is unable to bear compressive load. The spine can be likened to a flexible rod in that under compressive loading, it will buckle. If the rod has guy wires connected to it, like the rigging on a ship mast, the rod ultimately experiences more compression but is able to bear much more compressive load because it is stiffened and more resistant to buckling. The co-contracting musculature of the lumbar spine (the flexible beam) can perform the role of stabilizing guy wires (the truss) to each lumbar vertebra bracing against buckling. Work by Crisco and Panjabi[84] has begun to quantify the influence of muscle architecture and the necessary coactivation on stability of the lumbar spine. The architecture of the lumbar erector spinae is especially suited for this role.[26] To invoke this antibuckling and stabilizing mechanism when lifting, one could justify lightly co-contracting the musculature to minimize the potential of spine buckling.

MORE ON STABILITY AND MOTOR CONTROL: HOW DO PEOPLE HURT THEIR BACKS WHILE PICKING UP A PENCIL?

Although injury from large exertions is understandable, explanation of how people injure their backs performing rather benign-appearing tasks is more difficult—but the following is worth considering. Continuing the considerations about stabilization from the previous paragraph, a number of years ago, we were investigating the mechanics of power lifters' spines while they lifted extremely heavy loads using videofluoroscopy for a sagittal view of the lumbar spine.[85] The range of motion of the power lifters' spines was calibrated and normalized to full flexion by first asking them to flex at the waist and support the upper body against gravity with no load in the hands. During their lifts, although they outwardly appeared to have a flexed spine, in fact, the lumbar joints were 2 to 3 degrees per joint from full flexion, explaining how they could lift such magnificent loads (up to 210 kg) without sustaining the injuries that we suspect are linked with full lumbar flexion. During the execution of a lift, however, one lifter reported discomfort and pain. On examination of the videofluoroscopy records, one of the lumbar joints (specifically, the L4–L5 joint) reached the full flexion calibrated angle, while all other joints maintained their static position (2 to 3 degrees from full flexion). This is the first report in the scientific literature that we know of documenting proportionately more rotation occurring at a single lumbar joint, and it would appear that this occurrence was due to an inappropriate sequencing of muscle forces (or a temporary loss of motor control wisdom).

This motivated the work of our colleague and former graduate student, Dr. Jacek Cholewicki, to investigate and continuously quantify stability of the lumbar spine throughout a reasonably wide variety of loading tasks.[52] Generally speaking, it appears that the occurrence of a motor control error that results in a temporary reduction in activation to one of the intersegmental muscles—for example, a lamina of longissimus, iliocostalis, or multifidus—could allow rotation at just a single joint to the point where passive, or other, tissue could become irritated or even more traumatically injured. Cholewicki noted that the risk of such an event is greatest when there are high forces in the large muscles with simultaneous low forces in the small intersegmental muscles (a possibility in the case of the power lifter) or when all muscle forces are low, such as during a low-level exertion. Thus, a mechanism is proposed, based on motor control error resulting in temporary inappropriate neural activation, that explains how injury might occur during extremely low load situations, for example, picking up a pencil from the floor after a long day at work performing a very demanding job.

PREVENTING INJURY: WHAT DOES THE WORKER NEED TO KNOW?

Workers are often told to bend the knees and keep the back straight in an effort to minimize the risk of injury. This demonstrates an overly simplistic view of injury prevention because very few jobs can be performed this way and it is physiologically costly.[86] Rather, work may be designed to incorporate some of the principles developed in the previous sections of this chapter; for example, avoid end range of lumbar motion, design work to vary so that loads are rotated among the various supporting tissues to minimize the risk of accumulated deformation, allow time for tissues to restore their unloaded-rested geometry after the application of prolonged loads when creep has occurred before performing demanding tasks, avoid prolonged sitting, and keep the loads close to the low back. (A much more developed list may be found in McGill and Norman.[87])

USING BIOMECHANICS TO BUILD BETTER REHABILITATION PROGRAMS FOR PATIENTS WITH LOW-BACK INJURY

Rehabilitation of the injured low back involves exercise prescription to stress both damaged tissue and healthy supporting tissues and to foster repair; the key is to avoid excessive loading, which can exacerbate existing structural weakness. Once again, blending the understanding of the biomechanics of injury with clinical art assists the clinician in choosing the optimal load—neither too much nor too little.

It is important to understand the applications, and conversely the limitations, of scientific laboratory approaches for investigating tissue loading in vivo and in vitro. Because the low-back system is an extremely complex mechanical structure, and direct measurement of tissue forces in vivo is not feasible, the only tenable option for tissue load prediction is to use sophisticated modeling approaches. Several issues must be addressed, however, including the need for anatomic detail, a method to solve for the inherent indeterminacy from so many unknown forces among the significant load-bearing structures, and development of methods that enable the prediction of loads in deep (and inaccessible) muscles and supporting ligaments. Although these issues are outside the scope of this chapter, the interested reader is urged to consult Juker and colleagues,[35] McGill,[39] and Cholewicki and McGill[52] for a description of the scientific methods used to develop the following program.

TOWARD DEVELOPING SCIENTIFICALLY JUSTIFIED LOW-BACK REHABILITATION EXERCISES

Exercises in this section have been selected and evaluated based on tissue-loading evidence and the knowledge of how injury occurs to specific tissues (described in the original scientific publications[35, 88, 89]). In fact, some integrated components of this section were adapted from my chapter in The American College of Sports Medicine textbook *Resource Manual for Guidelines for Exercise Testing and Prescription.*[90]

Choosing exercises has not always been a scientific endeavor. The following example illustrates the need for quantitative analysis for evaluating the safety of certain exercises. We have all been aware of the principle to perform sit-ups and other flexion exercises with the knees flexed—but on what evidence? Several hypotheses have suggested that this disables or changes the line of action of the psoas. Recent MRI-based data[91] demonstrated that the psoas line of action does not change as a result of lumbar or hip posture (except at L5–S1) because the psoas laminae attach to each vertebra and "follow" the changing orientation of spine. There is no doubt, however, that the psoas is shortened with the flexed hip, modulating force production. But the question remains: is there a reduction in spine load with the legs bent?

In a recent study,[92] I examined 12 young men, with the laboratory technique described previously, and observed no major difference in lumbar load as the result of bending the knees (average moment of 65 N m in both straight legs and

bent knees; compression, 3230 N with straight legs, 3410 N with bent knees; shear, 260 N with straight legs, 300 N with bent knees). Compressive loads in excess of 3000 N certainly raise questions of safety. This type of quantitative analysis is necessary to demonstrate that the issue of performing sit-ups using bent knees or straight legs is probably not as important as the issue of whether to prescribe sit-ups at all! There are better ways to challenge the abdominals.

Several exercises are required to train all the muscles of the lumbar torso, and the exercises that best suit the individual depend on a number of variables, such as fitness level, training goals, and history of previous spinal injury. Depending on the purpose of the exercise program, however, several principles apply. For example, an individual beginning a postinjury program is better advised to avoid loading the spine throughout the range of motion, whereas a trained athlete may indeed achieve higher performance levels by doing so. Selection of the following exercises was biased toward safety—minimizing spine loading during muscle challenge. Therefore, a neutral spine (neutral lordosis) is emphasized while the spine is under load—neither hyperlordotic or hypolordotic. A general rule is to preserve the normal low-back curve (similar to that of upright standing) or some variation that minimizes pain. Although in the past performing a "pelvic tilt" when exercising has been recommended, this is not justified because the pelvic tilt increases spine tissue loading when the spine is no longer in static-elastic equilibrium; therefore, it is probably unwise to recommend the pelvic tilt when challenging the spine.

ISSUES OF FLEXIBILITY

Training to optimize spine flexibility depends on the person's injury history and exercise goal. Generally, for the patient with a back injury, spine flexibility should not be emphasized until the spine has stabilized and has undergone strength and endurance conditioning—some patients may never reach this stage! Despite the notion held by some, there are little quantitative data to support a major emphasis on trunk flexibility to improve back health and lessen the risk of injury. In fact, some exercise programs that have included loading of the torso throughout the range of motion (in flexion and extension, lateral bend, or axial twist) have had negative results,[93, 94] and greater spine mobility has been, in some cases, associated with low-back trouble.[95, 96] Furthermore, flexibility of the spine has been shown to have little predictive value for future low-back trouble.[94, 97] The

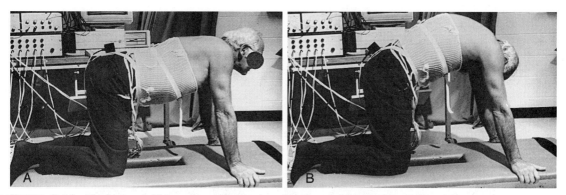

FIGURE 5–19 The "cat stretch" is performed by slowly cycling through full spine flexion (A) to full extension (B). Spine mobility is emphasized rather than "pressing" at the end range of motion. This exercise provides motion for the spine with very low loading of the intervertebral joints.

most successful programs appear to emphasize trunk stabilization through exercise with a neutral spine[98] but emphasize mobility at the hips and knees. Bridger and colleagues[99] demonstrate advantages for sitting and standing, whereas McGill and Norman[87] outline advantages for lifting.

For these reasons, specific torso flexibility exercises should be limited to unloaded flexion and extension for those concerned with safety but perhaps not for those interested in specific athletic performance (of course, spine flexibility may be of greater desirability in athletes who have never suffered back injury). The spine may be cycled

through full flexion and extension in a slow, smooth motion (Fig. 5–19). Hip and knee flexibility may be achieved with the following maneuvers, emphasizing a neutral spine throughout: hip mobility—standing hip extension, standing hip flexion; hip mobility, strength, and endurance—slow lunges (Figs. 5–20 and 5–21).

ISSUES OF STRENGTH AND ENDURANCE

The link between lower muscle strength and endurance performance in patients with previous

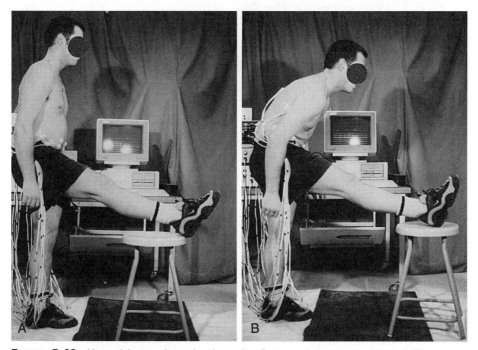

FIGURE 5–20 Hip mobility is enhanced with standing flexion and extension positions. A, The correct neutral spine. B, An incorrect, flexed spine.

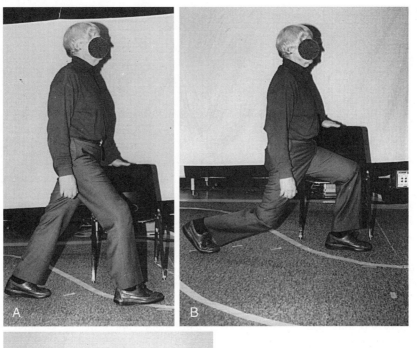

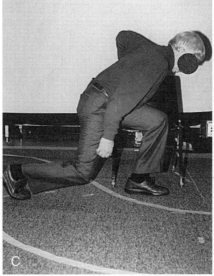

FIGURE 5–21   Hip mobility, strength, and endurance are challenged with slow lunges. *A,* The torso remains upright throughout the lunge effort. *B,* Emphasis is placed on a neutral spine during hip exercises to focus the stretch over the hip and knee joints. *C,* The incorrect, flexed spine.

back injuries is well documented. In fact, few longitudinal studies have linked reduced strength and endurance with the risk of a subsequent first-time low-back injury. The few studies available suggest that endurance has a much greater prophylactic value than strength.[100] Furthermore, it would appear that emphasis placed on endurance should precede specific strengthening exercise in a graduated progressive exercise program (i.e., longer-duration, lower-effort exercises).

Aerobic Exercise

The mounting evidence supporting the role of aerobic exercise both in reducing the incidence of low-back injury[101] and in treating low-back injury patients[102] is compelling. Recent investigation into loads sustained by the low-back tissues during walking[54] confirm very low levels of supporting passive tissue load coupled with mild, but prolonged, activation of the supporting musculature.

Epidemiologic evidence also sheds light on the effects of aerobic exercise. A large study[103] examined age-related changes to the lumbar spines of elderly people as a function of lifelong activity level; those who were runners had no differences in spine changes measured from MRI images, whereas weight lifters and soccer players were characterized with more disk degeneration and bulges.

The Abdominals (Anterior and Lateral) and Quadratus Lumborum

There is no single abdominal exercise that challenges all of the abdominal musculature—requiring the prescription of more than a single exercise. Calibrated intramuscular and surface EMG evidence[35, 92] suggests that the various types of curl-ups challenge mainly the rectus abdominis because psoas and abdominal wall (internal and external oblique, transverse abdominis) activity is low. Sit-ups (both straight-leg and bent-knee) are characterized by higher psoas activation and higher low-back compression, whereas leg raises cause even higher activation and also spine compression (Table 5–9).

Several relevant observations were made regarding abdominal exercises in our investigations. The challenge to psoas is lowest during curl-ups, followed by higher levels during the horizontal isometric side support, whereas bent-knee sit-ups

were characterized by larger psoas activation than straight-leg sit-ups, through to the highest psoas activity observed during leg raises and hand-on-knee flexor isometric exertions. Note that the "press-heels" sit-up, which has been hypothesized to activate hamstrings and neurally inhibit psoas, actually increased psoas activation. Normalized EMG data in Table 5–9 are provided for comparative purposes. (Some athletes intentionally wish to train psoas and will find these data informative; low-back injury patients must be more selective.)

One exercise not often performed but appearing to have merit is the horizontal side support because it challenges the lateral obliques without high lumbar compressive loading.[89] In addition, this exercise produces high activation levels in the quadratus lumborum, which appears to be a significant stabilizer of the spine[40] (as previously noted). Graded activity in the rectus abdominis and each of the components of the abdominal wall change with each of these exercises, demonstrating that there is no single best task for the collective abdominal muscles. Clearly, curl-ups excel at activating the rectus abdominis but produce relatively lower oblique activity. Several other clinically relevant findings from these two data sets include notions that psoas activation is dominated by hip flexion demands and that psoas activity is not consistent with either lumbar sagittal moment or spine compression demands. We question the often-cited notion that psoas is a lumbar

TABLE 5–9 **Subject Averages of Electromyogram Activation Normalized to 100% of Maximum Voluntary Contraction***

ABDOMINAL TASKS	QUADRATUS LUMBORUM	PSOAS 1$_i$	PSOAS 2$_i$	EOi	IOi	TAi	RA	RF	ES
Straight-leg sit-ups		15 (12)	24 (7)	44 (9)	15 (15)	11 (9)	48 (18)	16 (10)	4 (3)
Bent-knee sit-ups	12 (7)	17 (10)	28 (7)	43 (12)	16 (14)	10 (7)	55 (16)	14 (7)	6 (9)
Press-heel sit-ups		28 (23)	34 (18)	51 (14)	22 (14)	20 (13)	51 (20)	15 (12)	4 (3)
Bent-knee curl-up	11 (6)	7 (8)	10 (14)	19 (14)	14 (10)	12 (9)	62 (22)	8 (12)	6 (10)
Bent-knee leg raise	12 (6)	24 (15)	25 (8)	22 (7)	8 (9)	7 (6)	32 (20)	8 (5)	6 (8)
Straight leg raise	9 (2)	35 (20)	33 (8)	26 (9)	9 (8)	6 (4)	37 (24)	23 (12)	7 (11)
Isometric hand-to-knee									
LH-RK		16 (16)	16 (8)	68 (14)	30 (28)	28 (19)	69 (18)	8 (7)	6 (4)
RH-LK		56 (28)	58 (16)	53 (12)	48 (23)	44 (18)	74 (25)	42 (29)	5 (4)
Cross curl-up									
RS—across	6 (4)	5 (3)	4 (4)	23 (20)	24 (14)	20 (11)	57 (22)	10 (19)	5 (8)
LS—across	6 (4)	5 (3)	5 (5)	24 (17)	21 (16)	15 (13)	58 (24)	12 (24)	5 (8)
Isometric side support	54 (28)	21 (17)	12 (8)	43 (13)	36 (29)	39 (24)	22 (13)	11 (11)	24 (15)
Dynamic side support		26 (18)	13 (5)	44 (16)	42 (24)	44 (33)	41 (20)	9 (7)	29 (17)
Push-up from feet	4 (1)	24 (19)	12 (5)	29 (12)	10 (14)	9 (9)	29 (10)	10 (7)	3 (4)
Push-up from knees		14 (11)	10 (7)	19 (10)	7 (9)	8 (8)	19 (11)	5 (3)	3 (4)

*Mean and standard deviation (in parentheses) are given. Note psoas channels, external oblique (EO), internal oblique (IO), and transverse abdominals (TA) are intramuscular electrodes (i), whereas rectus abdominis (RA), rectus femoris (RF), and erector spinae (ES) are surface electrodes.
LH-RK, left hand–right knee; RH-LK, right hand–left knee; RS, right shoulder; LS, left shoulder.

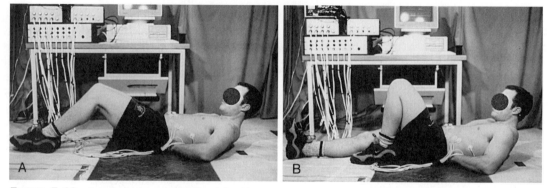

FIGURE 5–22   A, In the curl-up, the head and shoulders are raised off the ground with the hands under the lumbar region to help stabilize the pelvis and support the neutral spine. B, A variation is to bend only one leg while the other, straight leg assists in pelvic stabilization and preservation of a neutral lumbar curve.

spine stabilizer; quadratus lumborum activity is consistent with lumbar sagittal moment and compression demands, suggesting a larger role in stabilization; and psoas activation is relatively high (greater than 25% MVC) during push-ups, suggesting cautious concern for the low-back injury patient.

A wise choice for abdominal exercises in the early stages of training or rehabilitation would consist of several variations of curl-ups for the rectus abdominis, and isometric, horizontal side support (with the body supported by the knees and upper body supported by one elbow on the floor) exercises to challenge the abdominal wall in a way that imposes minimal compressive penalty on the spine. The level of challenge with the isometric, horizontal side support exercises can be increased by supporting the body with the feet rather than the knees. Specific recommended ab-

dominal exercises are shown—the curl-up with the hands on the low back to stabilize the pelvis and assist in preservation of a neutral lordosis (lumbar curvature), and the horizontal isometric side support (again with the spine in a neutral posture) using either the knees or the feet for support (Figs. 5–22 and 5–23).

The Back Extensors

We have been searching for methods to activate the extensors with minimal spine loading,[88] given that most traditional extensor exercises are characterized by high spine loads, which result from externally applied compressive and shear forces (from either free weights or resistance machines). It appears that the single leg extension hold, while on the hands and knees (Fig. 5–24), minimizes external loads on the spine but produces spine

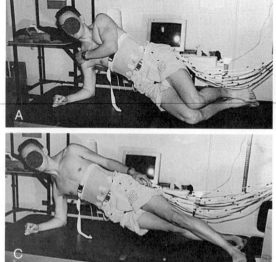

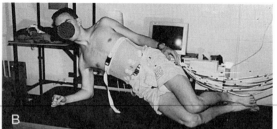

FIGURE 5–23   The horizontal isometric side support. Supporting the lower body with the knees on the floor reduces the demand further for those who are more concerned with safety. Supporting the body with the feet increases the muscle challenge but also the spine load. Progression of challenge is indicated, with the lowest in A and highest in C.

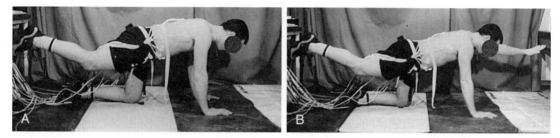

FIGURE 5–24   *A*, Single-leg extension holds, while on the hands and knees, produce mild extensor activity and lower spine compression (<2500 N). *B*, Raising the contralateral arm increases extensor muscle activity but also spine compression to levels higher than 3000 N. (From Callaghan J, Gunning J, McGill SM: Relationship between lumbar spine load and muscle activity during extensor exercises. Phys Ther 78[1]:8–18, 1998.)

extensor moment (and small isometric twisting moments), activating the extensors (one side of the lumbar extensors about 18% MVC). Activation is sufficiently high on one side of the extensors to facilitate training, but the total spine load is reduced because the contralateral extensors are producing lower forces (lumbar compression is less than 2500 N). Switching legs trains both sides of the extensors.

In total, seven tasks were analyzed to facilitate comparison of various extensor tasks.[88] Simultaneous leg extension with contralateral arm raise increases the unilateral extensor muscle challenge (about 27% MVC in one side of lumbar extensors and 45% MVC in the other side of thoracic extensors) but also increases lumbar compression to well more than 3000 N (see Fig. 5–24). The often-performed exercise of lying prone on the floor and raising the upper body and legs off the floor is contraindicated for anyone at risk of low-back injury or reinjury (Fig. 5–25). In this task, the lumbar region pays a high compression penalty to a hyperextended spine (about 4000 N or higher), which transfers load to the facets and crushes the interspinous ligament (noted earlier as an injury mechanism).

Should Abdominal Belts Be Worn?

The average patient must be confused when observing both elite lifting athletes and back injury patients wearing abdominal belts. Several years ago, I conducted a review of the effects of belt wearing[104] and summarized the following: those who have never had a previous back injury appear to have no additional protective benefit from wearing a belt; it would appear that those who have had an injury while wearing a belt risk a more severe injury; belts appear to give people the perception they can lift more and may in fact enable them to lift more; and belts appear to increase intraabdominal pressure and blood pressure; belts appear to change the lifting styles of some people to either decrease the loads on the spine or increase the loads on the spine. In summary, given the assets and liabilities of belt wearing, they are not recommended for routine exercise participation.

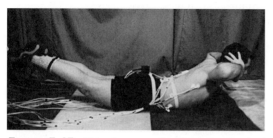

FIGURE 5–25   This often-prescribed extensor exercise is contraindicated for most people because of the extended posture (and facet and anulus loading) and high spine compression load of 4000 to 6000 N. (From Callaghan J, Gunning J, McGill SM: Relationship between lumbar spine load and muscle activity during extensor exercises. Phys Ther 78[1]:8–18, 1998.)

NOTES FOR EXERCISE PRESCRIPTION

The exercise professional must design exercise programs to meet a wide variety of objectives. The following is a list of general caveats to assist in achieving the best prescription (this list was adapted from my chapter in the American College of Sports Medicine publication[90]):

1. Although there is a common belief among some experts that exercise sessions should be performed at least three times per week, it appears that low-back exercises have the most beneficial effect when performed daily.[105]

2. The "no pain, no gain" axiom does not apply when exercising the low back, particularly when applied to weight training, and scientific and clinical wisdom would suggest the opposite is true.

3. Although specific low-back exercises have been rationalized in this chapter, general exercise programs that also combine cardiovascular components (such as walking) have been shown to be more effective in both rehabilitation and injury prevention.[102] The exercises shown here constitute only a component of the total program.

4. Diurnal variation in the fluid level of the intervertebral disks (disks are more hydrated early in the morning after rising from bed) changes the stresses on the disk throughout the day. It would be unwise to perform full-range spine motion while under load, shortly after rising from bed.[17]

5. Low-back exercises performed for maintenance of health need not emphasize strength. High-load, low-repetition tasks, rather than more repetitions of less demanding exercises, will assist in the enhancement of endurance and strength. There is no doubt that back injury can occur during seemingly low-level demands (such as picking up a pencil) and that the risk of injury from motor control error can occur. Although it appears that the chance of motor control errors, resulting in inappropriate muscle forces, increases with fatigue, there is also evidence documenting the changes in passive tissue loading with fatiguing lifting.[106] Given that endurance has more protective value than strength,[100] strength gains should not be overemphasized at the expense of endurance.

6. There is no such thing as an ideal set of exercises for all patients. An individual's training objectives must be identified (e.g., rehabilitation, injury risk reduction, optimization of general health and fitness, or maximization of athletic performance) and the most appropriate exercises chosen. Although science cannot evaluate the optimal exercises for each situation, the combination of science and clinical experience must be used to enhance low-back health.

7. Patience and perseverance are important. Increased function and reduction of pain may not occur for 3 months.[107]

Acknowledgments: I wish to acknowledge the contributions of several colleagues to the collection of works reported here: Daniel Juker, MD; Craig Axler, MSc; Jacek Cholewicki, PhD; Michael Sharratt, PhD; John Seguin, MD; Vaughan Kippers, PhD; and in particular, Robert Norman, PhD. Financial support from the Natural Science and Engineering Research Council, Canada has made this series of work possible.

References

1. Roberts S, Menage J, Urban JPG: Biochemical and structural properties of the cartilage endplate and its relationship to the intervertebral disc. Spine 14:166, 1989.
2. Gallois J, Japoit T: Architecture intérieure des vertèbres du point de vue statique et physiologique. Rev Chir (Paris) 63:688, 1925.
3. Nachemson AL: Lumbar interdiscal pressure. Acta Orthop Scand Suppl 43, 1960.
4. Nachemson A: The load on lumbar discs in different positions of the body. Clin Rel Res 45:107, 1966.
5. Brinckmann P, Biggemann M, Hilweg D: Prediction of the compressive strength of human lumbar vertebrae. Clin Biomech 4(suppl 2), 1989.
6. Yingling VR, McGill SM: Mechanical properties and injuries resulting from anterior and posterior shear loading of the spine at different load rates. *In* Proceedings of the American Society for Biomechanics, Atlanta, October 17–19, 1996, pp 267–268.
7. Farfan HF: Mechanical disorders of the low back. Philadelphia, Lea & Febiger, 1973.
8. Roaf R: A study of the mechanics of spinal injuries. J Bone Joint Surg 42B:810, 1960.
9. Fyhrie DP, Schaffler MB: Failure mechanisms in human vertebral cancellous bone. Bone 15(1):105–109, 1994.
10. McGill SM: Low back exercises: Prescription for the healthy back and when recovering from injury. *In* American College of Sports Medicine: Resource Manual for Guidelines for Exercise Testing and Prescription, 3rd ed. Baltimore, Williams & Wilkins, 1998.
11. Bogduk N, Engel R: The menisci of the lumbar zygapophyseal joints: A review of their anatomy and clinical significance. Spine 9:454, 1984.
12. Bedzinski R: Application of speckle photography methods to the investigations of deformation of the vertebral arch. *In* Little EG (ed): Experimental Mechanics. New York, Elsevier, 1992.
13. Dickey JP, Pierrynowski MR, Bednar DA: Deformation of vertebrae in vivo: Implications for facet joint loads and spinous process pin instrumentation for measuring sequential spinal kinematics. Presented at the Canadian Orthopaedic Research Society, Quebec City, May 25, 1996.

14. Hardcastle P, Annear P, Foster D: Spinal abnormalities in young fast bowlers. J Bone Joint Surg 74B(3):421, 1992.

15. Cripton P, Berlemen U, Visarino H, et al: Response of the lumbar spine due to shear loading. *In* Injury Prevention Through Biomechanics. Detroit, Wayne State University, May 4–5, 1995, p 111.

16. Markolf KL, Morris JM: The structural components of the intervertebral disc. J Bone Joint Surg 56A(4):675, 1974.

17. Adams MA, Dolan P: Recent advances in lumbar spinal mechanics and their clinical significance. Clin Biomech 10(1):3, 1995.

18. Adams MA, Hutton WC: Prolapsed intervertebral disc: A hyperflexion injury. Spine 7:184, 1982.

19. Adams MA, Hutton WC: Gradual disc prolapse. Spine 10:524, 1985.

20. Adams P, Muir H: Qualitative changes with age of proteoglycans of human lumbar discs. Ann Rheum Dis 35:289, 1976.

21. King AI: Injury to the thoraco-lumbar spine and pelvis. *In* Nahum AM, Melvin JW (eds): Accidental Injury, Biomechanics and Presentation. New York, Springer-Verlag, 1993.

22. Gordon SJ, Yang KH, Mayer PJ, et al: Mechanism of disc rupture: A preliminary report. Spine 16:450, 1991.

23. Videman T, Nurminen M, Troup JDG: Lumbar spinal pathology in cadaveric material in relation to history of back pain, occupation and physical loading. Spine 15(8):728, 1990.

24. Wilder DG, Pope MH, Frymoyer JW: The biomechanics of lumbar disc herniation and the effect of overload and instability. J Spinal Disord 1(1):16, 1988.

25. Goel VK, Monroe BT, Gilbertson LG, Brinckmann P: Interlaminar shear stresses and laminae—separation in a disc: Finite element analysis of the L3–L4 motion segment subjected to axial compressive loads. Spine 20(6):689, 1995.

26. Bogduk N: A reappraisal of the anatomy of the human lumbar erector spinae. J Anat 131(3):525, 1980.

27. Macintosh JE, Valencia F, Bogduk N, Munro RR: The morphology of the human lumbar multifidus. Clin Biomech 1:196, 1986.

28. Macintosh JE, Bogduk N: The morphology of the lumbar erector spinae. Spine 12(7):658, 1987.

29. McGill SM, Patt N, Norman RW: Measurement of the trunk musculature of active males using CT scan radiography: Duplications for force and moment generating capacity about the L4/L5 joint. J Biomech 21(4):329, 1988.

30. McGill SM, Santaguida L, Stevens J: Measurement of the trunk musculature from T6 to L5 using MRI scans of 15 young males corrected for muscle fibre orientation. Clin Biomech 8:171, 1993.

31. McGill SM, Juker D, Axler CT: Correcting trunk muscle geometry obtained from MRI and CT scans of supine postures for use in standing postures. J Biomech 29:643–646, 1996.

32. Nitz AJ, Peck D: Comparison of muscle spindle concentrations in large and small human epaxial muscles acting in parallel combinations. Am Surg 52:273–277, 1986.

33. McGill SM, Norman RW: Effects of an anatomically detailed erector spinae model on L4/L5 disc compression and shear. J Biomech 20(6):591, 1987.

34. Sirca A, Kostevc V: The fibre type composition of thoracic and lumbar paravertebral muscles in man. J Anat 141:131, 1985.

35. Juker D, McGill SM, Kropf P, Steffen T: Quantitative intramuscular myoelectric activity of lumbar portions of psoas and the abdominal wall during a wide variety of tasks. Med Sci Sports Exerc 30(2):301–310, 1998.

36. Belanger M: Personal communication. University of Quebec at Montreal, 1996.

37. McGill SM: A revised anatomical model of the abdominal musculature for torso flexion efforts. J Biomech 29(7):973, 1996.

38. McGill SM: Electromyographic activity of the abdominal and low back musculature during the generation of isometric and dynamic axial trunk torque: Implications for lumbar mechanics. J Orthop Res 9:91, 1991.

39. McGill SM: A myoelectrically based dynamic 3-D model to predict loads on lumbar spine tissues during lateral bending. J Biomech 25(4):395, 1992.

40. McGill SM, Juker D, Kropf P: Quantitative intramuscular myoelectric activity of quadratus lumborum during a wide variety of tasks. Clin Biomech 11(3):170, 1996.

41. Heylings DJ: Supraspinous and interspinous ligaments of the human lumbar spine. J Anat 125:127, 1978.

42. Bogduk N, Twomey LT: Clinical anatomy of the lumbar spine. New York, Churchill Livingstone, 1987.

43. Sharma M, Langrama NA, Rodriguez J: Role of ligaments and facets in lumbar spine stability. Spine 20(8):887, 1995.

44. Noyes FR, De Lucas JL, Torvik PJ: Biomechanics of ligament failure: An analysis of strain-rate sensitivity and mechanisms of failure in primates. J Bone Joint Surg 56A:236, 1994.

45. Rissanen PM: The surgical anatomy and pathology of the supraspinous and interspinous ligaments of the lumbar spine with special reference to ligament ruptures. Acta Orthop Scand Suppl 46, 1960.

46. Carr D, Gilbertson L, Frymoyer J, et al: Lumbar paraspinal compartment syndrome: A case report with physiologic and anatomic studies. Spine 10:816, 1985.

47. Styf J: Pressure in the erector spinae muscle during exercise. Spine 12:675, 1987.

48. Gracovetsky S, Farfan HF, Lamy C: Mechanism of the lumbar spine. Spine 6(1):249, 1981.

49. Ashton-Miller JA, Schultz AB: Biomechanics of

the human spine and trunk. *In* Parrdolf KB (ed): Exercise and Sport Science Reviews, vol 16. American College of Sports Medicine Series. New York, MacMillan, 1988.

50. Spencer DL, Miller JAA, Schultz AB: The effects of chemonucleolysis on the mechanical properties of the canine lumbar disc. Spine 10:555, 1985.

51. Kirkaldy-Willis WH, Burton CV: Managing low back pain, 3rd ed. New York, Churchill Livingstone, 1992.

52. Cholewicki J, McGill SM: Mechanical stability of the in vivo lumbar spine: Implications for injury and chronic low back pain. Clin Biomech 11(1):1, 1996.

53. Potvin J, Norman RW, McGill S: Reduction in anterior shear forces on the L4/L5 disc by the lumbar musculature. Clin Biomech 6:88, 1991.

54. Callaghan JP, Patla A, McGill SM: 3D Analysis of Spine Loading During Gait. Atlanta, American Society for Biomechanics, October 17–19, 1996.

55. Troup JDG, Leskinen TPJ, Stalhammear HR, Kuorinka IA: A comparison of intra-abdominal pressure increases, hip torque, and lumbar vertebral compression in different lifting techniques. Hum Factors 25(5):517, 1983.

56. Thomson KD: On the bending moment capability of the pressurized abdominal cavity during human lifting activity. Ergonomics 31(5):817, 1988.

57. Bearn JG: The significance of the activity of the abdominal muscles in weight lifting. Acta Anat 45:83, 1961.

58. Grew ND: Intraabdominal pressure response to loads applied to the torso in normal subjects. Spine 5(2):149, 1980.

59. Ekholm J, Arborelius UP, Nemeth G: The load on the lumbosacral joint and trunk muscle activity during lifting. Ergonomics 25(2):145, 1982.

60. Krag MH, Byrne KB, Gilbertson LG, Haugh LD: Failure of intraabdominal pressurization to reduce erector spinae loads during lifting tasks. *In* Proceedings of the North American Congress on Biomechanics, Montreal, August 25–27, 1986, p 87.

61. Nachemson AL, Morris JM: In vivo measurements of intradiscal pressure. J Bone Joint Surg 46A:1077, 1964.

62. Nachemson A, Andersson GBJ, Schultz AB: Valsalva manoeuvre biomechanics: Effects on lumbar trunk loads of elevated intra-abdominal pressure. Spine 11(5):476, 1986.

63. McGill SM, Norman RW: Reassessment of the role of intraabdominal pressure in spinal compression. Ergonomics 30(11):1565, 1987.

64. Lucas D, Bresler B: Stability of the ligamentous spine. Tech. Report No. 40, Biomechanics Laboratory, University of California, San Francisco, 1961.

65. Tesh KM, Dunn J, Evans JH: The abdominal muscles and vertebral stability. Spine 12(5):501, 1987.

66. Macintosh JE, Bogduk N, Gracovetsky S: The biomechanics of the thoracolumbar fascia. Clin Biomech 2:78, 1987.

67. McGill SM, Norman RW: The potential of lumbodorsal fascia forces to generate back extension moments during squat lifts. J Biomed Eng 10:312, 1988.

68. Bogduk N, Macintosh JE: The applied anatomy of the thoracolumbar fascia. Spine 9:164, 1984.

69. Hukins DWL, Aspden RM, Hickey DS: Thoracolumbar fascia can increase the efficiency of the erector spinae muscles. Clin Biomech 5(1):30, 1990.

70. Carter DR, Hayes WC: The comprehensive behavior of bone as a two-phase porous structure. J Bone Joint Surg 58A:954, 1977.

71. Adams MA, Hutton WC, Stott JRR: The resistance to flexion of the lumbar intervertebral joint. Spine 5:245, 1980.

72. McGill SM, Brown S: Creep response of the lumbar spine to prolonged lumber flexion. Clin Biomech 7:43, 1992.

73. Dontigny RL: Function and pathomechanics of the sacroiliac joint. Phys Ther 65:35–44, 1985.

74. Resnick D, Niwayama G, Georgen TG: Degenerative disease of the sacroiliac joint. Invest Radiol 19:608, 1975.

75. McGill SM: A biomechanical perspective of sacro-iliac pain. Clin Biomech 2:145–151.

76. McGill SM, Norman RW: Partitioning of the L4/L5 dynamic moment into disc, ligamentous and muscular components during lifting. Spine 11(7):666, 1986.

77. McGill SM, Kippers V: Transfer of loads between lumbar tissues during the flexion relaxation phenomenon. Spine 19(19):2190, 1994.

78. Reilly T, Tynell A, Troup JDG: Circadian variation in human stature. Chronobiol Int 1:121, 1984.

79. Adams MA, Dolan P, Hutton WC: Diurnal variations in the stresses on the lumbar spine. Spine 12(2):130, 1987.

80. McKenzie RA: Prophylaxis in recurrent low back pain. N Z Med J 89:22, 1979.

81. Krag MH, Seroussi RE, Wilder DG, Pope MH: Internal displacement distribution from in vitro loading of human thoracic and lumbar spinal motion segments: Experimental results and theoretical predictions. Spine 12(10):1001, 1987.

82. McGill SM, Brown S: Creep response of the lumbar spine to prolonged lumber flexion. Clin Biomech 7:43, 1992.

83. Davis PR: The causation of herniae by weight-lifting. Lancet 2:155, 1959.

84. Crisco JJ, Panjabi MM: Postural biomechanical stability and gross muscular architecture in the spine. *In* Winters J, Woo S (eds): Multiple Muscle Systems. New York, Springer-Verlag, 1990, p 438.

85. Cholewicki J, McGill SM: Lumbar posterior ligament involvement during extremely heavy

lifts estimated from fluoroscopic measurements. J Biomech 25(1):17, 1992.

86. Garg A, Herrin G: Stoop or squat: A biomechanical and metabolic evaluation. Am Inst Ind Eng Trans 11:293, 1979.

87. McGill SM, Norman RW: Low back biomechanics in industry: The prevention of injury. *In* Grabiner MD (ed): Current Issues of Biomechanics. Champaign, IL, Human Kinetics, 1992.

88. Callaghan J, Gunning J, McGill SM: Relationship between lumbar spine load and muscle activity during extensor exercises. Phys Ther 78(1):8–18, 1998.

89. Axler CT, McGill SM: Low back loads over a variety of abdominal exercises: Searching for the safest abdominal challenge. Med Sci Sports Exerc 29(6):804–811, 1997.

90. McGill SM: Low back exercises: Prescription for the healthy back and when recovering from injury. *In* American College of Sports Medicine: Resource Manual for Guidelines for Exercise Testing and Prescription, 3rd ed. Baltimore, Williams & Wilkins, 1998.

91. Santaguida L, McGill SM: The psoas major muscle: A three-dimensional mechanical modelling study with respect to the spine based on MRI measurement. J Biomech 28(3):339, 1995.

92. McGill SM: The mechanics of torso flexion: Situps and standing dynamic flexion manoeuvres. Clin Biomech 10(4):184, 1995.

93. Malmivaara A, Hakkinen U, Aro T, et al: The treatment of acute low back pain: Bed rest, exercises, or ordinary activity? N Engl J Med 332:351, 1995.

94. Nachemson A: Newest knowledge of low back pain: A critical look. Clin Orthop 279:8, 1992.

95. Biering-Sorensen F: Physical measurements as risk indicators for low back trouble over a one year period. Spine 9:106, 1984.

96. Burton AK, Tillotson KM, Troup JDG: Variation in lumbar sagittal mobility with low back trouble. Spine 14(6):584, 1989.

97. Battie MC, Bigos SJ, Fischer LD, et al: The role of spinal flexibility in back pain complaints within industry: A prospective study. Spine 15(8):768, 1990.

98. Saal JA, Saal JS: Nonoperative treatment of herniated lumbar intervertebral disc with radiculopathy: An outcome study. Spine 14(4):41, 1989.

99. Bridger RS, Orkin D, Henneberg M: A quantitative investigation of lumbar and pelvic postures in standing and sitting: Interrelationships

with body position and hip muscle length. Int J Ind Ergonom 9:235, 1992.

100. Luoto S, Heliovaara M, Hurri H, Alaranta M: Static back endurance and the risk of low back pain. Clin Biomech 10(6):323, 1995.

101. Cady LD, Bischoff DP, O'Connell ER, et al: Strength and fitness and subsequent back injuries in firefighters. J Occup Med 21(4):269, 1979.

102. Nutter P: Aerobic exercise in the treatment and prevention of low back pain. State Art Rev Occup Med 3:137, 1988.

103. Videman T, Sarna S, Crites-Battie M, et al: The long term effects of physical loading and exercise lifestyles on back-related symptoms, disability, and spinal pathology among men. Spine 20(b):669, 1995.

104. McGill SM: Abdominal belts in industry: A position paper on their assets, liabilities and use. Am Ind Hyg Assoc J 54(12):752, 1993.

105. Mayer TG, Gatchel RJ, Kishino N, et al: Objective assessment of spine function following industrial injury: A prospective study with comparison group and one-year follow up. Spine 10(6):482, 1985.

106. Potvin JR, Norman RW: Can fatigue compromise lifting safety? *In* Proceedings of the Second North American Congress on Biomechanics, August 24–28, 1992, p 153.

107. Manniche C, Hesselsoe G, Bentzen L, et al: Clinical trial of intensive muscle training for chronic low back pain. Lancet Dec. 24/31:1473, 1988.

108. White AA, Panjabi MM: Clinical Biomechanics of the Spine. Philadelphia, JB Lippincott, 1978.

109. Pearcy MJ, Portek J, Shepherd J: Three dimensional x-ray analysis of normal measurement in the lumbar spine. Spine 9:294, 1984.

110. Pearcy MJ, Tibrewal SB: Axial rotation and lateral bending in the normal lumbar spine measured by three-dimensional radiography. Spine 9:582, 1984.

111. Shultz AB, Warwick DN, Berkson MH, Nachemson AL: Mechanical properties of human lumbar spine motion segments. I. Response in flexion, extension, lateral bending and torsion. J Biomech Eng 101:46, 1979.

112. Berkson MH, Nachemson AL, Shultz AB: Mechanical properties of human lumbar spine motion segments. II. Responses in compression and shear: Influence of gross morphology. J Biomech Eng 101:53, 1979.

113. McGlashen KM, Miller JAA, Shultz AB, Anderson GBJ: Load displacement behaviour of the human lumbosacral joint. J Orthop Res 5:488, 1987.

CHAPTER 6

BIOMECHANICS OF THE SHOULDER COMPLEX

Elsie Culham and Judith Laprade

The shoulder complex consists of the humerus, clavicle, and scapula and the joints that link them into a functional articulated unit. Although glenohumeral stability is provided by the capsular ligamentous structures and the dynamic action of the rotator cuff musculature surrounding the shoulder, the mobility is governed largely by the structure of the shallow glenoid, which affords a large degree of motion. Ultimately, the three bones and four joints of the shoulder complex work interdependently to position the hand in space and allow intricate gross and skilled functions to be performed. The four functional articulations that contribute to this essential joint motion are the scapulothoracic joint, the sternoclavicular joint, the acromioclavicular joint, and the glenohumeral joint. The coracoacromial arch and the head of the humerus compose a fifth functional articulation, which plays an important role in shoulder function and is commonly included in the description of the complex. It is important to understand the structure, mechanics, and function of each component of the complex before the integrated dynamic function of the shoulder complex can be fully appreciated.

STERNOCLAVICULAR JOINT

JOINT STRUCTURE

The sternoclavicular joint is the only articulation connecting the upper limb and the axial skeleton. This is a synovial joint between the inferior portion of the bulbous medial end of the clavicle and the superolateral aspect of the manubrium and the cartilage of the first rib. The articular surfaces are covered with fibrocartilage and are saddle shaped;

the clavicular surface is concave anteroposteriorly and convex cephalocaudally.[1, 2] The superior portion of the medial end of the clavicle extends above the manubrium and forms the border of the sternal notch (Fig. 6–1).

An intraarticular disk runs downward from the nonarticular superomedial aspect of the clavicle to the first costal cartilage near its junction with the sternum. The circumference of the disk is attached to the capsule, completely dividing the joint into two separate cavities.[2] The inferior portion of the disk is thinner than the superior aspect, and its attachment is weaker and easily torn.[1, 3]

The sternoclavicular joint is inherently stable and rarely dislocates. However, the relative contribution of the joint capsule, ligaments, and disk to joint stability has not been extensively studied. The joint is enclosed by the fibrous capsule, which is reinforced on all sides by ligaments. The superior capsule is reinforced by the interclavicular ligament, which connects the clavicles, and ante-

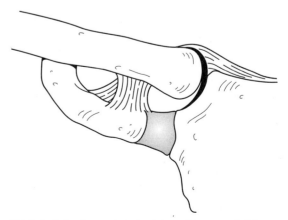

FIGURE 6–1 Sternoclavicular joint and interposed disk.

rior and posterior sternoclavicular ligaments reinforce the anterior and posterior capsule. Bearn[3] determined, based on cadaver experimentation, that stability of the joint is primarily due to the strong joint capsule and supporting ligaments. The posterior superior aspect of the capsule was the thickest portion and was found to be the primary mechanism responsible for maintaining the normal 10-degree upward angulation of the clavicle in the coronal plane. Division of the joint capsule, leaving the disk intact, resulted in depression of the lateral end of the clavicle below that of the medial end.[3] The addition of a load, equivalent to the weight of the arm, to the lateral end of the clavicle resulted in rupture of the inferior attachment of the disk.

The costoclavicular ligament runs superiorly and laterally from the superior surface of the first rib and costal cartilage to the inferior surface of the clavicle. It has two components: an anterior part, which passes upward and laterally, and a posterior part, which runs upward and medially. The ligament strongly binds the medial end of the clavicle to the first rib and prevents medial displacement of the clavicle over the sternum.[4] This ligament also limits elevation and protraction of the clavicle at the sternoclavicular joint during arm elevation.

KINEMATICS

Scapulothoracic motion occurs primarily at the sternoclavicular joint.[5] Although the articular surfaces are saddle shaped, the joint functions as a ball-and-socket joint with 3 degrees of freedom (Fig. 6–2). Movements are limited by ligaments and compression of the joint surfaces.[1] Elevation and depression occur primarily between the medial end of the clavicle and the articular disk. It is estimated that 45 degrees of elevation and 5 degrees of depression occur,[6] the latter movement being limited by the first rib. In the movements of protraction and retraction, the disk and clavicle move as a unit on the sternum. Moseley[6] estimated that 15 degrees of movement occur in each direction, whereas Abbott and Lucas[4] stated that 35 degrees of clavicular protraction occurs at the sternoclavicular joint. The clavicle is also capable of rotating around its long axis, with dorsal axial rotation occurring during the final stages of upper extremity elevation. Abbott and Lucas[4] stated that 50 degrees of rotation are possible; however, Bearn[3] reported 25 degrees of rotation based on cadaver experimentation. Dempster[1] also reported 25 to 30 degrees of axial rotation of the clavicle at the sternoclavicular joint.

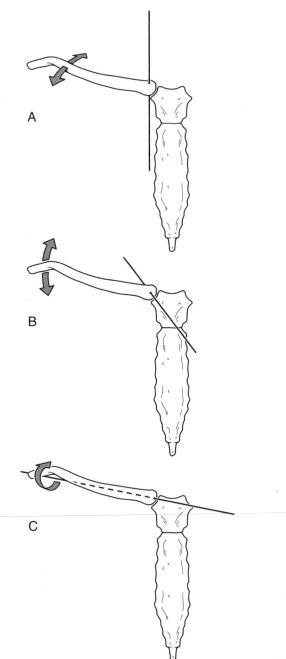

FIGURE 6–2 Kinematics of the sternoclavicular joint. *A,* Anteroposterior rotation around a vertical axis. *B,* Elevation and depression around an anteroposterior axis. *C,* Rotation around the long axis of the clavicle.

ACROMIOCLAVICULAR JOINT

JOINT STRUCTURE

A small oval convex articular facet on the lateral end of the clavicle articulates with a concave facet on the acromion process of the scapula at the acromioclavicular joint.[7] The joint line is oblique, running inferiorly and medially, and the lateral end of the clavicle rises above the acromion. Thus, there is a tendency for the acromion to be driven under the lateral end of the clavicle when forces are applied through the joint. Fibrocartilage covers the joint surfaces,[2] and an intraarticular disk may partially or completely divide the joint cavity into two components.[6]

Stability is provided by superior and inferior acromioclavicular ligaments, which reinforce the joint capsule. The coracoclavicular ligament is a primary stabilizing structure of the joint and the major suspensory ligament of the scapula (Fig. 6–3). This ligament lies medial to the joint and has two distinct portions, often separated by a bursa or fat pad. The trapezoid ligament, the anterolateral component, runs laterally and slightly upward from the superior aspect of the coracoid process to the trapezoid line on the inferior surface of the clavicle.[2] The conoid ligament is posterior and medial to the trapezoid. Its fibers run more vertically from the superior aspect of the coracoid process to the conoid tubercle located on the inferior surface of the clavicle posteriorly.[2]

Fukuda and associates[8] studied the relative contribution of the ligaments to stability of the acromioclavicular joint in cadavers using load-displacement tests combined with sequential sectioning of the ligaments. Experiments involved anterior, posterior, and superior movement of the sternal end of the clavicle on a fixed acromion; anterior, posterior, and superior displacement of the distal clavicle on the acromion; axial rotation of the clavicle around its long axis; and compression and distraction. The acromioclavicular ligament was found to be primarily responsible for resisting posterior displacement of the distal clavicle on the acromion and posterior axial rotation. This ligament was also responsible for restraining superior displacement of the distal clavicle at small loads; the conoid ligament became increasingly important as the load increased. Similarly, anterior displacement was resisted by both the acromioclavicular and conoid ligaments. The conoid ligament provided the most constraint to anterior movement of the sternal end of the clavicle on the acromion, whereas all three ligaments resisted posterior movement. The acromioclavicular and conoid provided resistance to upward rotation of the sternal end of the clavicle, with the conoid assuming a greater role as the load increased. The trapezoid ligament provided significant restraint only to axial compressive loading.

KINEMATICS

The acromioclavicular joint also functions as a ball-and-socket joint and has 3 degrees of freedom (Fig. 6–4). Movements occurring around a vertical axis through the joint result in rotation of the scapula around the lateral end of the clavicle, a motion termed *scapular winging*. If conventional terminology for motion at the glenohumeral joint were applied, as advocated by Dempster,[1] this motion would be equivalent to internal and external rotation. Abbott and Lucas[4] described 15 degrees of motion around a vertical axis. Rotation around a sagittal axis results in upward and downward rotation of the scapula on the distal clavicle, a movement termed *abduction and adduction* using Dempster's terminology. Movement of the scapula around a frontal axis through the acromioclavicular joint causes tipping or tilting of the scapula in the sagittal plane, or flexion and extension of the scapula. The amount of movement in this plane is limited by the contact between the scapula and thorax.

Although significant motion has been described around these axes in the acromioclavicular joint in cadaver experiments, little motion occurs at this joint in vivo.[5, 9] The clinical significance of this is that the acromioclavicular joint, unlike the sternoclavicular joint, can be fused without loss of upper extremity function.[5]

Acromioclavicular joint separations are common, accounting for about 12% of all injuries to the shoulder girdle.[10] They occur most often in young athletic males, with the most common mechanism of injury being a fall in which the adducted shoulder strikes the ground or a firm object.[11] With this type of fall, the scapula is

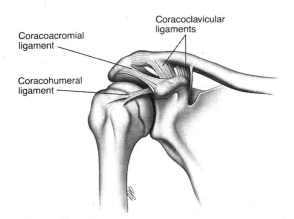

FIGURE 6–3 Ligaments arising from the coracoid process: the acromioclavicular, coracohumeral, and coracoclavicular, a primary stabilizer of the acromioclavicular joint. (From Neer CS II: Shoulder Reconstruction. Philadelphia, WB Saunders, 1990. With permission from Robert Demarest.)

Coracoclavicular ligaments

Coracoacromial ligament

Coracohumeral ligament

driven in an inferior direction relative to the clavicle.[11] Injuries of this type, in which only the acromioclavicular joint ligaments are either sprained or disrupted, are classified as type I and type II injuries, respectively.[10] In type III injuries, both the acromioclavicular and coracoclavicular ligaments are ruptured, and the acromion moves inferiorly in relation to the clavicle. Types IV and V injuries are more severe and result in damage to the trapezius and deltoid muscles.

Types I and II injuries can generally be treated conservatively with a reduction in activity and stabilization with a sling.[12, 13] Treatment of type III injuries is more controversial, but there is some evidence that outcomes are as good or better with conservative versus surgical management.[12, 13] Types IV and V injuries require open reduction and surgical repair with stabilization of the acromioclavicular joint with or without repair of the acromioclavicular and coracoclavicular ligaments.[11] Alternatively, the lateral clavicle is fixed to the coracoid process with screws, wire loops, or other materials.

In rare instances, a force directed to the distal clavicle may drive it inferiorly such that it lodges under the acromion or coracoid process.[11] The acromioclavicular and coracoclavicular ligaments are ruptured in this type of injury.[10] This is classified as a type VI dislocation and requires surgical repair.

SCAPULOTHORACIC COMPLEX

SCAPULAR POSITION

The scapula is a thin, flat triangular bone that lies on the posterolateral aspect of the thorax over ribs two to seven.[14, 15] It has no bony or ligamentous attachment to the axial skeleton, other than through the acromioclavicular and sternoclavicular joints. The axioscapular muscles, including the trapezius, serratus anterior, and rhomboid major and minor, and the levator scapulae play a role in maintaining scapular position.[2] The concave anterior surface of the scapula is separated from the convex external surface of the thorax by the subscapularis and serratus anterior muscles, which glide over one another during movement.

The plane of the scapula is approximately at right angles to the plane of the glenoid,[16] and at rest it lies obliquely, 30 to 45 degrees anterior to the coronal plane.[14, 17, 18] Objective measures of the resting position of the scapula, in the plane of the scapular spine, have been obtained using an electromagnetic system.[19] The scapular spine, represented by a line joining the angle of the acro-

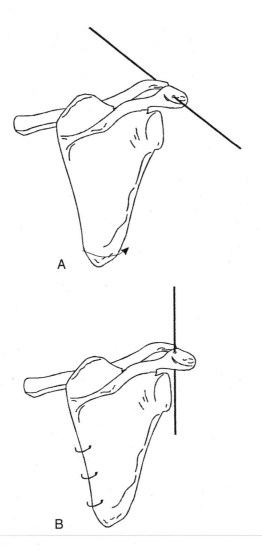

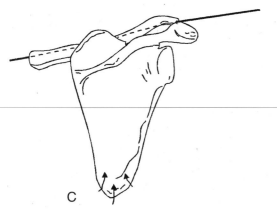

FIGURE 6–4 Kinematics of the acromioclavicular joint. *A,* Rotation around an anteroposterior axis (scapular abduction and adduction). *B,* Rotation around a vertical axis (scapular winging). *C,* Rotation around a mediolateral axis (scapular tilt).

mion and the root, formed a mean angle of 30.2 degrees to the coronal plane in healthy women younger than 40 years of age. The coronal plane was defined as a line connecting the roots of the right and left scapular spines.[19]

The scapula is tilted forward slightly in the sagittal plane.[19, 20] The average angle of forward inclination of the medial border of the scapula was 9.0 degrees in healthy women younger than 40 years of age.[19]

In the coronal plane, the medial border of the scapula is oriented vertically. The mean lateral angle formed between the medial border of the scapula and a horizontal axis was 91.3 degrees in women younger than 40 years of age[19] (Fig. 6–5). Basmajian and Bazant[21] stated that when the scapula is correctly oriented on the thorax, the glenoid fossa faces anteriorly, laterally, and upward. These authors further suggested that the upward orientation of the glenoid fossa provided a "locking mechanism," which prevented downward subluxation of the humeral head on the glenoid. Subsequent radiographic studies, however, have confirmed that in the relaxed standing position, the glenoid fossa has a slight downward inclination in most normal shoulders.[18, 22] Glenoid tilt, the angle of a line connecting the superior and inferior glenoid tubercles relative to the vertical, was measured from radiographs taken in the scapular plane

in standing. The average downward tilt, measured in 52 healthy male subjects, was 5.29 degrees.[22] Similarly, Poppen and Walker[18] reported an average downward tilt of 4.7 degrees.

KINEMATICS

The scapula can rotate and move linearly on the thorax from its resting position. Motions generally do not occur independently of one another, and all motion must occur at the sternoclavicular or acromioclavicular joint or both. Generally, three rotatory motions and two translatory motions of the scapula are described. Upward and downward movements of the scapula on the rib cage are translatory movements termed *elevation* and *depression*. Translation of the scapula toward and away from the vertebral column has been called adduction and abduction, respectively, by some authors.[16]

Rotation of the scapula around a sagittal axis results in upward or downward tilt of the glenoid fossa. This movement has been labeled both abduction or adduction[1] and upward or downward rotation.[16] Full elevation of the upper extremity requires about 60 degrees of scapular rotation in this plane, which results in progressive upward tilt of the glenoid fossa, thus providing a base on which the humeral head moves.[23] From 0 to about 80 degrees of arm elevation, scapular rotation is predominantly a result of elevation of the clavicle at the sternoclavicular joint. The middle phase of arm elevation, described by Bagg and Forrest,[23] occurs between 80 and 140 degrees of total arm elevation. This is described as the most stressful phase of arm elevation and is the phase when most scapular rotation occurs.[20, 23] The scapular rotation is due to continued elevation of the clavicle at the sternoclavicular joint and limited rotation of the scapula on the clavicle at the acromioclavicular joint.[23]

In the final phase of arm elevation in the scapular plane, clavicular elevation becomes increasingly limited by tension in the costoclavicular ligament[16, 24] as the powerful scapular muscles continue to rotate the scapula upward. The amount of movement of the scapula on the clavicle at the acromioclavicular joint is limited by the coracoclavicular ligament.[25] The tension generated in this ligament, as the coracoid process moves away from the clavicle, causes a dorsal rotation of the clavicle around its long axis.[4, 24, 26, 27] Because the clavicle is crank shaped, this long axis rotation causes the acromial end of the clavicle to elevate further, carrying the scapula with it.[24, 26, 28] According to Neer,[29] rupture of the coracoclavicular ligaments in acromioclavicular separation injuries

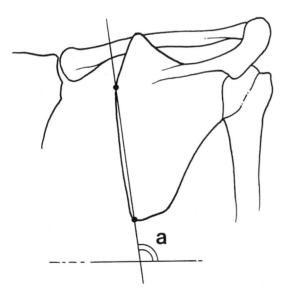

FIGURE 6–5 Scapular position in the plane of the scapula. The mean angle between the medial border of the scapula and the horizontal (a) was 91.3 degrees in women younger than the age of 40 years (n = 34). (From Culham E, Peat M: Functional anatomy of the shoulder compex. J Orthop Sports Phys Ther 18:342, 1993, with permission of the Orthopaedic and Sports Sections of the American Physical Therapy Association.)

can disrupt this mechanism. If these ligaments are not intact, the scapula may not rotate sufficiently during arm elevation, resulting in impingement of the greater tuberosity against the acromion process. van der Helm[30] postulated that absence of the conoid ligament would lead to increased torsional stress in the acromioclavicular joint and potentially to joint damage.

The instant center of rotation of the scapula (ICR) varies throughout arm elevation, its position indicating where the motion is primarily occurring. Based on radiographic evidence, Dvir and Berme[24] reported that the ICR was near the root of the scapular spine during the first 90 to 100 degrees of arm elevation, and at the acromioclavicular joint during the final phase of elevation. Similarly, Bagg and Forrest[23] found the ICR of the scapula to be at or near the root of the scapular spine during the first 80 degrees of arm elevation. Thereafter, the ICR moved along the scapular spine toward the acromioclavicular joint as the arm was elevated between 80 and 140 degrees, and reached the acromioclavicular joint in the final phases of elevation. Poppen and Walker[18] reported a somewhat different pattern of movement of the ICR. In this study, the ICR was found to be initially located near the center of the scapula, moving superiorly and medially during the first 60 degrees of arm elevation and thereafter moving superiorly and laterally toward the acromioclavicular joint.

Rotation of the scapula in other planes has been less extensively studied. Poppen and Walker[18] described rotation of the scapula around a coronal axis during arm elevation in the scapular plane that resulted in movement of the superior angle of the scapula away from the body wall. Forty degrees of motion were measured from radiographs during arm elevation.[18] van der Helm[30] also described upward and posterior movement of the clavicle and ventral movement of the inferior angle of the scapula during coronal plane abduction in a finite element model. This movement is generally described as scapular *tipping* or *tilting*.

Protraction and retraction occur around a vertical axis. *Protraction*, defined as forward movement of the scapula around the thoracic wall, combines linear translation away from the vertebral column, rotation of the scapula around the end of the clavicle (winging), and anterior movement of the lateral end of clavicle.[2] The reverse of these combined motions results in scapular retraction. Abbott and Lucus[4] describe 50 degrees of scapular protraction, 35 degrees due to anterior movement of the clavicle at the sternoclavicular joint and 15 degrees due to scapular rotation on the clavicle at the acromioclavicular joint.

KINETICS OF SCAPULAR MOTION

Axioscapular Musculature

Trapezius and Serratus Anterior Muscles

Upward rotation of the scapula during arm elevation is brought about by the upper and lower portions of trapezius combined with the serratus anterior muscle, particularly the powerful lower digitations.[23, 31, 32] These muscles constitute the scapular force couple (Fig. 6–6). The upper trapezius, forming the superior component of the force couple, has a supportive as well as a rotatory function. The lower fibers of trapezius and lower digitations of serratus form the inferior component. The serratus anterior, owing to its large moment arm, is capable of producing large moments around the sternoclavicular joint and is considered the most important component of the force couple.[30]

Electromyographic (EMG) activity has been monitored in these muscles during elevation in both the coronal and sagittal planes.[27, 33, 34] Both trapezius and serratus anterior are active throughout arm elevation in both planes, reaching peak activity at maximal elevation. Upper trapezius has

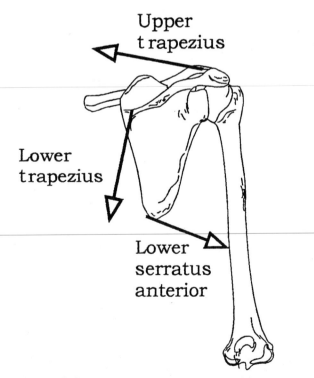

FIGURE 6–6 Scapular force couple consisting of the upper and lower trapezius and the lower serratus anterior muscles.

been found to be more active in coronal plane abduction than in sagittal plane elevation[35] and was reported to be particularly active in the first 60 degrees of coronal plane abduction. This component of the force couple has a large moment arm around a sagittal axis through the sternoclavicular joint during this phase of coronal plane elevation.[30] Lower trapezius was found to be the more active during abduction than during flexion, whereas serratus anterior is more active during sagittal plane flexion.[27, 30, 33] It was proposed that the decrease in lower trapezius activity during flexion allowed the scapular protraction needed for elevation in this plane. Both Inman and colleagues[27] and Weidenbauer and Mortenson[33] reported that the lower trapezius was most active during the latter stages of elevation in both planes. Similarly, van der Helm[30] reported minimal activity in lower trapezius below 90 degrees of elevation in the coronal plane.

Bagg and Forrest[31] studied EMG activity of the scapular rotators during elevation in the scapular plane. The upper trapezius and lower serratus anterior were active throughout arm elevation, with activity gradually increasing, particularly in the upper ranges of elevation. Little activity was observed in the lower trapezius until after 90 degrees of elevation, with a sharp rise in activity thereafter. These authors proposed that migration of the ICR of the scapula toward the acromioclavicular joint during the middle phase of elevation would result in an increase in the moment arm of lower trapezius, thus improving its mechanical advantage. The lower trapezius is therefore better able to

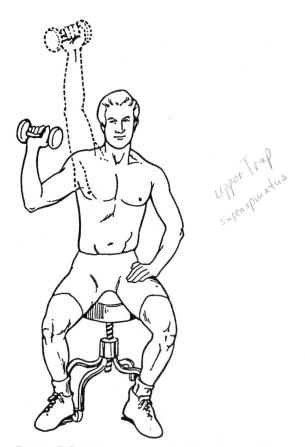

FIGURE 6–8   Military press exercise. (From Townsend H, Jobe F, Pink M, Perry J: Electromyographic analysis of the glenohumeral muscles during a baseball rehabilitation program. Am J Sports Med 19:264, 1991.)

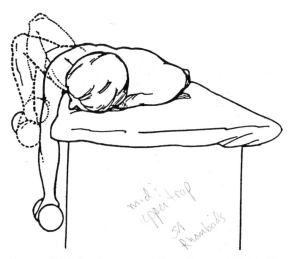

FIGURE 6–7   Rowing exercise. (From Townsend H, Jobe F, Pink M, Perry J: Electromyographic analysis of the glenohumeral muscles during a baseball rehabilitation program. Am J Sports Med 19:264, 1991.)

assist upper trapezius and serratus anterior during the phase when the most scapular rotation is occurring.

Activity in these muscles has also been studied in healthy subjects performing rehabilitation exercises to determine which exercises most effectively recruited these muscles.[34] Rowing (Fig. 6–7) and the military press (Fig. 6–8) best recruited the upper trapezius. Coronal plane abduction, rowing, horizontal abduction in prone with the humerus in a neutral or external rotation (Fig. 6–9), and sagittal plane flexion all resulted in significant activity in the lower trapezius. All exercises were done with a light weight in the hand. High levels of activity occurred in the middle and lower fibers of serratus anterior during elevation of the arm in the sagittal, coronal, and scapular planes. The press-up (Fig. 6–10) and the push-up exercises (Fig. 6–11) also resulted in high levels of activity in this muscle.

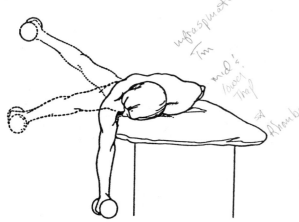

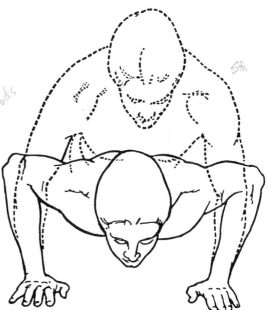

FIGURE 6–9 Horizontal abduction exercise with the arm in internal rotation. The same exercise was performed with the arm in neutral and external rotation. (From Townsend H, Jobe F, Pink M, Perry J: Electromyographic analysis of the glenohumeral muscles during a baseball rehabilitation program. Am J Sports Med 19:264, 1991.)

FIGURE 6–11 Push-up exercise. (From Townsend H, Jobe F, Pink M, Perry J: Electromyographic analysis of the glenohumeral muscles during a baseball rehabilitation program. Am J Sports Med 19:264, 1991.)

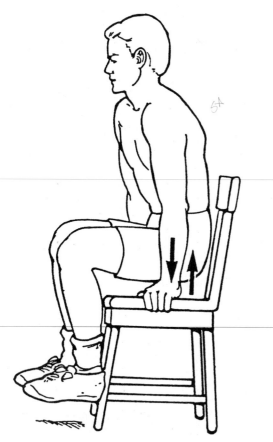

FIGURE 6–10 Press-up exercise. (From Townsend H, Jobe F, Pink M, Perry J: Electromyographic analysis of the glenohumeral muscles during a baseball rehabilitation program. Am J Sports Med 19:264, 1991.)

Middle Trapezius and Rhomboid Muscles

EMG studies demonstrate that the middle trapezius is active throughout elevation of the upper extremity in both the coronal[27] and scapular planes.[31] Peak activity during coronal plane abduction occurred at 90 degrees of elevation, with activity reaching a plateau or decreasing slightly beyond that level.[27] Conversely, during scapular plane abduction, low levels of activity were reported below 90 degrees; the activity level increased beyond 90 degrees and peaked at maximum elevation.[31] Much lower levels of middle trapezius activity were recorded during elevation of the upper extremity in the sagittal plane.[27, 30] Inman and colleagues[27] suggested that the middle trapezius functions to stabilize the scapula during coronal plane abduction. Activity must be reduced during sagittal plane elevation to allow protraction of the scapula around the thorax.[27]

The rhomboids, like the middle trapezius, are most active during coronal plane abduction, with lower levels of activity during sagittal plane flexion.[27, 30] van der Helm[30] stated that during elevation in the coronal plane, rhomboid activity acts to counterbalance activity in the upper serratus anterior, with both muscles acting to stabilize the root of the scapular spine on the thorax. In both the coronal and sagittal planes, peak activity occurred at the end of range.[27]

In the study of rehabilitation exercises conducted by Moseley and coauthors,[34] horizontal abduction with the humerus in neutral rotation (see Fig. 6–9) resulted in high levels of activity in both the rhomboid and middle trapezius muscles. High levels of activity were also found in the middle trapezius during humeral extension in prone position (Fig. 6–12) and during rowing exercise (see Fig. 6–7). Rhomboids were recruited during elevation in the coronal and scapular planes (light weight in hand) and during the rowing exercise.

GLENOHUMERAL JOINT

ARTICULAR SURFACES

The glenohumeral joint is a synovial, multiaxial ball-and-socket joint between the head of the humerus and glenoid cavity of the scapula. The head of the humerus is much larger than the glenoid cavity, and thus only a portion of the head articulates with the fossa in any position of the joint. The glenohumeral index, calculated by dividing the maximal transverse diameter of the glenoid by the maximal transverse diameter of the humeral head, was found to average 57.5 in 50 normal shoulders.[36] Lower values of this index have been reported in shoulders with recurrent anterior dislocation; however, the difference was due to erosion of the anterior glenoid margin and labrum resulting from recurrent trauma rather than to developmental dysplasia of the glenoid fossa.[36, 37]

The humeral head forms a portion of a sphere, with deviations from sphericity of less than 1% of the radius.[38] The head faces medially, superiorly, and posteriorly with respect to the shaft of the bone.[15, 16] The angle of inclination, the angle between an axis through the humeral neck and head

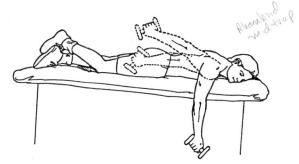

FIGURE 6–12   Humeral extension in prone lying. (From Townsend H, Jobe F, Pink M, Perry J: Electromyographic analysis of the glenohumeral muscles during a baseball rehabilitation program. Am J Sports Med 19:264, 1991.)

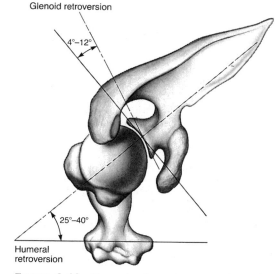

FIGURE 6–13   Humeral and scapular retrotorsion angles. (From Neer CS II: Shoulder Reconstruction. Philadelphia, WB Saunders, 1990. With permission from Robert Demarest.)

and the humeral shaft in the frontal plane, varies from 130 to 150 degrees.[14] In the transverse plane, the humeral head and neck are rotated posteriorly 25 to 40 degrees with respect to an axis through the humeral epicondyles[36, 37] (Fig. 6–13). This is called the *angle of torsion* or *retrotorsion*.[37] It has been suggested that a high retrotorsion angle may contribute to recurrent anterior dislocation.[39] Retrotorsion angle, however, measured radiographically and with computed tomography, did not differ in shoulders with anterior instability compared with normal shoulders.[36, 37]

The glenoid fossa has been described as pear shaped.[40] The superoinferior dimensions of the glenoid fossa averaged 39 mm in 140 cadaver shoulders.[40] The average anteroposterior dimension of the lower portion of the glenoid was 29 mm.[40] The articular cartilage of the glenoid is thicker peripherally than centrally, whereas the cartilage on the humeral head is slightly thicker centrally.[38] Soslowsky and colleagues[38] reported that the glenoid fossa with articular cartilage formed a portion of a sphere with a radius of curvature within 3 mm of that of the corresponding humeral head. Thus, although the bone surface of the glenoid is flatter than that of the corresponding humeral head, the cartilage surface is not, and the mating surfaces of the humeral head and glenoid are more congruent than the bony architecture alone would indicate.[38]

Several studies have confirmed that the glenoid fossa is retrotilted with respect to the plane of the scapula in most normal shoulders[36, 37, 39] (see Fig.

6–13). Saha reported an average of 7.4 degrees of retrotilt of the fossa in relation to the plane of the scapula.[39, 41] This author[39] also suggested that a ventral tilt or anteversion of the glenoid was associated with anterior instability of the joint. However, no cases of anteversion were found in either stable or unstable shoulders at any level of the glenoid in a computed tomography study by Randelli and Gambrioli.[36] Brewer and associates[42] found that excessive retroversion was the primary cause associated with nontraumatic posterior instability of the shoulder.

GLENOID LABRUM

The glenoid labrum is a rim of fibrous tissue attached around the margin of the glenoid fossa. Its inner surface is covered with synovium; the outer surface is continuous with the periosteum of the scapular neck.[28] It is a flexible structure, allowing adaptation of its shape to accommodate rotation of the humeral head. Cooper and coauthors,[43] in an anatomic and histologic study, found that the labrum consisted of primarily fibrous tissue, confirming findings of an earlier study by Moseley and Övergaard.[44] Fibrocartilage bridged the region between hyaline articular cartilage and the fibrous labrum.[43] Differences were identified in the superior and inferior aspects of the labrum. The superior and superoanterior labrum was loosely attached to the glenoid rim by thin elastic connective tissue. The most superior portion inserted into the biceps tendon distal to its insertion onto the supraglenoid tubercle. The inferior portion of the labrum consisted of inelastic fibrous tissue, which was firmly attached to the glenoid margin, resembling an extension of the articular cartilage.[43]

It is generally accepted that the glenoid labrum deepens the glenoid cavity.[7, 45, 46] This hypothesis was supported by a study of 25 cadaver shoulders in which the labrum was found to contribute about half of the total depth of the fossa.[47] The labrum and glenoid margin combined to create a socket that was 9 mm deep on average in a superoinferior direction and 5 mm deep in an anteroposterior direction.[47] Lippitt and Matsen[48] reported lower values of 4.9 mm on average in the superoinferior plane and 2.2 mm in an anteroposterior direction. These authors also investigated the ability of the glenoid concavity to resist translatory forces applied to the humeral head in a cadaver study.[48] Compressive forces were applied to the humeral head, followed by increasing tangential forces, until the humeral head dislocated over the glenoid rim. Average maximal translatory forces that could be resisted in the superoinferior direction were twice that resisted in an anteroposterior direction. The degree of stability was related to the depth of the concavity and to the degree of compression between the humeral head and the glenoid. Removal of the labrum resulted in a 20% reduction in the resistance to translatory forces in both directions.[48]

Dislocation of the glenohumeral joint most commonly occurs in an anterior direction.[49] The most common position of dislocation is with the humerus in maximal external rotation with the arm in an overhead position. Acute dislocation results in avulsion of the anterior labrum and joint capsule from the rim of the glenoid (Bankart lesion) and, less commonly, in a fracture of the anterior rim of the glenoid.[49]

JOINT CAPSULE

The fibrous capsule originates from the labrum and from the margin of the glenoid fossa beyond the labrum. Laterally, it is attached to the circumference of the anatomic neck of the humerus. Inferiorly and medially, the attachment descends about ½ inch onto the shaft of the humerus.[2] The capsule forms a continuous structure connecting the two bones, except in the area of the biceps groove, where the biceps tendon exits the joint.[50] If the capsule is intact, little distraction of the joint surfaces is possible because of the negative intraarticular pressure within the joint.[50] Up to 2 cm of distraction could be obtained when the capsule of cadaver shoulders was opened or vented.[50] Similarly, puncture of the capsule in cadaver shoulders was found to result in significant subluxation of the humeral head[51] and increased anteroposterior translation of the humeral head on the glenoid during movement of the arm, emphasizing the importance of negative intraarticular pressure to joint stability.[52]

The anterior, superior, and posterior aspects of the capsule are reinforced by the tendons of the rotator cuff. Fibers of these tendons insert into the capsule, and separation of the tendons from the capsule is difficult.[53] It has been suggested that this tendinous insertion into capsule helps in retracting redundant portions of capsule during arm movements.[50] There is no reinforcement by the musculotendinous cuff in the interval between the anterior border of supraspinatus tendon and the superior border of the subscapularis tendon.[53] This triangular space, with the coracoid process forming the base, is called the *rotator interval*.[54] The capsule was found to be thickest in this region in a histologic study by Clark and associates.[50]

The inferior capsule is lax when the arm is adducted. Although this portion of the capsule is not crossed by tendons, Clark and associates[50] found that fibers of subscapularis and teres minor muscles inserted into the anterior and posterior aspects of the inferior capsule. A muscular portion of the long head of the triceps was also found to arise from the medial side of the inferior capsule.[50] In mechanical stress tests of glenohumeral joint capsule, Kaltsas[55] found the anteroinferior capsule to be the weakest area of capsule because this was the first region to rupture.

LIGAMENTS

Coracohumeral and Superior Glenohumeral Ligaments

The coracohumeral and superior glenohumeral ligaments reinforce the joint capsule in the rotator interval[56] (Fig. 6–14). The coracohumeral ligament has a broad origin from the lateral aspect of the base of the coracoid process[54, 57] (see Fig. 6–3). It runs obliquely downward and laterally. Ferrari[58] stated that the ligament divides into two components, which insert into the greater and lesser tuberosities, thus creating a tunnel through which

the biceps tendon passes.[58] Others describe insertion of the ligament into the capsule in the rotator interval and into supraspinatus and subscapularis tendons.[50, 57] Neer and colleagues[57] found that in most of the cadaver shoulders studied, the ligament did not have a distinct insertion into bone. Cooper and coauthors[53] stated that the coracohumeral ligament is a fold of anterior superior capsule that is more prominent when the humeral head is translated inferiorly and much less distinct with superior translation of the humeral head.

The smaller superior glenohumeral ligament originates from the base of the coracoid process and labrum adjacent to the supraglenoid tubercle and inserts into the humerus just above the lesser tuberosity. Although the ligament is readily identified in most shoulders,[58–60] its size is variable.[58, 60]

Cadaver studies indicate that the structures in the rotator interval limit inferior translation of the humeral head on the glenoid fossa in the adducted arm.[54, 56, 58] Bowen and Warren,[61] based on selective cutting and static translation experimentation in cadavers, concluded that the superior glenohumeral ligament was the primary restraint to inferior translation and that the coracohumeral liga-

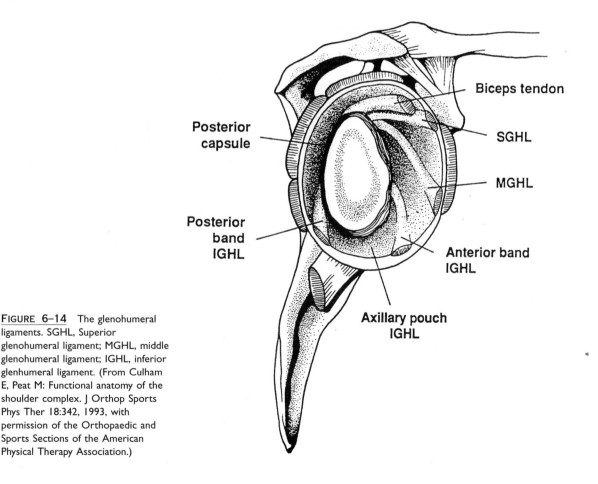

FIGURE 6–14 The glenohumeral ligaments. SGHL, Superior glenohumeral ligament; MGHL, middle glenohumeral ligament; IGHL, inferior glenhumeral ligament. (From Culham E, Peat M: Functional anatomy of the shoulder complex. J Orthop Sports Phys Ther 18:342, 1993, with permission of the Orthopaedic and Sports Sections of the American Physical Therapy Association.)

Posterior capsule

Posterior band IGHL

Biceps tendon

SGHL

MGHL

Anterior band IGHL

Axillary pouch IGHL

ment played little or no role. Conversely, Ferrari[58] and Nobuhara and Ikeda[56] found that the coracohumeral ligament was a major restraint to inferior translation.[56, 58]

Insufficiency of the rotator interval structures also leads to anteroposterior instability of the glenohumeral joint. Cadaver studies have demonstrated that the capsule and ligaments in the rotator interval must be sectioned, along with the posterior capsule, to produce posterior dislocation of the adducted arm.[62, 63] The coracohumeral ligament also functions to limit external rotation of the adducted humerus[57] as well as external rotation between 0 and 60 degrees of arm elevation and therefore is important in providing anterior stability during this phase of arm elevation.[58]

Middle Glenohumeral Ligament

The middle glenohumeral ligament is the most variable of the glenohumeral ligaments (see Fig. 6–14). O'Brien and associates[60] reported that it was deficient or absent in 4 of the 11 shoulders examined. It arises from the anterosuperior aspect of the labrum and margin of the glenoid fossa inferior to the superior glenohumeral ligament. The ligament passes laterally and inserts into the anterior aspect of the anatomic neck and lesser tuberosity of the humerus. It lies under the tendon of the subscapularis muscle and is intimately attached to it near its insertion into the lesser tuberosity.[58, 64] The middle and superior glenohumeral ligaments are separated by the subscapularis bursa.[58]

The middle glenohumeral ligament and subscapularis tendon contribute to anterior stability of the glenohumeral joint in the lower to middle ranges of abduction.[58, 59, 63, 65,58] Based on anatomic dissections of 100 cadaver shoulders, Ferrari[58] found that the middle glenohumeral ligament was a major anterior stabilizer between 60 and 90 degrees of elevation. Attenuation or absence of this ligament could lead to anterior instability in this part of the range.

Inferior Glenohumeral Ligament

The inferior glenohumeral ligament is crucial to shoulder stability, particularly in the upper ranges of elevation.[60, 66] The ligament attaches to the anterior, inferior, and posterior margins of the glenoid labrum and neck. It inserts into the neck of the humerus just below the articular margin.[59] Turkel and coauthors[59] described a thickened anterosuperior portion of the ligament, which they called the *superior band* (see Fig. 6–14). The remaining inferoposterior part of the ligament was termed

the *axillary pouch*. More recently, O'Brien and associates[60] described a thickened posterior band in addition to the anterior band and axillary pouch. Histologically, the anterior and posterior bands consisted of organized bundles of collagen fibers oriented in the coronal plane. The axillary pouch was thicker in comparison, but the collagen fibers were less organized.

All three components of the inferior glenohumeral ligament are important to joint stability. The anterior or superior band and axillary pouch tighten with elevation and external rotation, providing a broad buttress-like support for the anterior and inferior aspects of the joint in the middle and upper ranges of abduction.[59, 60] Deficiency in this part of the ligament may result in anterior subluxation and dislocation in this part of the range. Similarly, the posterior band and axillary pouch provide support for the humeral head posteriorly when the abducted arm is internally rotated.[60]

CORACOACROMIAL ARCH

The coracoacromial arch is formed by the acromion process, the coracoid process, and the coracoacromial ligament, the triangular ligament that runs upward, laterally, and slightly posteriorly from the coracoid to the acromion process[2, 67] (see Fig. 6–3). Together, these structures form an important protective arch over the glenohumeral joint and provide a secondary restraining socket for the humeral head, preventing upward dislocation. The space between the arch and the proximal humerus is called the *subacromial space* or the *supraspinatus outlet* (Fig. 6–15). This space is occupied by the supraspinatus tendon, the tendon of the long head of biceps, and the subacromial bursa.

One of the most common causes of chronic shoulder pain is impingement of the structures within the subacromial space in people with frequent overhead use of the upper extremity. The supraspinatus tendon and the tendon of the long head of the biceps are the structures most commonly affected. Neer[68] described three progressive phases of impingement: stage I, edema and hemorrhage; stage II, thickening and fibrosis of the bursa and tendinitis of the cuff; and stage III, rotator cuff tears, biceps rupture, and bone changes.

Neer[68] recognized that impingement occurred against the anterior edge and undersurface of the anterior third of the acromion and under the acromioclavicular joint, rather than under the lateral acromion as previously thought (Fig. 6–16). Most upper extremity functional activities occur with the arm in or anterior to the scapular plane. When elevation occurs in these planes, the supra-

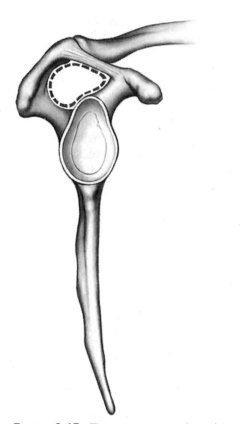

FIGURE 6-15 The supraspinatus outlet is the space beneath the anterior acromion, coracoclavicular ligament, and acromioclavicular joint. Narrowing of this space is the most common cause of impingement syndrome. (From Neer CS II: Shoulder Reconstruction. Philadelphia, WB Saunders, 1990. With permission from Robert Demarest.)

spinatus and biceps tendons pass under the anterior acromion, the acromioclavicular joint, and the coracoclavicular ligament.

Impingements have been classified as either outlet or nonoutlet in type. Outlet impingements are by far the more common and are a consequence of factors that result in a narrowing of the supraspinatus outlet. Variations in the shape and slope of the acromion, anterior acromial spurs, and a prominent acromioclavicular joint all can contribute to outlet impingement.[29] Three distinct acromial shapes were identified by Bigliani and associates[69, 70] in both cadaver and in vivo studies (Fig. 6–17). A type I or flat acromion was identified in 18% of 200 patients studied, a type II or curved acromion was found in 41%, and a type III or hooked acromion was identified in 41%.[69] A similar distribution was found in 140 cadaver shoulders. A type III acromion was more commonly associated with rotator cuff tears in both cadaver and living subjects. Of 35 patients who

underwent surgical repair of rotator cuff tears, 70% had a type III acromial shape.[69]

The slope of the acromion has also been implicated in outlet impingement syndrome.[29, 71] Anterior acromial spurs and a narrower supraspinatus outlet were associated with a flatter acromial slope[71] (Fig. 6–18).

Anterior acromial spurs at the attachment of the coracoacromial ligament can also narrow the supraspinatus outlet. These spurs may be due to chronic impact of the humerus on the ligament, resulting in development of a traction spur on the acromion. A prominent acromioclavicular joint or osteophytes on the undersurface the acromioclavicular joint also lead to narrowing of the outlet and can contribute to impingement.[29]

OSTEOKINEMATICS

The glenohumeral joint is a ball-and-socket synovial joint with 3 degrees of freedom. Much of the early research investigated glenohumeral motion in the anatomic planes of the body or, in other words, described humeral movement relative to the trunk rather than to the scapula. Internal and external rotation occur in the transverse plane, and the range available is dependent on the degree of elevation of the arm. Flexion and extension occur in the sagittal plane, and flexion is accompanied by some medial rotation.[72, 73] According to Gagey

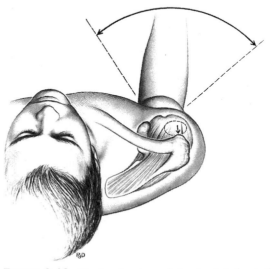

Arc of elevation

FIGURE 6-16 The functional arc of elevation is in front of, rather than lateral to, the body, and impingement occurs more commonly against the anterior one third of the acromion and undersurface of the acromioclavicular joint. (From Neer CS II: Shoulder Reconstruction. Philadelphia, WB Saunders, 1990.)

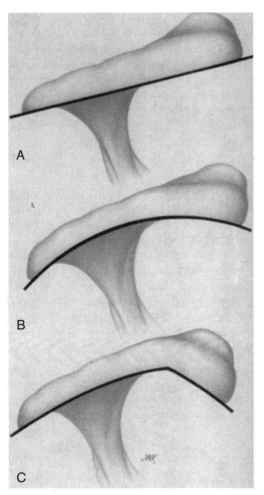

and 120 degrees when the humerus is allowed to externally rotate.[14, 45, 75]

It has long been recognized that the final humeral position is the same, regardless of the plane of elevation. The humeral epicondyle faces forward, and the humerus is in the plane of the scapula.[73, 76] This is the position of maximal osseoligamentous stability and greatest congruency between the articular surfaces. Little or no active rotation is possible with the humerus in this close-packed position.

Elevation of the humerus occurs naturally in the plane of the scapula (30 to 40 degrees anterior to the coronal plane) (Fig. 6–19). Johnston[73] argued that humeral motion should be described relative to the scapula rather than to the trunk, and the terms *scapular plane abduction* and *true abduction* were adopted to describe elevation in this plane. True flexion and extension occur in a plane at right angles to the plane of the scapula.

In scapular plane abduction, the deltoid and supraspinatus muscles are optimally aligned to abduct the humerus,[18, 73] and the glenohumeral joint capsule is not twisted. Little or no rotation of the humerus is required when elevation occurs in this plane. In the final stages of elevation in either the coronal or sagittal plane, increasing tension in components of the capsule and ligamentous complex occurs, necessitating movement of the humerus into the scapular plane to achieve full

FIGURE 6–17   Three distinct acromion shapes, flat *(A)*, curved *(B)*, and hooked *(C)*, as described by Bigliani and colleagues.[69, 70] (From Ticker JB, Bigliani LU: Impingement pathology of the rotator cuff. *In* Andrews JR, Wilk KE [eds]: The Athletic Shoulder. New York, Churchill Livingstone, 1994, p 124.)

and colleagues,[74] the medial rotation occurs because of increasing tension in the coracohumeral ligament as the humerus elevates in this plane. Abduction occurs in the coronal plane, and it is generally accepted that this movement must be accompanied by external rotation of the humerus. This external rotation was thought to be necessary for the greater tuberosity to pass under the acromion. More recent research suggests that the external rotation occurs because of increasing tension in the inferior capsule and glenohumeral ligament. Tension in this ligament limits coronal plane abduction to 60 to 90 degrees when the humerus is maintained in internal rotation during elevation in this plane.[45, 74, 75] The range of coronal plane abduction range increases to between 90

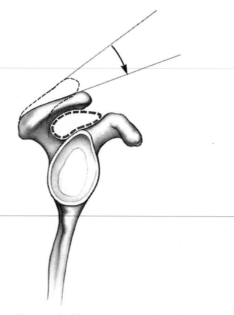

FIGURE 6–18   A flat acromial angle may result in a narrower supraspinatus outlet and cause impingement syndrome. (From Neer CS II: Shoulder Reconstruction. Philadelphia, WB Saunders, 1990. With permission from Robert Demarest.)

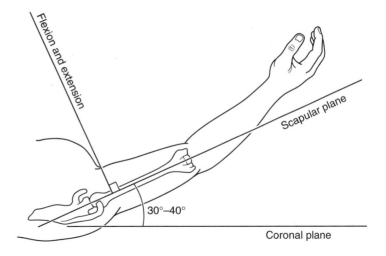

FIGURE 6–19 The arm is naturally elevated in the plane of the scapula rather than in the sagittal or coronal plane of the body. The capsule is not twisted when elevation occurs in this plane, and external humeral rotation is not needed for the greater tuberosity to clear the acromion. Flexion and extension occur in a plane at right angles to the scapular plane.

elevation. The range of elevation possible in the glenohumeral joint during scapular plane elevation varies from 100 to 115 degrees.[20, 22, 23]

ARTHROKINEMATICS

Translatory motion of the humeral head on the glenoid during upper extremity motion has been studied by several researchers.[18, 52, 77] Poppen and Walker[18] measured humeral translation on the glenoid in a radiographic study of 12 healthy subjects and 15 patients with abnormalities of the shoulder. During the first 30 to 60 degrees of arm elevation in the scapular plane, the humeral head moved upward on the glenoid about 3 mm in the healthy subjects. The authors hypothesized that this upward motion during early elevation served to correct the initial depression of the head in the dependent position. Through the remainder of elevation range, the humeral head was relatively centered on the glenoid, moving upward or downward an average of 1.09 mm. Excessive upward translation occurred in 7 subjects who had experienced a previous dislocation, had a rotator cuff tear, or had shoulder pain associated with previous trauma.

Howell and colleagues[77] studied glenohumeral mechanics during movement in the horizontal plane in 20 healthy subjects and 12 patients who had anterior instability. Measurements were made from radiographs taken with the subject in supine-lying position with the arm in varying positions of horizontal abduction and external rotation. In the healthy subjects, the humeral head remained centered on the glenoid during all horizontal plane movement, except when the arm was in maximal extension and external rotation (cocking phase of pitching). Movement into this position was accompanied by a 4-mm posterior translation of the humeral head on the glenoid. The head recentered

on the glenoid with movement into either flexion or internal rotation from this position. The maximal extension and external rotation range was less in subjects with anterior instability, and the posterior translation of the humeral head did not occur. Seven of the 12 subjects with instability demonstrated anterior translation of the head on the glenoid during maximal horizontal abduction without rotation and in submaximal abduction with full external rotation.

Similarly, Harryman and associates[52] reported posterior translation of the humeral head on the glenoid with extension and lateral rotation and anterior translation with flexion and medial rotation of the glenohumeral joint in a cadaver study. The degree of anterior translation on flexion increased after operative tightening of the posterior capsule.

These studies[52, 77] suggest that translation of the humeral head on the glenoid is related to tightening of the joint capsule as movement approaches the end of range of motion. Harryman and co-workers[52] suggested that as the capsule becomes taut, it forces the humeral head to translate in the direction of humeral movement. A taut anterior capsule in abduction and external rotation thus forces the humeral head to translate posteriorly on the glenoid. That posterior translation did not occur in subjects with anterior capsular laxity lends support to this hypothesis.

The data presented in these studies appear to contradict the translation or glide predicted by the concave–convex rule, which states that when a convex surface moves on a concave surface, the direction of the glide that accompanies the roll must be in the opposite direction to the roll. Accordingly, the humeral head should slide inferiorly during abduction, anteriorly during external rotation, and posteriorly during internal rotation. The research suggests that the direction of the glide is dictated by tautness in the capsule, at least as end range is approached. The direction of mobilization for stiffness may need to be reconsidered in view of these findings.

Excessive translation of the humeral head on the glenoid in patients with glenohumeral instability can lead to secondary impingement syndrome. Laxity of the static stabilizers (capsule and ligaments) is common in people who perform activities requiring repetitive overhead motion, as a result of the repetitive physical demands placed on the shoulder. This laxity can result in superior translation of the humeral head and impingement of the tendons of the cuff and biceps under the coracoacromial arch. Muscular fatigue of the humeral head depressors is also postulated to contribute to an increase in superior humeral head translation and impingement syndrome in swimmers.[78]

KINETICS

Scapulohumeral Musculature

Deltoid and Supraspinatus

The deltoid and supraspinatus muscles are generally considered the prime movers of humeral elevation regardless of the plane in which elevation occurs.[79–82] Inman and coauthors[27] demonstrated that both muscles are active throughout the range of elevation in both the coronal and sagittal planes. Deltoid activity increased throughout elevation to about 100 degrees of elevation and plateaued. The level of activity was greater when movement was performed in the coronal plane. Similarly, Scheving and Pauly[83] demonstrated that all three components of the deltoid were active during coronal and sagittal plane elevation, with the greatest amplitude occurring for the component of the muscle actually producing the motion (anterior deltoid in flexion and middle deltoid in abduction). It was hypothesized that simultaneous contraction of the other components assisted in stabilization of the humeral head on the glenoid fossa. McCann and colleagues[84] also reported posterior deltoid activity during elevation in the coronal plane but no contribution from this component during elevation in the scapular plane. Activity in both the middle deltoid and supraspinatus was considerably reduced when scapular plane elevation was performed with the elbow flexed rather than extended, and this exercise was recommended during the early postoperative period after total shoulder arthroplasty to reduce stress on healing tissues.[84]

Inman and coauthors[27] found that supraspinatus EMG activity increased during elevation in both planes, reaching a peak between 80 and 100 degrees. Activity decreased beyond this point in the range. Saha[39] reported a similar pattern of supraspinatus activity during elevation in the coronal plane. Peak activity occurred sooner when elevation was performed in the sagittal plane.[27]

The deltoid has the largest cross-sectional area of the scapulohumeral muscles and also has a greater moment arm than the supraspinatus. Thus, the deltoid exerts the largest moments around the glenohumeral joint and is more effective in elevation.[30] Wuelker and associates[85] demonstrated greater effectiveness of the deltoid in arm elevation in cadaver experimentation. The supraspinatus produced less rotational torque but high compression forces, necessary for stabilization of the humeral head on the glenoid.[85] van der Helm[30] also stated that the moments and forces exerted by the supraspinatus are small because of the small cross-sectional area and small moment arm and concluded that the supraspinatus contributed little to the abductor moment when elevation occurred in the coronal plane. Conflicting information was reported by Howel and colleagues.[81] In vivo studies of paralysis of either the suprascapular or axillary nerves resulted in a 50% reduction in torque produced during elevation in the scapular plane and sagittal plane flexion. The authors concluded that the deltoid and supraspinatus were responsible for 100% of the torque production in these planes of motion and that the supraspinatus and deltoid contributed equally to torque production.[81] The infraspinatus was not considered to have a role in abduction. Otis and associates,[86] however, concluded that the infraspinatus can contribute to abduction of the arm in the scapular plane based on the results of measures of moment arm length in cadavers. Similarly, van der Helm[30] reported that the infraspinatus could contribute to elevation in the sagittal plane and to the first 60 degrees of coronal plane abduction.

Although the deltoid is the prime mover for abduction, its removal because of tumor was found to result in only minimal loss of range of arm elevation in five patients.[87] Muscle strength measurements in both flexion and abduction revealed no greater than a 40% reduction compared with the contralateral limb in any of the positions measured.[87] Thus, other muscles, possibly including the biceps, coracobrachialis, and clavicular portion of the pectoralis major, are capable of assuming the role of the deltoid in arm elevation.

Townsend and colleagues[88] studied 17 exercises used in a rehabilitation program for baseball players using indwelling wire electrodes. The purpose of the study was to determine which exercises most effectively elicited activity in the shoulder musculature and therefore would be the best exercises for strengthening these muscles. Activity was measured as a percentage of that obtained during a maximal isometric contraction. Abduction in the scapular plane with the arm in internal rotation (thumb-down position) and a light weight in the hand resulted in high levels of activity in both the supraspinatus and middle deltoid muscles. The military press (see Fig. 6–8) resulted in the highest level of EMG activity in the supraspinatus muscle.

Infraspinatus, Teres Minor, and Subscapularis

The rotator cuff is the musculotendinous complex formed by the attachment to the capsule of the supraspinatus muscle superiorly, the subscapularis muscle anteriorly, and the teres minor and infraspinatus muscles posteriorly. These tendons blend intricately with the fibrous capsule. They are major active stabilizers of the glenohumeral joint and can be considered true dynamic ligaments.[27, 89] The capsule is less well protected inferiorly because the tendon of the long head of the triceps brachii muscle is separated from the capsule by the axillary nerve and the posterior circumflex humeral artery.[2]

With the arm at the side, the directional force of the deltoid muscle is almost vertical.[45, 64] Thus, most of the deltoid force will cause upward translatory motion of the humeral head, which if unopposed would cause the humeral head to contact the coracoacromial arch, resulting in impingement of soft tissues.[90] The action line of the infraspinatus, subscapularis, and teres minor muscles are such that each tends to have a rotatory component as well as a compressive force.[64, 90] Each also has a downward translatory component that offsets the upward translation force of the deltoid[32, 45, 85, 91] (Fig. 6–20).

Wuelker and associates,[85] based on cadaver experimentation, found that the supraspinatus did not contribute to the depressive forces on the humeral head. The infraspinatus, teres minor, and subscapularis thus form a force couple with the deltoid and act to stabilize the humeral head on the glenoid fossa, allowing the deltoid to act to abduct the humerus.[76, 91] The compressive and downward translation actions of these muscles are thought to be most important in the middle range of elevation when the capsule and ligaments are relatively lax.[92]

In studies on a mechanical model, Comtet and colleagues[79] determined that the depressor forces would be at their maximum between 60 and 80

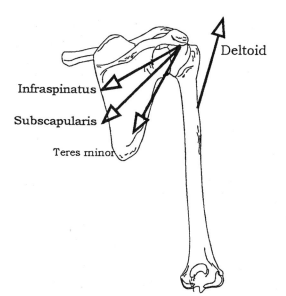

FIGURE 6–20 Force couple consisting of the deltoid, the primary abductor of the humerus, and the muscles of the musculotendinous cuff, which function to depress the humeral head and oppose the upward translatory force of the deltoid.

degrees of elevation and disappear beyond 120 degrees. Weakness or loss of the humeral head depressors may lead to increased superior migration of the humeral head during arm elevation, contributing to impingement of the supraspinatus and possibly the biceps tendons against the acromion process.[29] Thus, instability often coexists with impingement of subacromial structures. Strengthening of the rotator cuff muscles has been advocated to improve their efficiency as humeral head depressors.[91]

Inman and coauthors[27] studied the EMG activity of the subscapularis, infraspinatus, and teres minor muscles during elevation of the arm in the coronal and sagittal planes. All three muscles were found to work continuously throughout arm elevation in both planes. Teres minor and subscapularis activity peaked between 100 and 120 degrees of elevation and declined through the remaining elevation range. Subscapularis activity was greater when elevation was carried out in the coronal plane. Infraspinatus activity increased throughout the entire motion in the coronal plane. Greater activity was observed in this muscle during sagittal plane flexion, with two peaks of activity occurring at 60 and 120 degrees of elevation.[27]

van der Helm[30] predicted the contribution of the infraspinatus, teres minor, and subscapularis muscles to glenohumeral elevation using a finite element model. The model predicted that the teres minor would not contribute to either coronal or sagittal plane elevation. The infraspinatus contributed to sagittal plane elevation and the first 60 degrees of coronal plane abduction. The subscapularis was found to be the second most important (after deltoid) contributor to coronal plane abduction, owing to its large cross-sectional area and useful moment arm, but would not contribute to sagittal plane elevation.

The EMG activity of these muscles has also been studied during performance of rehabilitation exercises in healthy subjects using indwelling wire electrodes. Exercises that generated at least half the amount of activity obtained during a maximal isometric contraction were considered to be suitable choices for a strengthening program.[88] The most effective exercise for recruitment of the subscapularis was abduction in the scapular plane with the arm in internal rotation (thumb-down position) and a light weight in the hand. The exercise that generated the greatest EMG activity in the infraspinatus and teres minor was horizontal abduction of the arm in the prone-lying position with the humerus in external rotation and a light weight held in the hand. The same exercise with the arm in internal rotation also generated high levels of EMG activity in these muscles (see Fig. 6–9).

McCann and coauthors[84] reported moderate to high levels of EMG activity in the external rotators during resistive exercises performed with an elastic band below shoulder level and advocated this technique for strengthening after shoulder reconstruction. Similarly, Harms-Ringdahl and colleagues[93] advocated resisted external rotation exercises using a pulley apparatus to strengthen the infraspinatus muscle and determined the optimal patient positioning to maximize muscle strengthening without excessive joint loading.

Biceps Brachii

The tendon of the long head originates on the supraglenoid tubercle of the scapula, crosses over the anterolateral aspect of the glenohumeral joint, and passes through the intertubercular groove. The tendon lies within the joint capsule within its own synovial sleeve. The short head originates from the coracoid process. Furlani,[94] in an EMG study of healthy men, demonstrated that both heads of the biceps are active during free and resisted flexion of the shoulder with the elbow extended. Little activity was seen in either the long or short head during free or resisted shoulder abduction, and neither component contributed in medial or lateral rotation movements. The short head was active during resisted adduction in half of the 30 subjects tested.[94]

The biceps brachii is postulated to contribute to both superior and anterior stability of the glenohumeral joint. Kumar and coauthors,[95] in an in vitro study, measured the acromial humeral distance from radiographs with tension applied to one or both heads of the biceps, before and after division of the tendon of the long head. With the long head divided, application of tension to the short head resulted in upward migration of the humeral head on the glenoid. The authors concluded that the long head was an important stabilizer of the shoulder during activities involving elbow flexion and supination. Action of the cuff musculature was not simulated in this study, and it is unclear whether normal functioning of these muscles in vivo would compensate for loss of the long head of biceps. Neer[29] also postulated that rupture of the long head of the biceps could result in elevation of the humeral head during arm movements and a nonoutlet type of impingement of the humeral head against the acromion process.

The contribution of the long and short heads of the biceps to anterior stability has also been investigated in cadavers.[96, 97] Anterior translation forces were applied to the humeral head with the arm in 90 degrees of abduction and 60, 90, or 120 degrees of external rotation with and without loads applied to either the long or short head. Tension applied to both the long and short heads was found to decrease anterior translation of the head on the glenoid at 60 and 90 degrees of external rotation. The degree of anterior translation that occurred when anterior translation forces were applied at 120 degrees of external rotation was minimal, possibly because of the extreme tautness of the capsule in this position. Loading of the biceps tendons decreased anterior translation at this angle of external rotation only when a Bankart lesion (sectioning of the anteroinferior capsule) was present. The authors concluded that the biceps is an important anterior stabilizer, particularly when the anteroinferior capsule is compromised, and suggested that strengthening of the biceps was indicated for patients with chronic anterior shoulder instability.[96, 97] Glousman's[98] observation that EMG activity of the biceps was greater during the acceleration phase of pitching in subjects with unstable shoulders also suggests that the biceps may help to compensate for anterior instability.

Axiohumeral Musculature

Two muscles, latissimus dorsi and pectoralis major, connect the axial skeleton and humerus. The latissimus dorsi also has an attachment on the scapula and is capable of scapular adduction and depression as well as glenohumeral extension, adduction, and medial rotation.[83] The latissimus dorsi is particularly active in closed kinetic chain activities in which body weight is supported by the upper extremities, for example, when using crutches or doing a push-up. Contraction of the muscle during these activities results in elevation of the trunk in relation to the humerus.[32, 88] The sternal portion of pectoralis major also contributes to depression of the shoulder complex during upper extremity weight-bearing activities.[88] Both muscles were found to have high levels of EMG activity during a press-up exercise[88] (see Fig. 6–10) and during the pull-through phase of the free-style swim stroke.[99]

In open kinetic chain motions, both the clavicular and sternal portions of the pectoralis major assist the anterior deltoid in elevation of the humerus in the sagittal plane, with the clavicular portion being the more active.[83] The pectoralis major also contributes to adduction and resisted medial rotation of the humerus in open kinetic chain movements.[83] Both latissimus dorsi and pectoralis major may also contribute to the depressor forces on the humeral head.[88]

FORCES AT THE GLENOHUMERAL JOINT

Lippitt and Matsen[48] discussed the concept of concavity compression in maintaining glenohumeral joint stability throughout the range of motion. The concavity component related to the depth of the glenoid fossa and its surrounding labrum, as previously discussed. The compressive component referred to the degree to which forces compressing the humeral head into the glenoid fossa contribute to stability of the articulation. The degree to which compressive forces could limit translation of the humeral head on the glenoid was investigated using fresh-frozen cadaver shoulders, with the surrounding musculature resected. The magnitude and direction of applied compressive and translatory forces were measured using magnetic spatial sensors and force transducers.[48] Compressive forces of 50 and 100 N were applied at various points in the range of motion, followed by the application of translatory forces in each position. The higher compressive load resulted in increased resistance to translatory forces, leading the authors to conclude that the greater the compression, the more stable the joint. The authors suggested that, in vivo, the rotator cuff muscles and the biceps brachii are aligned such that they contribute to the compressive force of the humeral head on the glenoid. It was suggested that weakened or damaged cuff muscles might be less able to withstand translatory forces, leading to instability during movement.[48] The outer muscular sleeve, deltoid,

pectoralis major, and latissimus dorsi were postulated to contribute to this compression in some shoulder positions.

The magnitude and direction of forces at the glenohumeral joint have been estimated by several researchers.[27, 90, 100] Inman and coauthors[27] estimated the compressive forces due to activity in the deltoid and rotator cuff musculature during arm abduction in the coronal plane. A maximum compressive force of 50% body weight was estimated to occur at 90 degrees of abduction. Poppen and Walker[90] estimated the compressive, sheer, and resultant forces at the glenohumeral joint during scapular plane abduction with neutral rotation. The resultant force increased with elevation, reaching a peak of 0.89 times body weight at 90 degrees of elevation. The upward sheer force of the humeral head on the glenoid peaked at 0.42 times body weight at 60 degrees of elevation. The authors suggested that the greater compressive forces, compared with those reported by Inman and coauthors,[27] may have been related to a difference in assumptions regarding the resultant line of action of the depressor cuff muscle. Karlsson and Peterson,[100] using a computer model, predicted a resultant glenohumeral contact force of 600 N (0.8 times body weight) between 60 and 90 degrees of scapular plane elevation.

Three-dimensional biomechanical models have also been used to predict muscle forces around the glenohumeral joint.[101, 102] Predicted forces in the subscapularis, middle and anterior deltoid, supraspinatus, and infraspinatus ranged from 45 N (supraspinatus) to 167 N (middle deltoid) when the arm was held in 90 degrees of scapular plane abduction with the elbow extended. The same muscles were active during a maximal abduction effort, at 90 degrees of elevation, with forces increasing by 260%. The greatest forces were predicted for the middle and anterior deltoids (323 N and 434 N, respectively), whereas the posterior deltoid was inactive in both unloaded and loaded conditions. Subscapularis force was greatest during a resisted internal rotation effort with the arm in an abducted position (1725 N). Resisted external rotation in an abducted position generated forces of 175 N and 723 N for the supraspinatus and infraspinatus, respectively.

Maximal teres minor forces were predicted during a maximal external rotation effort with the arm in an adducted position. Force predictions for supraspinatus were 150% greater during maximal external rotation exertions than during maximal abduction exertion, and the authors suggested that reduction of internal rotation loading be considered in the prevention and rehabilitation of rotator cuff impairments. The posterior deltoid was active during internal rotation efforts in both the abducted and adducted positions and during external rotation efforts with the arm adducted. The force predicted for the middle deltoid during a maximal internal rotation effort in the abducted position exceeded that predicted for the resisted abduction effort at 90 degrees of scapular plane elevation.

Muscle forces have also been predicted at 15-degree intervals between 0 and 120 degrees of scapular plane elevation with a 1-kg weight in the hand. Force levels of up to 150 N were predicted for the middle and anterior deltoids, supraspinatus, infraspinatus, subscapularis, clavicular portion of the pectoralis major, biceps, and coracobrachialis during the movement. Greatest forces were predicted for the middle deltoid (150 N) at about 100 degrees of elevation. Zero or low levels of activity were predicted in the subscapularis during the early phase of elevation and for the supraspinatus and infraspinatus at higher elevation angles. These muscles demonstrated EMG activity throughout scapular plane elevation, and it was suggested that the activity was related to their role as humeral head stabilizers.

INTEGRATED FUNCTION OF THE SHOULDER COMPLEX

SCAPULOHUMERAL RHYTHM

Full elevation of the upper extremity results from the combination of scapular rotation, such that the glenoid fossa tilts progressively upward, and elevation of the humerus at the glenohumeral joint. Codman[103] introduced the term *scapulohumeral rhythm* to describe this integrated movement at the glenohumeral and scapulothoracic joints during upper extremity elevation. Glenohumeral and scapular motions were studied during arm elevation in the coronal and sagittal planes by Inman and coauthors.[27] Glenohumeral and scapular rotation were found to contribute a maximum of 120 and 60 degrees, respectively, to total arm motion. An initial scapular "setting phase" was described, in which the scapula moved medially or laterally or remained fixed. This phase constituted the first 30 degrees of abduction or first 60 degrees of flexion. Most of the motion during the setting phase occurred at the glenohumeral joint. The overall ratio of glenohumeral to scapular thoracic rotation throughout full elevation was 2:1.[27]

Scapulohumeral rhythm during arm elevation has been examined more recently during scapular plane elevation.[20, 22, 23] Total range of upper extremity elevation measured in these studies varied between 168 and 172 degrees, somewhat less than the 180 degrees described by Inman and coauthors.[27] Total scapular rotations of 58.6[20] and 63.8[23] degrees have been reported. Elevation at the glenohumeral joint varied from 103 to 113 degrees.[20, 22, 23]

The ratio of glenohumeral to scapulothoracic motion, measured during elevation in the scapular plane, was found to vary throughout the range and to be highly variable among subjects.[20, 22, 23, 104] Högfors and colleagues[104] reported that there was considerable variation in scapulohumeral relationship among subjects; however, the rhythm within a subject was stable and was unaffected by small loads held in the hand.

Glenohumeral motion predominates during initial arm elevation. A glenohumeral-to-scapulothoracic ratio as high as 7.29:1 has been reported during the first 30 degrees of elevation.[20] A ratio of 3.29:1 was reported by Bagg and Forrest[23] between 20 and 80 degrees of elevation. Scapular motion predominates between 80 and 140 degrees of total arm elevation. Glenohumeral-to-scapulothoracic ratios of 0.79:1[20] and 0.71:1[23] have been reported during this phase of elevation. Glenohumeral motion again predominates above 140 or 150 degrees of total arm motion.[20, 23] Bagg and Forrest[23] reported a glenohumeral-to-scapulothoracic ratio of 3.49:1 during this phase in subjects demonstrating the most typical pattern of movement.

Alteration in the normal scapulohumeral rhythm has not been extensively studied in subjects with shoulder pathology. It has been postulated that weakness or fatigue of the scapular rotators, particularly the serratus anterior, may contribute to shoulder instability related to a failure of these muscles to maintain a stable glenoid base for humeral movement.[98, 99, 105, 106] It has also been suggested that dysfunction of these muscles could lead to insufficient upward movement of the glenoid during overhead activities, resulting in secondary impingement of structures in the subacromial space.[98, 99] Glousman and associates[105] have indicated that the trapezius and serratus anterior may be more prone to fatigue than other muscles near the shoulder during activities requiring repetitive overhead motion, lending some support to these hypotheses.

Abnormal scapular motion has been identified in subjects with inferior and multidirectional instability of the glenohumeral joint using cineradiography.[107] Scapular motion and humeral motion were measured through arm elevation in the scapular plane in 11 subjects with instability and in 30 normal shoulders. The scapula did not rotate upward to the same degree in the subjects with instability as in those with normal shoulders.[107]

Similarly, Nobuhara and Ikeda[56] reported abnormal scapular motion in subjects with instability due to lesions of the capsule and ligaments in the rotator interval, and Poppen and Walker[18] found an abnormal glenohumeral-to-scapulothoracic ratio in 9 of 15 subjects with shoulder pathology.

Alterations in scapular mechanics and EMG activity in the scapular muscles has been identified in swimmers with shoulder pain.[108] Decreased activity in the serratus anterior was reported throughout the free-style stroke in swimmers with painful shoulders. A decrease in activity in the anterior and middle deltoids, rhomboids, and upper trapezius was also reported to be associated with a more medial hand placement during the early pull-through phase. It is unclear whether the altered mechanics and EMG activity contributed to the shoulder pathology or were related to an alteration in the stroke because of the pain.

Warner and colleagues[106] studied symmetry of scapulothoracic motion in 22 healthy subjects, 22 patients with anteroinferior instability, and 7 subjects with impingement syndrome using a Moire topographic analysis technique. Static tests involved holding a 4.5-kg weight in each hand with both arms held in a 90-degree forward flexed position with elbows extended for 5 seconds. For the dynamic tests, subjects lifted the same weight through 0 to 120 degrees of forward flexion bilaterally with elbows flexed to 60 degrees. Sixty-four percent of subjects with instability and 100% of those with impingement demonstrated some abnormality in the scapulothoracic motion during the dynamic flexion test. In the static test, the scapula was lower on the side of the unstable shoulder in the instability group compared with the contralateral side but was higher on the side of the lesion in the impingement group relative to the contralateral side. The differences in both the static and dynamic tests were attributed to weakness of the serratus anterior and trapezius muscles. Whether the alterations are primary or secondary is unknown.

In summary, full elevation and normal mechanics of the shoulder complex is dependent on simultaneous, coordinated motions of the scapulothoracic, sternoclavicular, acromioclavicular, and glenohumeral joints. Disruptions of any of the normal joint mechanics or altered joint structure can result in the development of clinical pathologies and disruption of function.

References

1. Dempster WT: Mechanisms of shoulder movement. Arch Phys Med Rehabil 46:49, 1965.
2. Warwick R, Williams P: Gray's Anatomy, 37th ed. London, Longman Group, 1989.
3. Bearn JG: Direct observations on the function of the capsule of the sternoclavicular joint in clavicular support. J Anat 101:159, 1967.
4. Abbott LC, Lucas DB: The function of the clavicle: Its surgical significance. Ann Surg 140:583, 1954.
5. Flatow EL: The biomechanics of the acromioclavicular, sternoclavicular, and scapulothoracic joints. Instr Course Lect 42:237, 1993.
6. Moseley HF: The clavicle: Its anatomy and function. Clin Orthop 58:17, 1968.
7. Moore KL: Clinically Oriented Anatomy. Baltimore, Williams & Wilkins, 1980.
8. Fukuda K, Craig EV, An K, et al: Biomechanical study of the ligamentous system of the acromioclavicular joint. J Bone Joint Surg 68A:434, 1986.
9. Rockwood CA Jr: Dislocations about the shoulder. In Rockwood CA Jr, Green DP (eds): Fractures. Philadelphia, JB Lippincott, 1975, p 624.
10. Herscovici D, Sanders R, DiPasquale T, Gregory P: Injuries of the shoulder girdle. Clin Orthop 318:54, 1995.
11. Richards R: Acromioclavicular joint injuries. Instr Course Lect 42:259, 1993.
12. Larson E, Bjerg-Nielsen A, Christensen P: Conservative or surgical treatment of acromioclavicular dislocation: A prospective, controlled randomized study. J Bone Joint Surg 68A:552, 1986.
13. Taft TN, Wilson FC, Oglesby JW: Dislocation of the acromioclavicular joint: An end-result study. J Bone Joint Surg 69A:1045, 1987.
14. Steindler A: Kinesiology of the Human Body Under Normal and Pathological Conditions. Springfield, IL, Charles C Thomas, 1955.
15. Kapandji IA: The Physiology of the Joints, vol 1: Upper Limb, 2nd ed. Edinburgh, E & S Livingstone, 1970.
16. Norkin CC, Levangie PK: Joint Structure and Function, 2nd ed. Philadelphia, FA Davis, 1992.
17. Bechtol CO: Biomechanics of the shoulder. Clin Orthop 146:37, 1980.
18. Poppen NK, Walker PS: Normal and abnormal motion of the shoulder. J Bone Joint Surg 58A:195, 1976.
19. Culham E, Peat M: Spinal and shoulder complex posture. I. Measurement Using the 3Space Isotrak. Clin Rehabil 7:309, 1993.
20. Doody SG, Freedman L, Waterland JC: Shoulder movements during abduction in the scapular plane. Arch Phys Med Rehabil 51:595, 1970.
21. Basmajian JV, Bazant FJ: Factors preventing downward dislocation of the adducted shoulder joint. J Bone Joint Surg 41A:1182, 1959.
22. Freedman L, Munro RR: Abduction of the arm in the scapular plane: Scapular and glenohumeral movements. J Bone Joint Surg 48A:1503, 1966.
23. Bagg SD, Forrest WJ: A biomechanical analysis of scapular rotation during arm abduction in the

scapular plane. Am J Phys Med Rehabil 67:238, 1988.

24. Dvir Z, Berme N: The shoulder complex in elevation of the arm: A mechanism approach. J Biomech 11:219, 1978.

25. Singleton MC: Functional anatomy of the shoulder: A review. J Am Phys Ther Assoc 46:1043, 1966.

26. Ljunggren AE: Clavicular function. Acta Orthop Scand 50:261, 1979.

27. Inman VT, Saunders JB, Abbott LC: Observations on the function of the shoulder joint. J Bone Joint Surg 26:1, 1944.

28. Peat M: Functional anatomy of the shoulder complex. Phys Ther 66:1855, 1986.

29. Neer CS: Shoulder Reconstruction. Philadelphia, WB Saunders, 1990.

30. van der Helm FCT: Analysis of the kinematic and dynamic behavior of the shoulder mechanism. J Biomech 27:527, 1994.

31. Bagg SD, Forrest WJ: Electromyographic study of the scapular rotators during arm abduction in the scapular plane. Am J Phys Med 65:111, 1986.

32. Perry J: Normal upper extremity kinesiology. Phys Ther 58:265, 1978.

33. Wiedenbauer MM, Mortenson OA: An electromyographic study of the trapezius muscle. Am J Phys Med 31:363, 1952.

34. Moseley JB, Jobe FW, Pink M, et al: EMG analysis of the scapular muscles during a shoulder rehabilitation program. Am J Sports Med 20:128, 1992.

35. Mathiassen SE, Winkel J: Electromyographic activity in the shoulder-neck region according to arm position and glenohumeral torque. Eur J Appl Physiol 61:370, 1997.

36. Randelli M, Gambrioli PL: Glenohumeral osteometry by computed tomography in normal and unstable shoulders. Clin Orthop 208:151, 1986.

37. Cyprien JM, Vasey HM, Burdet A, et al: Humeral retrotorsion and glenohumeral relationship in the normal shoulder and in recurrent anterior dislocation (scapulometry). Clin Orthop 175:8, 1983.

38. Soslowsky J, Flatow EL, Bigliani LU, Mow VC: Articular geometry of the glenohumeral joint. Clin Orthop 285:181, 1992.

39. Saha AK: Dynamic stability of the glenohumeral joint. Acta Orthop Scand 42:491, 1971.

40. Iannotti JP, Gabriel JP, Schneck SL, et al: The normal glenohumeral relationships. J Bone Joint Surg 74A:491, 1992.

41. Saha AK: Mechanics of elevation of glenohumeral joint: Its application in rehabilitation of flail shoulder in upper brachial plexus injuries and poliomyelitis and in replacement of the upper humerus by prosthesis. Acta Orthop Scand 44:668, 1973.

42. Brewer BJ, Wubben RC, Carrera GF: Excessive retroversion of the glenoid cavity: A cause of

non-traumatic posterior instability of the shoulder. J Bone Joint Surg 68A:724, 1986.

43. Cooper DE, Arnoczky SP, O'Brien SJ, et al: Anatomy, histology, and vascularity of the glenoid labrum. J Bone Joint Surg 74–A:46, 1992.

44. Moseley HF, Övergaard B: The anterior capsular mechanism in recurrent anterior dislocation of the shoulder: Morphological and clinical studies with special reference to the glenoid labrum and the gleno-humeral ligaments. J Bone Joint Surg 44B:913, 1962.

45. Lucas DB: Biomechanics of the shoulder joint. Arch Surg 107:425, 1973.

46. Perry J: Anatomy and biomechanics of the shoulder in throwing, swimming, gymnastics, and tennis. Clin Sports Med 2:247, 1983.

47. Howell SM, Galinat BJ: The glenoid-labral socket: A constrained articular surface. Clin Orthop 243:122, 1989.

48. Lippitt S, Matsen F: Mechanisms of glenohumeral joint stability. Clin Orthop 291:20, 1993.

49. Zarins B, McMahon MS, Rowe CR: Diagnosis and treatment of traumatic anterior instability of the shoulder. Clin Orthop 291:75, 1993.

50. Clark J, Sidles JA, Matsen FA III: The relationship of the glenohumeral joint capsule to the rotator cuff. Clin Orthop 254:29, 1990.

51. Kumar VP, Balasubramaniam P: The role of atmospheric pressure in stabilising the shoulder: An experimental study. J Bone Joint Surg 67B:719, 1985.

52. Harryman DT II, Sidles JA, Clark JM, et al: Translation of the humeral head on the glenoid with passive glenohumeral motion. J Bone Joint Surg 72A:1334, 1990.

53. Cooper DE, O'Brien SJ, Warren RF: Supporting layers of the glenohumeral joint. Clin Orthop 289:144, 1993.

54. Harryman DT, Sidles JA, Harris SL, Matsen FA III: The role of the rotatory interval capsule in passive motion and stability of the shoulder. J Bone Joint Surg 74A:53, 1992.

55. Kaltsas DS: Comparative study of the properties of the shoulder joint capsule with those of other joint capsules. Clin Orthop 173:20, 1983.

56. Nobuhara K, Ikeda H: Rotator interval lesion. Clin Orthop 223:44, 1987.

57. Neer CS, Satterlee CC, Dalsey RM, Flatow EL: The anatomy and potential effects of contracture of the coracohumeral ligament. Clin Orthop 280:182, 1992.

58. Ferrari DA: Capsular ligaments of the shoulder: Anatomical and functional study of the anterior superior capsule. Am J Sports Med 18:20, 1990.

59. Turkel SJ, Panio MW, Marshall JL, Girgis FG: Stabilizing mechanisms preventing anterior dislocation of the glenohumeral joint. J Bone Joint Surg 63A:1208, 1981.

60. O'Brien SJ, Neves MC, Arnoczky SP, et al: The anatomy and histology of the inferior

glenohumeral ligament complex of the shoulder. Am J Sports Med 18:449, 1990.

61. Bowen MK, Warren RF: Ligamentous control of shoulder stability based on selective cutting and static translation experiments. Clin Sports Med 10:757, 1991.

62. Schwartz E, Warren RF, O'Brien SJ: Posterior shoulder instability. Orthop Clin North Am 18:409, 1987.

63. Ovesen J, Nielsen S: Anterior and posterior shoulder instability: A cadaver study. Acta Orthop Scand 57:324, 1986.

64. Sarrafian SK: Gross and functional anatomy of the shoulder. Clin Orthop 173:11, 1983.

65. Ovesen J, Nielsen S: Stability of the shoulder joint: Cadaver study of stabilizing structures. Acta Orthop Scand 56:149, 1985.

66. Bigliani LU, Pollock RG, Soslowsky LJ, et al: Tensile properties of the inferior glenohumeral ligament. J Orthop Res 10:187, 1992.

67. Rothman RH, Marvel JP, Heppenstall RB: Anatomic considerations in the glenohumeral joint. Orthop Clin North Am 6:341, 1975.

68. Neer CS: Impingement lesions. Clin Orthop 173:70, 1983.

69. Bigliani LU, Ticker JB, Flatow EL, et al: The relationship of acromial architecture to rotator cuff disease. Clin Sports Med 10:823, 1991.

70. Bigliani LU, Morrison DS, April EW: The morphology of the acromion and rotator cuff impingement. Orthop Trans 10:228, 1986.

71. Aoki M, Ishii I, Usui M: The slope of the acromion and rotator cuff impingement. Orthop Trans 10:228, 1986.

72. Blakely RL, Palmer ML: Analysis of rotation accompanying shoulder flexion. Phys Ther 64:1214, 1984.

73. Johnston TB: The movements of the shoulder-joint: A plea for the use of the "plane of the scapula" as the plane of reference for movements occurring at the humero-scapular joint. Br J Surg 25:252, 1937.

74. Gagey O, Bonfait H, Gillot C, et al: Anatomic basis of ligamentous control of elevation of the shoulder (reference position of the shoulder joint). Surg Radiol Anat 9:19, 1987.

75. Cailliet R: Shoulder Pain. Philadelphia, FA Davis, 1966.

76. Saha AK: Mechanism of shoulder movements and a plea for the recognition of "zero position" of the glenohumeral joint. Clin Orthop 173:3, 1983.

77. Howell SM, Galinat BJ, Renzi AJ, Marone PJ: Normal and abnormal mechanics of the glenohumeral joint in the horizontal plane. J Bone Joint Surg 70A:227, 1988.

78. Allegrucci M, Whitney SL, Irrgang JJ: Clinical implications of secondary impingement of the shoulder in freestyle swimmers. J Orthop Sports Phys Ther 20:307, 1994.

79. Comtet JJ, Herberg G, Naasan IA: Biomechanical basis of transfers for shoulder paralysis. Hand Clin 5:1, 1989.

80. deLuca CJ, Forrest WJ: Force analysis of individual muscles acting simultaneously on the shoulder joint during isometric abduction. J Biomech 6:385, 1973.

81. Howell SM, Imobersteg AM, Seger DH, Marone PJ: Clarification of the role of the supraspinatus muscle in shoulder function. J Bone Joint Surg 68A:398, 1986.

82. Colachis SC, Strohm BR: Effect of suprascapular and axillary nerve blocks on muscle force in upper extremity. Arch Phys Med Rehabil 52:22, 1971.

83. Scheving LE, Pauly JE: An electromyographic study of some muscles acting on the upper extremity of man. Anat Rec 135:239, 1959.

84. McCann PD, Wootten ME, Kadaba MP, Bigliani LU: A kinematic and electromyographic study of shoulder rehabilitation exercises. Clin Orthop 288:179, 1993.

85. Wuelker N, Plitz W, Roetman B, Wirth CJ: Function of the supraspinatus muscle. Acta Orthop Scand 65:442, 1994.

86. Otis JC, Jiang CC, Wickeiwicz TL, et al: Changes in the moment arms of the rotator cuff and deltoid muscles with abduction and rotation. J Bone Joint Surg 76A:667, 1994.

87. Markhede G, Monastyrski J, Stener B: Shoulder function after deltoid removal. Acta Orthop Scand 56:242, 1985.

88. Townsend H, Jobe FW, Pink M, Perry J: Electromyographic analysis of the glenohumeral muscles during a baseball rehabilitation program. Am J Sports Med 19:264, 1991.

89. Broström L, Kronberg M, Nemeth G: Muscle activity during shoulder dislocation. Acta Orthop Scand 60:639, 1989.

90. Poppen NK, Walker PS: Forces at the glenohumeral joint in abduction. Clin Orthop 135:165, 1978.

91. Sharkey NA, Marder RA: The rotator cuff opposes superior translation of the humeral head. Am J Sports Med 23:270, 1995.

92. Speer KP: Anatomy and pathomechanics of shoulder instability. Clin Sports Med 14:751, 1995.

93. Harms-Ringdahl K, Arborelius UP, Ekholm J, et al: Shoulder externally rotating exercises with pulley apparatus. Scand J Rehabil Med 17:129, 1985.

94. Furlani J: Electromyographic study of the m. biceps bracii in movements at the glenohumeral joint. Acta Anat 96:270, 1976.

95. Kumar VP, Satku K, Balasubramaniam P: The role of the long head of biceps brachii in the stabilization of the head of the humerus. Clin Orthop 244:172, 1989.

96. Itoi E, Kuechle DK, Newman SR, et al: Stabilizing function of the biceps in stable and unstable shoulders. J Bone Joint Surg 75B:546, 1993.

97. Itoi E, Newman SR, Kuechle DK, et al: Dynamic anterior stabilizers of the shoulder with the arm in abduction. J Bone Joint Surg 76B:834, 1994.

98. Glousman R: Electromyographic analysis and its role in the athletic shoulder. Clin Orthop 288:27, 1993.

99. Nuber GW, Jobe FW, Perry J, et al: Fine wire electromyography analysis of muscles of the shoulder during swimming. Am J Sports Med 14:7, 1986.

100. Karlsson D, Peterson B: Towards a model for force predictions in the human shoulder. J Biomech 25:189, 1990.

101. Karlsson D, Peterson B: Towards a model for force predictions in the human shoulder. J Biomech 25:189, 1992.

102. Hughes RE, An K: Force analysis of rotator cuff muscles. Clin Orthop 330:75, 1996.

103. Codman EA: The Shoulder. Boston, Thomas Todd, 1934.

104. Högfors C, Peterson B, Sigholm G, Herberts P: Biomechanical model of the human shoulder joint. II. The shoulder rhythm. J Biomech 24:699, 1991.

105. Glousman R, Jobe F, Tibone J, et al: Dynamic electromyographic analysis of the throwing shoulder with glenohumeral instability. J Bone Joint Surg 70A:220, 1988.

106. Warner JJP, Micheli LJ, Arslanian LE, et al: Scapulothoracic motion in normal shoulders and shoulders with glenohumeral instability and impingement syndrome. Clin Orthop 285:191, 1992.

107. Ozaki J: Glenohumeral movements of the involuntary inferior and multidirectional instability. Clin Orthop 238:107, 1989.

108. Scovazzo ML, Browne A, Pink M, et al: The painful shoulder during freestyle swimming: An electromyographic cinematographic analysis of twelve muscles. Am J Sports Med 19:577, 1991.

CHAPTER 7

BIOMECHANICS OF NEUROLOGIC TREATMENT

Richard W. Bohannon

INTRODUCTION

For an individual to function effectively, he or she must be able to generate forces that are of appropriate magnitude and rapidity, are applied in the appropriate direction, and are coordinated. This chapter is concerned primarily, but not exclusively, with the ability of patients with neurologic disorders to generate forces (and therefore torques) of sufficient magnitude and rapidity to function. Prior to discussing the treatment of force production problems, the determinants, nature, and implications of such problems will be discussed. Topics relevant to the biomechanics of neurologic treatment but covered elsewhere in detail (e.g., posture and balance, and orthoses) will receive limited attention.

FORCE PRODUCTION BY PATIENTS WITH NEUROLOGIC DISORDERS

DETERMINANTS OF FORCE PRODUCTION

Muscles are the means by which the vast majority of forces are generated within humans. The forces have both a passive and an active element.

The passive component of muscle force reflects the contribution of the musculotendinous unit's elasticity and is reflected in the unit's passive length–tension curve. As the musculotendinous unit is elongated (stretched), its passive force increases curvilinearly.[1] After neurologic insults, particularly those involving the central nervous system, the musculotendinous unit can become increasingly resistant to stretch. This resistance, which is largely the consequence of changes in the musculotendinous unit, results in a shift of the length–tension curve to the left (Fig. 7–1).[2, 3] In mature mammals, the changes involve the shortening of the muscle belly secondary to a loss of sarcomeres in series.[4] This loss occurs in both innervated and denervated muscles.[5] In growing children, another source of increased stiffness is possible.[6] As children grow in stature, their muscles or associated tendons may not grow at a rate comparable to that of the bones to which they are attached. As a consequence, the muscle belly or tendon of the unit may become short relative to its associated bones.

The active component of muscle force reflects motor unit activity. The number of motor units activated, the frequency of motor unit activation, and the size of activated motor units are the major determinants of the force generated by a pool of motor units over a period of time. All of these factors can be altered in the presence of neurologic disorders. Lesions of either the central or peripheral nervous system can decrease the total volume of motor drive through a reduction in the number of motor units that can be activated[7–10] and the frequency with which they are activated.[11–13] These reductions can result from a destruction of motor nerves, a block of the conduction of motor axons, or a slowing of the velocity at which they conduct impulses. Fortunately, the body has means for compensating for the loss of motor unit drive. At the level of the motor unit, the body sometimes compensates for a loss of functioning units by expanding the territory of remaining motor units[9, 14–17] or by increasing the ratio of motor unit firing per unit of force.[18, 19] Another way in which the body compensates is by prolonging the duration that a pool of motor units is activated. In the presence of an inadequate magnitude of muscle drive, the duration of drive can be extended to

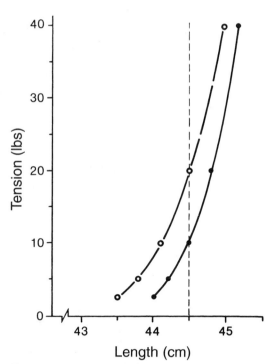

FIGURE 7–1 Passive length tension curves derived from the stretching of the gastrocnemius musculotendinous units of 14 patients with spastic hemiplegia. The left *(open circles)* curve represents the plegic side. The right *(closed circles)* curve represents the nonplegic side. The tension associated with a given length (e.g., 44.5 cm) is greater on the plegic side. (Adapted from Halar EM, Stolov WC, Venkatesh B, et al: Gastrocnemius muscle belly and tendon length in stroke patients and able-bodied persons. Arch Phys Med Rehabil 59:476, 1978.)

associated with spasms can affect the motor behavior in patients with central nervous system lesions.[24–26]

Spasticity, if defined as a velocity-dependent response to stretch, can be a problem only if an action is of sufficient velocity to evoke a stretch reflex. Although this is certainly possible,[27] it is probably less frequent than seems to be suggested by some authorities.[28] Research points to excessive coactivation as the more likely source of restraint. Although exaggerated coactivation is well documented in patients with central nervous system lesions,[29–31] it is not always present.[32–34] It is more likely to occur during concentric dynamic efforts, particularly those that are of a high speed or reciprocal nature.[30, 35] Overall, however, it appears that failures of patients with neurologic disorders to bring sufficient force to bear on the environment can be attributed primarily to reduced agonist drive rather than to excessive antagonist restraint.[32, 33, 36, 37]

NATURE OF MUSCLE FORCE PRODUCTION

Although an array of signs and symptoms can accompany neurologic disorders, particularly those of the brain, force production impairments are among the most prevalent. Particularly common are reductions in the maximum force that a person can bring to bear on the environment (strength). Associated with these reductions are decreases in the rate of force generation and speed of movement. The ability to sustain adequate force production over time (endurance) can also be reduced.

Impairments in Muscle Strength

Impairments in the force that patients with neurologic disorders are able to bring to bear on the environment are apparent during both clinical testing and functional activities. The results of studies describing these impairments in some of the more common neurologic disorders follow.

Stroke is among the most prevalent of neurologic diagnoses accompanied by impairments in muscle strength. During clinical testing, these impairments are most overt in the limb muscles contralateral to the lesion, with the upper extremity of that side thought to be more affected than the lower extremity.[38, 39] In the upper extremity of the side contralateral to the lesion, the actions of the hand are usually weaker than the actions that are generated more proximally (e.g., elbow flexion or shoulder abduction).[40] A lesser but well-documented weakness is often present in the limb muscles of the side ipsilateral to the lesion as

generate the force necessary to move a mass through a required distance.[20, 21]

The forces that muscles are able to bring to bear on the environment depend on the combined effects of passive and active components and represent the resultant effects of agonist and antagonist muscles. The torques of any action, therefore, are the summed effect of mobilizing torques generated by agonists minus restraining torques generated by antagonists. Although the agonist activation associated with any muscle action tends to be accompanied by a concomitant activation of the antagonist, the latter is typically of minimal magnitude.[22, 23] In patients with central nervous system lesions, antagonist restraint is often increased. The restraint can be from the passive or active elements. Restraint originating from active elements can be the consequence of spasms, spasticity, or excessive coactivation. Spasms, which are short-duration involuntary muscle contractions, can be provoked by a muscle stretch but can result from other stimuli as well. The involuntary contractions well. This weakness appears to be greater in more proximal limb actions (e.g., shoulder abduction or hip flexion).[38] The muscles of the trunk are also affected by stroke. Impairments have been documented in lateral and forward flexion and in rotation.[41, 42] Although the weakness after stroke tends to be greater in some actions than in others, there is a degree of generalizability to the weakness.[43] Thus, a patient who is weaker than another patient in one action is likely to be weaker in other actions as well. Strength impairments diminish spontaneously with time, with the greatest improvements occurring in the first several months after stroke[44]; the ultimate strength realized is strongly related to the strength retained very soon after the stroke.[39, 45] Improvements in strength occur bilaterally in the limbs[39, 46] as well as in the trunk.[47] Figure 7–2 illustrates the relationship between the knee-extension strengths of the paretic and nonparetic sides obtained on initial and final assessment.

Not as common as stroke but also depressing limb muscle strength are other intracranial lesions, such as traumatic brain injury and intracranial tumors.[48, 49] Both, like stroke, have the potential to impair the strength of limb muscles contralateral and ipsilateral to the brain lesion, with this potential documented in patients with traumatic brain injuries.[48] Although strength tends to increase over time after a traumatic brain injury, the strength of patients with intracranial tumors can increase or decrease depending on the nature of the tumor and interventions directed at it. Cerebral palsy is another neurologic disorder of the brain with

which impairments in muscle strength are associated.[50–53] The distribution of these impairments is a major factor in the classification of the disorder (e.g., diplegia versus hemiplegia). There is no published evidence that the impairments tend to ameliorate naturally over time.

Spinal cord injuries represent another major diagnostic group with which impairments in muscle strength are an expected occurrence, the magnitude of the impairments being dependent on the neurologic level and completeness of the lesion.[54] Strength increases somewhat after the acute stage of the injury, but the ultimate strength demonstrated by patients with spinal cord injury is dependent on their strength soon after injury.[55–57]

Both multiple sclerosis[58–60] and amyotrophic lateral sclerosis[61] are characterized by muscle weakness that worsens with time. The deterioration in strength in multiple sclerosis is variable, whereas the deterioration accompanying amyotrophic lateral sclerosis tends to be precipitous and predictable.

Of the several forms of muscle disease that result in muscle weakness, Duchenne's muscular dystrophy has probably been studied the most. Unlike healthy boys whose strength increases as they mature and gain height and weight, boys with Duchenne's muscular dystrophy tend to get weaker as they age.[62–64] Consequently, they demonstrate a growing gap in strength relative to age-matched boys as they get older.

Acute cases of poliomyelitis are essentially nonexistent in the developed world today. There are, nonetheless, numerous survivors of the polio epidemics that occurred earlier in this century. Patients who appeared to have regained most or all of their premorbid strength are demonstrating, decades later, emerging deficits in muscle performance.[65, 66] Particularly susceptible to such deficits (postpolio syndrome) are older patients whose original poliomyelitis was more severe.[66] Although postpolio syndrome is an unfortunate reality for many polio survivors, strength does not necessarily decrease inexorably, at least not over a period of several years.[67] Decreases in strength tend to be insidious.

Muscle weakness is a hallmark sign of Guillain-Barré syndrome. Fortunately, most patients affected by this disease recover substantially or completely. Most realize their maximum strength impairment within 3 weeks. The extent of and time required for recovery is predictable from "muscle weakness at maximum."[68]

Parkinson's disease is but one neurologic disorder in which the primary impairment is not typically considered to be weakness. Nevertheless, patients with Parkinson's disease frequently dem-

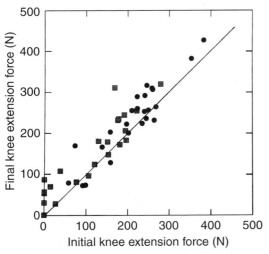

FIGURE 7–2 Scatterplot illustrating the relationship between paretic *(squares)* and nonparetic *(circles)* knee extension force measurements obtained on initial and final assessment from patients with stroke.

onstrate muscle weakness in the limbs and trunk.[69–73] That weakness is apparently related to some of the other more stereotypical motor signs (e.g., bradykinesia).[72]

Impairments in Rate of Force Generation and Speed of Movement

Impairments in the rate of force production have been documented in patients with stroke,[74, 75] Parkinson's disease,[72, 74–76] and multiple sclerosis.[58] Such impairments, however, are probably not limited to patients with these diagnoses. The relationship between rate of force generation and strength in patients with a variety of neurologic disorders suggests that impairments in the two force variables are reflecting a common underlying limitation.[72, 74, 75]

Patients with neurologic disorders as diverse as stroke,[34, 77–79] Parkinson's disease,[80, 81] cerebral palsy,[50, 52] and spinal cord injury[82] have been shown to demonstrate decreases in speed of movement. Research results are inconsistent but provide some evidence that these speed impairments are related to impairments in muscle strength, at least in patients with stroke.[34, 37, 77, 78] Thus, patients who have greater muscle weakness are likely to have lower maximum movement velocities.

Impairments in Muscle Endurance

Patients with weakness secondary to neurologic disorders are often unable to sustain their performance at activities requiring muscle force production over an extended time. Whether these patients are judged to be truly lacking in muscle endur-ance, however, depends in part on the manner in which their endurance is characterized. Studies in which a fatigue index (percentage decline in maximum force or torque) has been used to describe endurance are variable in their results. Some investigations have shown a greater percentage decline in neurologic patients than in healthy subjects.[83–85] Others have not shown greater declines.[86–90] What is more certain is that patients who are weak tend to decline to a required force more quickly. Whether or not their rate of decline differs from that of healthy subjects, patients who are weak reach the required threshold of force more quickly because they are closer to that threshold to start with (Fig. 7–3). Being weaker, the patients have less reserve separating their initial maximum and threshold forces.[91]

IMPLICATIONS OF MUSCLE FORCE PRODUCTION

Impairments in muscle force production are important because of their implications for the performance of functional activities. Historically, these implications were questioned by authorities who suggested that muscle weakness is not a central cause of dysfunction in patients with certain neurologic disorders.[28] Nevertheless, the implications should be self-evident. Although most functional activities do not require a great deal of strength, they do require force levels that are sufficient to accelerate or decelerate the mass of the body and its segments or to respond appropriately to external forces. In the absence of such muscularly generated forces, the person becomes dependent on assistance from other people or

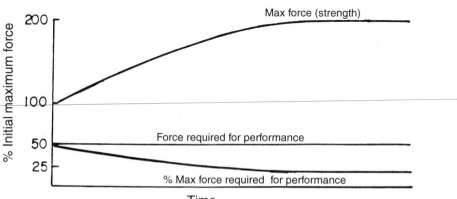

FIGURE 7–3 Illustration of the relationship between muscle strength and endurance. Note that greater strength results in a relative reduction in demand, which results in greater absolute endurance. (Reprinted by permission from Sale DG: Testing strength and power. In MacDougall JD, Wenger HA, Green HJ [eds]. Physiological Testing of the High-Performance Athlete, 2nd ed. Champaign, IL, Human Kinetics, 1991, pp 22–24.)

equipment. The importance of muscle force pro- duction to function has been confirmed by studies of statistical relationships involving clinical mea- surements and by biomechanical investigations. A brief review of this research follows.

Studies of Statistical Relationships

Numerous studies have revealed that muscle force production, particularly when expressed as strength, is related statistically to functional per- formance. Such studies have employed an array of muscle strength–measuring procedures and a variety of functional measures, either multicompo- nent or specific. Although research on relation- ships does not prove cause and effect, it does provide evidence for the validity of strength mea- surements among patients with neurologic disor- ders.

Multicomponent indexes characterizing the functional limitations of patients with neurologic disorders have been shown repeatedly to correlate significantly with the patients' muscle strength. This relationship has been pointed out most often among patients with stroke; their strength has been found to correlate with the Barthel Index,[92–98] Frenchay Arm Test,[44] and Sickness Impact Profile scores.[99] In one study involving the Barthel In- dex,[92] the correlations between initial measures of strength and final measures of function (r = 0.53 and 0.58, respectively) were particularly remark- able; they were only slightly less than the correla- tions between initial and final measures of func- tion (r = 0.64 and 0.65, respectively).[92] The muscle strength of patients with spinal cord inju- ries has also been noted to correlate with func- tional index scores, for example, with the Barthel Index, Functional Independence Measure, and Quadriplegia Index of Function.[57, 100, 101]

Patient performance at specific functional activ- ities can also be explained by measurements of muscle strength. This has been demonstrated most often in regard to various aspects of gait. Whether patients are weak as a consequence of stroke[102–108] (Fig. 7–4), muscular dystrophy,[62] myelomeningo- cele,[109] spinal cord injury,[110–112] poliomyelitis,[113] or cerebral palsy[51] does not seem to matter; their weakness is predictive of walking performance. Muscle weakness also explains limitations in pa- tient performance at transfers,[114, 115] bed mobil- ity,[116] dressing,[115, 117] stair climbing,[118] and wheel- chair propulsion.[115, 119, 120]

Biomechanical Investigations

Primarily through research involving forceplates or weighing scales, the forces that patients are

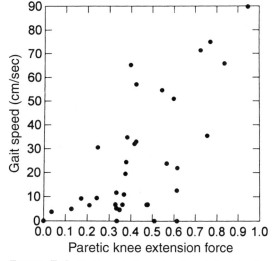

FIGURE 7–4   Scatterplot illustrating the relationship of paretic knee extension force (expressed as a ratio of normal) and comfortable gait speed (r = 0.74) in 35 patients with stroke.

able to generate have been linked to their perfor- mance at specific tasks. Chief among these tasks are the sit-to-stand maneuver, standing, and walk- ing.

Sit to Stand

Studies of the sit-to-stand maneuver have provided much insight into how people go about making a transition from one position to the other. The transition involves a movement of the person's center of mass in both the anterior and vertical directions[121] (Fig. 7–5). The movement, of course, is driven by muscular forces. Research on patients with stroke reveals findings that might be expected of people with lower extremity weakness that is greater on one side than the other. That is, the patients tend to take longer to attain standing than do matched control subjects.[121–123] When attaining standing in a natural fashion, the patients typically bear more weight through their nonparetic lower extremity.[121–123] Although it is logical that they would favor a "better" extremity during spontane- ous standing, they are able to increase their sym- metry with attention to it and training.[124, 125] The increase in symmetry, however, is not necessarily retained upon the cessation of training.[126]

Standing

Like studies of the sit-to-stand maneuver, most studies of force during standing have been con- ducted on patients with stroke. These studies also

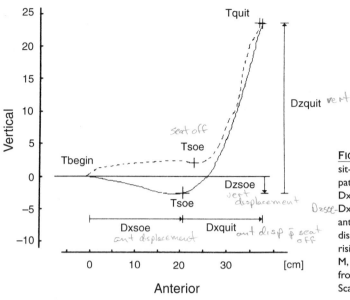

FIGURE 7–5 Movement of center of mass during sit-to-stand by a healthy subject (solid line) and a patient with hemiparesis (broken line). Tsoe, seat off; Dxsoe, anterior displacement before seat off; Dxsoe, vertical displacement before seat off; Dxquit, anterior displacement after seat off; Dzquit, vertical displacement after seat off; Tbegin, beginning of rising; Tquit, end of rising. (From Hesse S, Schauer M, Malezic M, et al: Quantitative analysis of rising from a chair in healthy and hemiparetic subjects. Scand J Rehabil Med 26:161, 1994.)

show a preference by patients for weight bearing through the nonparetic lower extremity during comfortable standing.[127–132] This asymmetry does not appear to be fixed; the patients are able to adjust their weight bearing both laterally and in an anteroposterior direction.[102, 133–136] Maximum weight bearing through or weight shifting toward the paretic lower extremity, however, is also reduced.[102, 133–136]

Walking

Weight Shifting. A person who is standing and wishes to initiate walking by taking a step must first shift weight away from the extremity that is to be lifted and advanced. Research involving forceplates has shed light on this process. The research has shown that in healthy subjects, most of the lateral force (about 4% of body weight) that shifts weight away from the uplifting lower extremity and onto the stance lower extremity is generated by the uplifting extremity before lift-off.[137, 138] In patients with stroke, most of the lateral shifting force is generated by the uplifting lower extremity only when that extremity is the nonparetic lower extremity. Most of the lateral shifting force preceding the lifting of the paretic lower extremity is generated by the nonparetic lower extremity, which remains on the ground. Thus, in patients with stroke, the nonparetic lower extremity is responsible for most of the lateral shifting force accompanying gait initiation regardless of which extremity is lifted first.[139, 140] The ability of patients with stroke to shift weight effectively is important but often compromised. Von

Schroeder and colleagues[140] concluded that "abnormal gait was due to difficulty in moving the body over the unstable limb." Pai and associates[141] found that in subjects they tested, 50% of the weight transfers to the nonparetic side were unsuccessful, and 80% of the weight transfers to the paretic side were unsuccessful (from a failure either to hold or to shift far enough).

Other Aspects of Walking. Biomechanical research reveals far more about gait than its initiation and problems with weight shifting. The research explains why patients with neurologic disorders walk slowly, and it also describes mechanical specifics of their ambulatory behavior.

Determinants of Gait Speed. A biomechanical explanation of the decreased walking speed demonstrated by patients with neurologic disorders begins with factors determining walking speed in people who are apparently healthy. Studies of healthy subjects demonstrate that muscle activity (as measured by electromyography) increases with increased speed.[142, 143] Net measures of moments, work, and power at the hip, knee, and ankle have also been shown to co-vary with gait speed. Winter[144] documented work and power bursts that decreased progressively as gait cadence went from fast to natural to slow. Winter and White[145] found a correlation of −0.94 between peak knee power and walking or jogging velocity. This led them to conclude the existence of a cause-and-effect relationship of neurologic origin. They wrote that "power or moment profiles represent the final output of the neuromuscular system, and therefore any discussion must take into account the organization of the CNS." It should not be surprising, therefore, that patients with pathologic[71, 102, 104, 110, 113, 146, 147] or experimental[148] lesions resulting in muscle weakness walk slower than normal and that the walking speed of patients with stroke tends to correlate significantly with the moments, work, and power generated at the lower extremity joints.[149, 150]

Mechanical Specifics of Walking. In addition to gross deficits in speed, specific deviations or deficits related to force are present in the gait of patients with neurologic disorders. These deviations have been examined most thoroughly in patients with stroke.

Weight loading and ground reaction forces have been the focus of numerous studies. Able-bodied subjects tend to demonstrate periods of lower extremity loading (stance) that are symmetric between sides. That is, the duration of left and right stance are essentially equal. After neurologic disorders that result in primarily unilateral weakness (e.g., stroke), the stance duration of the unaffected side is notably prolonged relative to the stance duration of the affected side and relative to the stance duration of able-bodied subjects.[147, 151] Double stance is also markedly prolonged.[147] Such behaviors might be expected to accompany a patient's reliance on the stronger of two lower extremities. In able-bodied people, the stance phase of gait is associated with a double-peaked vertical ground reaction force curve. The first peak of the curve, which accompanies weight acceptance, is distinct from the second peak, which accompanies push-off.[152, 153] The magnitude of the vertical ground reaction force, which exceeds body weight, increases with an increased speed of walking. Among patients with stroke, the ground reaction pattern is often changed; neither the double peaks nor the interpeak trough is necessarily present.[152, 154] The ground reaction force associated with weight acceptance is greater on the affected side than on the unaffected side, but the force associated with push-off is significantly less on the affected than on the unaffected side. The difference between sides in the magnitude of the ground reaction force is less in patients with greater motor recovery after stroke. Morita and coauthors[154] reported a correlation of 0.731 between the stage of motor recovery and a measure of vertical ground reaction force symmetry. Patients with Parkinson's disease also demonstrate abnormal vertical ground reaction force curves.[155] When patients are ambulating with a shuffling gait, their force curves are characterized by narrow, single peaks. When the patients become frozen in their gait, the amplitude and duration of the curves diminishes markedly as they cease shifting their weight completely from one foot to the other.

Given the decreased strength, reduced walking speed, and relationship between force-associated variables and gait speed present in patients with neurologic disorders, it should not be surprising that the patients demonstrate reduced joint moments, work, and power during gait itself. In patients who have experienced stroke, the joint moments, work, and power are reduced on the affected compared with the unaffected side. Specifically different are positive moments, work, and power at the ankle, negative work at the knee, and both positive and negative work at the hip.[149, 150]

INTERVENTIONS FOR IMPROVING FORCE PRODUCTION

Force production can be increased by interventions that have an immediate or nearly immediate effect or by training interventions that increase force production over a prolonged course of therapy. Both categories of interventions are addressed here. Interventions that might be considered physical, however, are emphasized.

INTERVENTIONS CAPABLE OF PRODUCING IMMEDIATE EFFECTS

Muscle Stretch

Chief among the techniques that can have a prompt effect on muscle force are those involving muscle stretch. Three such techniques are mentioned here.

The first technique involves merely putting a muscle in an elongated position so that it can generate more force. Although this behavior exists in able-bodied subjects,[156, 157] it has particular importance to patients with neurologic disorders.[158] By adjusting the position of the joints that a muscle crosses, the muscle can be lengthened and its force increased. Although there are many circumstances in which this helps neurologic patients to function, I will describe only three. First, a person with a weak grasp after a spinal cord injury may realize a useful augmentation of grip strength when the long finger flexors are put on stretch by splinting the wrist in extension. Second, a person who has difficulty using a lower extremity to propel a wheelchair after a stroke may gain a beneficial supplementation of knee flexion strength by leaning slightly forward rather than slouching back in the wheelchair seat. Doing so puts a greater stretch on the hamstrings, allowing the patient to pull back more vigorously with the propelling lower extremity. Third, a patient who is unable to lift a trailing lower extremity onto a bed while the lower extremity already on the bed is fully extended (Fig. 7–6A) may be able to do so if the contralateral hip and knee are first flexed (Fig. 7–6B). This maneuver tilts the pelvis posteriorly[159] and flattens the back. As a consequence, the hip flexors are lengthened and are enabled to create more force.

A second technique involving stretch calls on the stretch-shortening cycle. When a muscle undergoes active shortening (a concentric contraction) immediately after it has undergone active lengthening (an eccentric contraction), the concentric force is greater than if not preceded by the eccentric action.[160] The benefits of the stretch-shortening cycle are readily apparent in able-bodied subjects, for example, during jumping. In patients who are weak, however, the use of the stretch-shortening cycle is probably more crucial.[161] One important use of the stretch-shortening cycle is during the sit-to-stand maneuver. A patient who has difficulty attaining standing from sitting when the task is performed very slowly may be more independent when the trunk is flexed forward quickly before rising is attempted. By

preceding hip extension (which accompanies lift-off) with forward motion of the trunk, the hamstrings are activated eccentrically before being activated concentrically to extend the hips.[162]

A third technique involves a quick stretch of a muscle involved in an activity. Therapists sometimes provide such stretches manually in an effort to facilitate a desired movement.[163] The stretch can be applied by a quick pull on a segment that is counter to its intended direction of movement or by one or more taps on the tendon or belly of a muscle involved in a movement. That such "facilitation" techniques influence movement in patients with central nervous system lesions is easily verified. Tapping may even have a small short-duration residual effect on a muscle's force-producing capability.[164] The problem is that stretch facilitation involves an external input by another person. Patients themselves can employ muscle-elongating postures and the stretch-shortening cycle.

Other Interventions

Several other interventions can affect muscle force while they are being applied. Of particular note

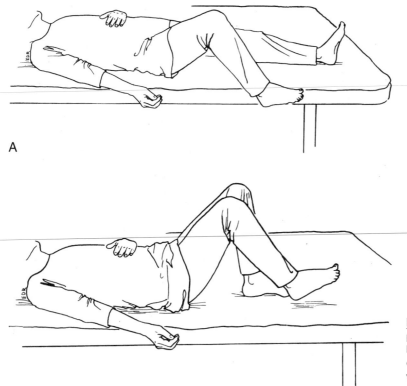

A

B

FIGURE 7–6 Line drawings from photographs of a patient with hemiparesis lifting his paretic lower extremity onto a bed. He was unable when the contralateral hip was extended (A) but able when the contralateral hip was flexed (B).

are electrical stimulation, vibration, and cutaneous stimulation.

Functional electrical stimulation can markedly augment the force generated by the muscles of patients with central nervous system lesions. The augmentation has been demonstrated during numerous activities, both in patients with stroke and in those with spinal cord injury. Among patients with stroke, tetanizing current has been used primarily to augment muscle force during gait. The ankle dorsiflexors are probably the muscle group most often stimulated during gait. Their stimulation can increase foot clearance during swing, counteract excessive inversion during swing and stance, increase gait speed, and decrease the energy demand of walking.[165–167] By activating numerous different muscle groups in a coordinated sequence, multichannel stimulation can affect numerous aspects of gait favorably (e.g., inadequate hip and knee flexion during swing, excessive knee flexion during stance, and inadequate push-off).[168] Electrical stimulation has also been used to improve muscle function in the upper extremity of patients with stroke. Stimulation of the supraspinatus and posterior deltoid can be used to reduce shoulder subluxation.[169] Merletti and colleagues[170] found that multichannel stimulation of the upper extremity allowed performance of tasks "that were impossible without stimulation." Among patients with spinal cord injury, electrical stimulation has been used most often to elicit contractions of the quadriceps femoris. Stimulation of the quadriceps has been used to assist patients with spinal cord injury to stand,[171–173] walk,[174, 175] and cycle.[176] Other muscles, however, have been stimulated in conjunction with or in lieu of the quadriceps femoris to help the patients to cycle and walk.[175–177] Electrical stimulation has also been employed to activate the upper extremity muscles of patients with tetraplegia.[178]

Vibration, much like tapping, can result in the potentiation of voluntary force production by muscles that are paretic after central nervous system lesions.[179] Although there is some short-term carry-over of vibration,[179] patients who are treated over time with vibration do not demonstrate strength increases beyond those realized by patients not treated with vibration.[180]

Cutaneous stimulation applied by at least two techniques has been shown to facilitate muscular activity in patients with hemiparesis. Cutaneous stimulation through rapid brushing has been reported by Matyas and associates[181] to increase isometric knee extension and flexion forces but not isometric dorsiflexion force. Neeman and Neeman[182] have attributed increases in the active elbow flexion range of a patient with hemiparesis to cutaneous stimulation provided by application of orthokinetic cuffs to the patient's paretic upper extremity.[182] Orthokinetic cuffs have also been applied to patients with cerebral palsy and poliomyelitis with positive results.[183, 184]

INTERVENTIONS PRODUCING LASTING IMPROVEMENTS IN MUSCLE FORCE PRODUCTION

Interventions aimed at increasing the forces that muscles can bring to bear on the environment typically focus on the amelioration of strength impairments through voluntary exercise. Other interventions target antagonist restraint. These therapies can be applied alone or in combination and can be supplemented with other treatments.

Voluntary Exercise for Increasing Muscle Force Production

It is now beyond question that the muscle force–producing capacity of able-bodied subjects can be increased when they participate in exercise regimens of adequate intensity, frequency, and duration. That voluntary exercise programs can promote improved motor performance in patients with a variety of neurologic conditions is also supported by considerable evidence.

Historically, authorities on the rehabilitation of patients with brain lesions did not recommend the training of strength among such patients.[28] The results of research, however, suggest that the patients can benefit from exercise programs of sufficient frequency, intensity, and duration. Numerous positive outcomes have been described among patients with stroke. More than 20 years ago, Inaba and colleagues[185] found that patients who participated in progressive resistance exercise (isotonic leg presses) increased significantly more in strength than patients undergoing an active exercise regimen or training in activities of daily living. The resistance-trained patients were also significantly more likely after 1 month to improve in activities of daily living than patients in active exercise or activities of daily living training groups. More recently, repetitive resisted flexion and extension of the fingers has been reported by Bütefisch and coauthors[186] to lead to increased strength, velocity, and acceleration in the hand. Sharp and Brouwer[187] found that isokinetic training of the hemiparetic knee resulted in improvements in both knee muscle strength and gait velocity.

Engardt and coworkers[188] also demonstrated that isokinetic training of the knee muscles is beneficial. Whether trained concentrically or eccentrically, their subjects who had experienced a stroke (on average) more than 2 years previously improved in paretic knee extension strength. Only the eccentric training group, however, increased in both concentric and eccentric strength on the paretic side compared with the nonparetic side. Only the eccentrically trained group realized a "nearly symmetrical body weight distribution" between lower extremities when achieving standing from sitting. Electromyographic studies of patients with spastic paresis offer an explanation for the apparent superiority of eccentric training.[189] Compared with concentric efforts, eccentric efforts are accompanied by a higher level of agonist activation and a lower level of antagonist activation. Knutsson and associates[189] concluded that "the stretch imposed on antagonists in concentric contractions dampens voluntary activation of agonists through reciprocal inhibition" and that "stretch imposed upon agonists in eccentric contractions facilitates voluntary activation."

Research supportive of the use of resistance training is not limited to adults with brain lesions. Patients with cerebral palsy have also been shown to respond favorably to resistance exercise.[51, 190–194] Investigations of their response demonstrate increases in strength and, in separate studies, improved gait[193] and wheelchair propulsion.[194]

Strength training has also been established to be effective for patients with neurologic disorders or problems outside the brain. Among such disorders are spinal cord injury, neuromuscular disease, and poliomyelitis. Resistance exercises have been shown to be effective for increasing the strength of patients with spinal cord lesions[194–195] and for improving their wheelchair propulsion performance.[194–196] Isotonic exercise has been found to augment the strength of multiple actions in patients with neuromuscular disorders.[197] Postpoliomyelitis patients also appear also to respond favorably and without adverse effects to nonfatiguing resistance training.[198–200] Even patients with myositis may benefit from progressive resistance exercise.[201]

Regardless of the neurologic disorder, the issue of action specificity should be taken into account when enrolling patients in a strengthening regimen. Not all actions entail the same degree of muscle activation, and training a muscle in one action may not optimize its improvement in another. Electromyography can clarify the degree to which muscles are activated during specific activities.[202–203] Although the research related to specificity of training has typically involved healthy subjects, it points to the importance of the goal of training. If, for example, the goal is to increase muscle performance under closed-chain

conditions, the training should probably be closed chain.[204, 205] Similarly, if the goal is to increase muscle performance under ballistic conditions, the training should at least be oriented ballistically.[206]

Interventions Targeting Antagonist Restraint

Because antagonist restraint can contribute to decreases in the force of muscle actions, interventions aimed at reducing the restraint are sometimes employed in an effort to improve the motor performance of patients with neurologic disorders. Positive effects have been demonstrated for such interventions.

One way that antagonist restraint can be reduced is by the lengthening of the antagonist. This is often accomplished surgically, particularly in children with cerebral palsy.[3, 207, 208] The effects of such lengthening on voluntary muscle force have been quantified by Reimers.[209, 210] He showed that ankle dorsiflexion strength increased more than 200% in 52 patients with cerebral palsy who underwent surgical elongation of the triceps surae a median of 14 months before and that knee extension strength increased by a median 22% in 38 patients with cerebral palsy who underwent surgical elongation of the hamstring muscles. Antagonists can also be lengthened by casting and stretching. Casting of the ankle to stretch the plantar-flexors markedly increases passive dorsiflexion and reduces resistance to dorsiflexion in patients with brain lesions.[6, 211, 212] Prolonged stretching of muscles can lead to notable increases in passive joint range of motion.[213–215] Stretching of the hip adductor muscles has also been reported to result in increased voluntary hip abduction in adults with spastic paraparesis.[215] Odéen reported an average increase of 255% in voluntary abduction after a mean of about 4 months of 30-minute stretches performed two to five times daily.[215]

Other ways of reducing antagonist restraint, at least in cases in which the restraint is due to spasticity or excessive coactivation, are through the administration of pharmacologic agents and nerve sections. Pharmacologic agents can be administered systemically or through injections into the antagonists or the nerves supplying them. The latter include injections of phenol or alcohol, and more recently botulinum toxin. In addition to reducing tone, these injections have been shown repeatedly to improve passive range of motion and in some cases to increase active range of motion.[216–223] Keenan,[216] for example, reported that patients increased an average 25 degrees in wrist extension after the motor points of their spastic wrist flexors were injected with phenol.[216] Pierson and colleagues[218] described a mean gain in active range of motion of 17 degrees in an array of different upper and lower extremity joints affected by spasticity.

The results of research addressing the functional consequences of pharmacologic injections are equivocal.[216-223] The reduction of antagonist restraint has been accomplished through two types of nerve sections: selective peripheral neurotomy and selective posterior rhizotomy. An example of the first is the partial section of the mixed tibial nerve that Féve and associates[224] described. That section resulted in a reduction in ankle plantar-flexor muscle tone and a significant (mean, 7.5 degrees) increase in active ankle dorsiflexion range of motion.[225, 226] All patients' gaits improved. The second involved the partial sectioning of posterior (sensory) roots. Steinbok and coauthors[225] compared patients with spastic cerebral palsy who underwent the procedure and physical therapy with a group that received only physical therapy. The patients whose treatment included rhizotomy showed greater reductions in spasticity and greater increases in passive range of motion. Muscle strength did not improve differentially between treatments, but the Gross Motor Function Measure did; at 9 months, it had increased 11.3% in the patients receiving the rhizotomy but only 5.2% in the patients receiving physical therapy alone. Thomas and colleagues[226] reported that the gait of children with spastic diplegia was improved a year after dorsal rhizotomy.

Supplements to Voluntary Exercise Interventions

Although they can be used in isolation, electrical stimulation, acupuncture, and biofeedback are typically used as supplements to voluntary exercise interventions. As such, they can be used individually or in combination.

Electrical stimulation, which can be employed for its immediate effects, can also be employed over an extended period to improve muscle performance. It has been found in numerous studies to be efficacious when so employed with patients who were paretic after stroke. Large strength increases have been reported by Levin and Hui Chan (ankle dorsiflexion force increased up to 820%)[227] and Merletti and colleagues (ankle dorsiflexion moment increased about 300%).[228] Substantial increases in voluntary movement amplitude have been noted by Smith (multiple limb joint movements increased 67% to 480%)[229] and Lagassé and Roy (elbow extension range increased 28 to 105 degrees).[230] Electrical stimulation in combination with positional feedback has been shown to increase muscle performance at the knee and wrist. Winchester and associates[231]

documented that isometric knee extension torque increased 479% in a combination treatment group but 166% in a control group. Bowman and coauthors[232] described significant increases in both wrist extension torque and selective range of motion. The torque increased 280% when measured with the wrist at 30 degrees of extension.

Evidence supporting the application of electrical stimulation in cases of cerebral palsy is also available but limited. A few studies have provided support for very-low-intensity "therapeutic electrical stimulation."[233, 234]

Considerable research has been conducted on the response of spinal cord injury patients to the longitudinal application of functional electrical stimulation. Much of this research, like that of Barr and coworkers[235] and Rabischong and Ohanna,[236] has specified how functional electrical stimulation can increase evoked muscular output in patients with intact peripheral innervation and motor complete paraplegia. Functional electrical stimulation, however, has also been shown to increase the voluntary strength of patients with motor incomplete cord injuries.[178]

Although most of the research supporting the use of electrical stimulation has focused on patients with lesions of the brain and spinal cord, its efficacy with other types of neurologic patients has been demonstrated. One particularly interesting application has been to cases of Bell's palsy. By using eutrophic electrical stimulation, Farragher and colleagues[237] reported remarkable responses in patients with "apparently intractable" Bell's palsy. They employed a facial paralysis recovery index to document improved muscle performance in the patients.

There is considerable support for the use of acupuncture to treat patients with neurologic disorders, particularly stroke. Naeser and associates[238] showed that patients with stroke receiving acupuncture treatment for hand paresis experienced a "good response defined as improvement in at least four of six hand tests after 20 or 40 acupuncture treatments." They observed significant improvements in the patients' grip and pinch strength and timed hand dexterity. The positive results of acupuncture appear to be limited by the extent of brain damage accompanying the stroke.[238, 239] The benefits, however, extend to postural control and function[239-242] (Fig. 7-7).

Researchers performing meta-analyses of the effectiveness of electromyographic biofeedback for patients with stroke, those to whom the procedure is probably most often applied, have come to differing conclusions. Schleenbaker and Mainous[243] suggested that such feedback "is an effective tool for neuromuscular reeducation in the

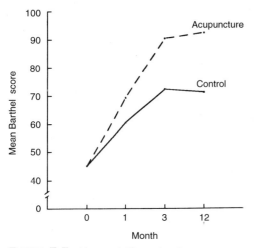

FIGURE 7–7 Line graph illustrating the greater recovery of function (Barthel scores) following stroke in a group of patients treated with acupuncture compared with a control group. (Graph generated from data reported by Johansson and colleagues.[242])

hemiplegic stroke patient." Glanz and coworkers,[244] on the other hand, concluded that "results of pooling available randomized control trials do not support the efficacy of biofeedback in restoring the range of motion of hemiparetic joints." Since the publication of these two analyses, Intiso and colleagues[245] completed a study that led them to conclude that "electromyographic biofeedback technique increases muscle strength and improves recovery of functional locomotion in patients with hemiparesis and foot-drop after cerebral ischemia." Although their sample size was small, their findings are compelling. If electromyographic biofeedback is to be applied, research suggests that it can be employed to augment agonist activation without concern for reducing the activation of the antagonist.[36, 37]

COMPENSATIONS FOR REDUCED FORCE PRODUCTION

Whether or not the force production of neurologic patients can be increased immediately or over time, compensations or adjustments can be employed to their advantage. These compensations take three major forms: altered techniques, the modification of demands, and the provision of assistive devices. Such compensations have been mentioned in passing earlier; they are elaborated on here.

ALTERED TECHNIQUES

There are many alternative techniques for accomplishing functional tasks. In the presence of mus-

cle weakness, patients with neurologic disorders may have to employ techniques that differ from those employed by people with normal strength. The use of interventions that rely on muscle strength have been mentioned previously. Beyond these alternatives, patients can use methods that rely on the muscle strength that they retain and maneuvers that optimize the effects of leverage. Numerous such methods exist. Three, however, provide particularly useful examples of the effectiveness of altered technique. The first involves rolling in patients with stroke. Patients with stroke have difficulty rolling toward their nonplegic side. Bohannon[115] showed that a significant number of patients with stroke increased in their independence at this task after being taught to use leverage (i.e., specific placement of their extremities) to their advantage. The second example of using altered technique can be found in patients with tetraplegia who lack sufficient triceps brachii strength to extend the elbow against gravity and can employ the anterior deltoid and upper pectoral muscles. These muscles can be used to lock the elbow while the hand is fixed and enable transfers.[246, 247] Third, patients with muscle disease and other neurologic disorders resulting in lower extremity weakness sometimes rely on the upper extremities and altered sequences of lower extremity and trunk maneuvers to arise from sitting.[248] One such maneuver, seen often in patients with Duchenne's muscular dystrophy, is Gowers' maneuver, in which patients push with their upper extremities on their thighs (Fig. 7–8).

MODIFICATION OF DEMANDS

Because force equals mass times acceleration and the force-producing capacity of the muscles of patients with neurologic disorders is frequently reduced, the demand for force from the muscles must often be reduced if the patients are to manage functionally. One way of reducing the demand is to reduce the body's mass,[249, 250] which has a tendency to increase in some patients with neurologic disorders. Another way of reducing the demand for force is to provide a means of reducing the force requirements on weak muscles. Assistive devices, discussed in the next section, are one way of reducing force requirements. In addition, assistance from other people and equipment serves this purpose. Clearly, there are many patients who can manage functionally if assistance is provided to move a body segment (e.g., the lower extremity off the bed when going from supine to sitting) or to supplement their efforts against gravity (e.g., during sit to stand or the unilateral stance phase of gait). An example of demand-reducing equipment

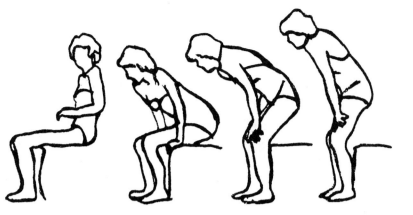

FIGURE 7–8 Line drawing of sit-to-stand technique in which the patient uses the upper extremities on her thighs to achieve standing. (From Butler PB, Nene AV, Major RE: Biomechanics of transfer from sitting to the standing position in some neuromuscular diseases. Physiotherapy 77:521, 1991.)

employed lately with good success, both during application of the equipment and afterward, is a weight-unloading harness during gait on a treadmill.[251–255] The buoyancy of water can also supplement patients' antigravity efforts.[256, 257] During sit to stand, the demand on the lower extremities can be reduced considerably by elevating the height of the seat from which a patient is rising.[258–261]

Arborelius and associates[261] found that the mean maximum knee extension moment was 60% lower when rising from a higher rather than a standard-height seat. Weiner and colleagues[260] reported that when the chair height increased from 17 to 22 inches, the number of nursing home residents in their study who were able to rise successfully nearly doubled. The demand on the lower extremities during sit to stand can also be reduced through the use of arm rests.[261, 262] Pneumatic or spring-loaded seating surfaces, although not used extensively, are capable of reducing the load on the lower extremities during sit to stand.[263, 264]

PROVISION OF ASSISTIVE DEVICES

A variety of assistive devices are available to increase the independence or performance level of patients during functional activities. Entire books have been written on this subject, which has been touched on elsewhere in this chapter and in Chapter 10. This section addresses in a cursory fashion only three categories of devices that can compensate for the reduction in muscle force production that so often accompanies neurologic pathology. The categories are wheelchairs, gait-assistive devices, and lower extremity orthoses.

Wheelchairs

Wheelchairs are often prescribed for patients with extremity and trunk muscle weakness secondary to

neurologic pathology. Even when patients possess enough strength to walk with an assistive device and orthoses, a wheelchair may be safer or more efficient.[265, 266] Patients with severely impaired lower extremity and trunk strength but adequate upper extremity strength can use their upper extremities to propel a wheelchair.[267, 268] Patients with insufficient extremity strength on one side (e.g., after stroke) can use the extremities of their stronger side to propel the chair, although for some hemiparetic patients this is too difficult or impossible.[269, 270] For patients with weakness of all four extremities and the trunk, a powered chair may be best, even if they can manage a standard chair.[271, 272]

Gait-Assistive Devices

Gait-assistive devices (i.e., walkers, crutches, and canes) are the most frequently prescribed of patient aides.[273] They can assist patients with neurologic disorders in two ways: they can increase stability by expanding a patient's base of support, and they can enable a patient to reduce the load placed through a weak lower extremity during stance.

That walkers, crutches, and canes can increase a patient's stability should be self-evident. Needless to say, gait-assistive devices can increase stability only if they are on the ground and the forces applied through them by a patient's upper extremity or extremities are properly directed. Patients with considerable postural instability may benefit from a device that does not have to be lifted to be advanced, that is, a wheeled walker. For patients lacking sufficient upper extremity strength to handle a walker (e.g., those with hemiparesis), a platform can sometimes be attached for the weaker upper extremity (Fig. 7–9). Provision of such a walker for a patient of mine with ataxia and hemiparesis of 30 years' duration resulted

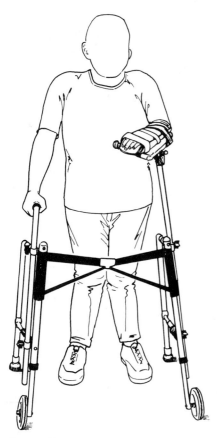

FIGURE 7–9 Line drawing of a patient with hemiparesis using a rolling platform walker.

in her ambulating more than 200 meters without assistance. She was unable to walk even a meter without assistance when using a hemiwalker or quad cane. Crutches and canes can also increase stability.[274, 275] One research study, however, was able to verify a stabilizing effect only while patients stood with canes; increased stability could not be verified during walking.[274] In their investigation of patients with stroke, Milczarek and colleagues[275] found that canes resulted not only in reduced mediolateral and anteroposterior sway but also in a shift in the center of pressure toward the cane side. Contrary to what might be expected, a four-footed cane was no more stabilizing than a single joint cane.

Some patients with neurologic disorders are not able to bear full weight through a weak lower extremity; it lacks sufficient extensor strength to support the weight.[102, 136] Consequently, they cannot advance their contralateral lower extremity. One possible solution to this problem is for the patients to use the upper extremities and an assistive device to unload the weak extremity. Walkers can be used for this purpose, and if the demand

for unloading is not too great, crutches or canes can be used.[276, 277] When crutches or canes are used unilaterally, better unloading is achieved when the device is placed on the side contralateral to the weak lower extremity.[276] Of course, in many cases, it is not possible to do otherwise. After a stroke, for example, many patients would lack sufficient strength in the upper extremity of the weak side to employ a cane or crutch. The degree to which an assistive device can be used to unload a weak lower extremity can be affected by the gait pattern with which it is used.[276]

Lower Extremity Orthoses

Clearly, orthoses are a practical way of compensating for weakness in patients with neurologic disorders. Although not limited in application to the lower extremities, it is there that they are employed most often. Orthoses are used either to stabilize structures with inadequate muscle support or to enable patients to complete or improve patterns of movement with which they are having difficulty. A multicomponent orthosis may accomplish both and can be supplemented with interventions already addressed, such as electrical stimulation.

An obvious example of stabilization is provided by long leg braces, which prevent the knees from giving way while a patient with lower extremity weakness stands or walks.[266, 278–280] An ankle that is unstable due to muscle weakness or imbalance can be stabilized by an orthosis.[281, 282] In patients with instability or inadequate control of both the knee and ankle after stroke, an orthosis with both knee and ankle components can be used to reduce genu recurvatum.[283]

The benefits of orthoses for the completion or improvement of movement patterns is probably most apparent in gait. During the swing phase of normal gait, the non–weight-bearing extremity is functionally shortened and advanced by active hip flexion, knee flexion, and ankle dorsiflexion. One of the most common applications of orthoses is to assist ankle dorsiflexion during swing among patients with stroke. Such assistance improves the mechanics of swing and initial stance as well as cadence, step length, gait speed, ambulatory distance, and oxygen consumption during gait.[281, 282, 284–289]

SUMMARY

Although biomechanics is relevant to the treatment of patients with a variety of pathologies and disorders, the muscle weakness that is so prevalent among patients with neurologic problems makes biomechanics an issue of particular importance in their treatment. This chapter has provided a cursory review of relevant background information as well as a basis for specific interventions to correct or compensate for the weakness that affects the function of patients with neurologic disorders.

References

1. Gajdosik RL, Guiliani CA, Bohannon RW: Passive compliance and length of the hamstring muscle of healthy men and women. Clin Biomech 5:23, 1990.
2. Halar EM, Stolov WC, Venkatesh B, et al: Gastrocnemius muscle belly and tendon length in stroke patients and able-bodies persons. Arch Phys Med Rehabil 59:476, 1978.
3. Tardieu G, Tardieu C: Cerebral palsy: Mechanical evaluation and conservative correction of limb joint contractures. Clin Orthop 219:63, 1987.
4. Tabary JC, Tabary C, Tardieu C, et al: Physiological and structural changes in the cat's soleus muscle due to immobilization at different lengths by plaster casts. J Physiol 224:231, 1972.
5. Goldspink G, Tabary C, Tabary JC, et al: Effect of denervation on the adaptation of sarcomere number and muscle extensibility to the functional length of the muscle. J Physiol 236:733, 1974.
6. Tardieu G, Tardieu C, Colbeau-Justin P, Lespargot A: Muscle hypoextensibility in children with cerebral palsy. II. Therapeutic implications. Arch Phys Med Rehabil 63:103, 1982.
7. Dantes M, McComas A: The extent and time course of motoneuron involvement in amyotrophic lateral sclerosis. Muscle Nerve 14:416, 1991.
8. Bromberg MB, Forshew DA, Nau KL, et al: Motor unit number estimation, isometric strength, and electromyographic measures in amyotrophic lateral sclerosis. Muscle Nerve 16:1213, 1993.
9. Lenman JAR: Quantitative electromyographic changes associated with muscular weakness. J Neurol Neurosurg Psychiatry 22:306, 1959.
10. McComas AJ, Sica REP, Upton ARM, Aguilera N: Functional changes in motoneurons of hemiparetic muscles. J Neurol Neurosurg Psychiatry 36:183, 1973.
11. Edström L, Grimby L, Hannerz J: Correlation between recruitment order of motor units and muscle atrophy pattern in upper motor neuron lesion significance of spasticity. Experentia 29:560, 1973.
12. Jakobsson F, Grimby L, Edström L: Motoneuron activity and muscle fibre type composition in hemiparesis. Scand J Rehabil Med 24: 115, 1992.
13. Brown WF: Negative symptoms and signs of peripheral nerve disease. *In* Brown WF, Bolton CF (eds): Clinical Electromyography, 2nd ed. Boston, Butterworth-Heinemann, 1993, p 95.
14. McComas AJ, Sica REP, Campbell MJ, Upton ARM: Functional compensation in partially denervated muscles. J Neurol Neurosurg Psychiatry 34:453, 1971.
15. Tollbäck A, Borg J, Borg K, Knutsson E: Isokinetic strength, macro EMG and muscle biopsy of paretic foot dorsiflexors in chronic neurogenic paresis. Scand J Rehabil Med 25:183, 1993.
16. Rodriguez AA, Agre JL, Harmon RL, et al: Electromyographic and neuromuscular variables in post-polio subjects. Arch Phys Med Rehabil 76:989, 1995.
17. Stalberg E, Grimby G: Dynamic electromyography and muscle biopsy changes in a 4-year follow-up: Study of patients with a history of polio. Muscle Nerve 18:699, 1995.
18. Miller RG, Sherratt M: Firing rates of human motor units in partially denervated muscle. Neurology 28:1241, 1978.
19. Reiners K, Herdmann J, Freund H-J: Altered mechanisms of muscular force generation in lower motor neuron disease. Muscle Nerve 12:647, 1989.
20. Angel RW: Electromyographic patterns during ballistic movement of normal and spastic limbs. Brain Res 99:387, 1975.
21. Hallett M, Khoshbin S: A physiological mechanism of bradykinesia. Brain 103:301, 1990.
22. Solomonow M, Guzzi A, Baratta R, et al: EMG force model of the elbows antagonistic muscle pair. Am J Phys Med 65:223, 1986.
23. Amiridis IG, Martin A, Morlon B, et al: Co-activation and tension-regulating phenomena during isokinetic knee extension in sedentary and highly skilled humans. Eur J Appl Physiol 73:149, 1996.
24. Little JW, Micklesen P, Umlauf R, Britell C: Lower extremity manifestations of spasticity in chronic spinal cord injury. Am J Phys Med Rehabil 68:32, 1989.
25. Kawamura J, Ise M, Tagami M: The clinical features of spasms in patients with a cervical cord injury. Paraplegia 27:222, 1989.
26. Fowler HL, Warmoth J, Nabizadeh A, Schein-berg L: Rapid conversion from extensor to fixed flexor posture of the lower extremities in multiple sclerosis. J Neurol Rehabil 2:159, 1988.
27. Corcos DM, Gottlieb GL, Penn RD, et al: Movement deficits caused by hyperexcitable stretch reflexes in spastic humans. Brain 109:1043, 1986.
28. Bobath B: Adult Hemiplegia: Evaluation and Treatment, 3rd ed. Oxford, Heinemann Medical Books, 1997.
29. Hammond MC, Fitts SS, Kraft GH, et al: Co-contraction in the hemiparetic forearm quantitative EMG evaluation. Arch Phys Med Rehabil 69:348, 1988.
30. Knutsson E, Måartensson A: Dynamic motor capacity in spastic paresis and its relation to

prime mover dysfunction, spastic reflexes and antagonist co-activation. Scand J Rehabil Med 12:93, 1980.

31. Levin MF, Hui-Chan C: Ankle spasticity is inversely correlated with antagonist voluntary contraction in hemiparetic subjects. Electroenceph Clin Neurophysiol 34:415, 1994.

32. Tang A, Rymer WZ: Abnormal force–EMG relations in paretic limbs of hemiparetic human subjects. J Neurol Neurosurg Psychiatry 44:690, 1981.

33. Fellows SJ, Kaus C, Ross HF, Thilmann AF: Agonist and antagonist EMG activation during isometric torque development at the elbow in spastic hemiparesis. Electroenceph Clin Neurophysiol 93:106, 1994.

34. Fellows SJ, Kaus C, Thilmann AF: Voluntary movement at the elbow in spastic hemiparesis. Ann Neurol 36:397, 1994.

35. Duncan P: The effect of a prior quadriceps contraction on knee flexor torque in normal subjects and multiple sclerosis patients with spastic paraparesis. Physiother Pract 3:11, 1987.

36. Gowland C, de Brain H, Basmajian JV, et al: Agonist and antagonist activity during voluntary upper-limb movement in patients with stroke. Phys Ther 72:624, 1992.

37. Wolf SL, Catlin PA, Blanton S, et al: Overcoming limitations in elbow movement in the presence of antagonist hyperactivity. Phys Ther 74:826, 1994.

38. Bohannon RW, Andrews AW: Limb muscle strength is impaired bilaterally after stroke. J Phys Ther Sci 7:1, 1995.

39. Bohannon RW: Muscle strength changes in hemiparetic stroke patients during inpatient rehabilitation. J Neurol Rehabil 2:163, 1988.

40. Colebatch JG, Gandevia SC: Distribution of muscular weakness in upper motor neuron lesions affecting the arm. Brain 112:749, 1989.

41. Bohannon RW, Cassidy D, Walsh S: Trunk muscle strength is impaired multidirectionally after stroke. Clin Rehabil 9:47, 1995.

42. Tanaka S, Hachisuka K, Ogata H: Trunk rotatory muscle performance in post-stroke hemiplegic patients. Am J Phys Med Rehabil 76:366, 1997.

43. Bohannon RW: Internal consistency of dynamometer measurements in healthy subjects and stroke patients. Percept Motor Skills 81:1113, 1995.

44. Sunderland A, Tinson D, Bradley L, Langton Hewer R: Arm function after stroke: An evaluation of grip strength as a measure of recovery and a prognostic indicator. J Neurol Neurosurg Psychiatry 52:1267, 1989.

45. Bohannon RW, Smith MB: Upper extremity strength deficits in hemiplegic stroke patients: Relationship between admission and discharge and time since onset. Arch Phys Med Rehabil 68:155, 1987.

46. Nakamura R, Watanabe S, Handa T, Morohashi I: The relationship between walking speed and muscle strength for knee extension in hemiparetic stroke patients: A follow up study. Tohoku J Exp Med 154:111, 1988.

47. Bohannon RW: Recovery and correlates of trunk muscle strength after stroke. Int J Rehabil Research 18:162, 1995.

48. Smutok MA, Grafman J, Salazar AM, et al: Effects of unilateral brain damage on contralateral and ipsilateral upper extremity function in hemiplegia. Phys Ther 69:195, 1989.

49. Walker GC, Cardenas DD, Guthrie MR, et al: Fatigue and depression in brain-injured, patients correlated with quadriceps strength and endurance. Arch Phys Med Rehabil 72:467, 1991.

50. Brown JK, van Rensburg F, Walsh G, et al: A neurological study of hand function of hemiplegic children. Dev Med Child Neurol 29:287, 1987.

51. Damiano DL, Vaughan CL, Abel MF: Muscle response to heavy resistance exercise in children with spastic cerebral palsy. Dev Med Child Neurol 37:731, 1995.

52. Brown JK, Rodda J, Walsh EG, Wright GW: Neurophysiology of lower-limb function in hemiplegic children. Dev Med Child Neurol 33:1037, 1991.

53. Van den Berg-Emons RJG, van Baak MA, de Barbanson DC, et al: Reliability of tests to determine peak aerobic power, anaerobic power and isokinetic muscle strength in children with spastic cerebral palsy. Dev Med Child Neurol 38:1117, 1996.

54. Maynard FM, Bracken MB, Creasey G, et al: International standards for neurological and functional classification of spinal cord injury. Spinal Cord 35:226, 1997.

55. Schwartz S, Cohen ME, Herbison GJ, Shah A: Relationship between two measures of upper extremity strength: Manual muscle test compared to hand-held myometry. Arch Phys Med Rehabil 73:1063, 1992.

56. Herbison GJ, Isaac Z, Cohen ME, Ditunno JF: Strength post-spinal cord injury: Myometer vs manual muscle test. Spinal Cord 34:543, 1996.

57. Saboe LA, Darrah JM, Pain KS, Guthrie J: Early predictors of functional independence 2 years after spinal cord injury. Arch Phys Med Rehabil 78:644, 1997.

58. Armstrong LE, Winant DM, Swasey PR, et al: Using isokinetic dynamometry to test ambulatory patients with multiple sclerosis. Phys Ther 63:1274, 1982.

59. Chen W-Y, Pierson FM, Burnett CN: Force-time measurements of knee muscle functions of subjects with multiple sclerosis. Phys Ther 67:934, 1987.

60. Ponichtera TA, Rodgers MM, Glaser RM, et al: Concentric and eccentric isokinetic lower extremity strength in persons with multiple sclerosis. J Orthop Sports Phys Ther 16:114, 1992.

61. Andres PL, Finison LJ, Conlon T, et al: Use of composite scores (megascores) to measure deficit

in amyotrophic lateral sclerosis. Neurology 38:405, 1988.

62. Scott OM, Hyde SA, Goddard C, Dubowitz V: Quantitation of muscle function in children: A prospective study in Duchenne muscular dystrophy. Muscle Nerve 5:291, 1982.

63. Allsop KG, Ziter FA: Loss of strength and functional decline in Duchenne's dystrophy. Arch Neurol 38:406, 1981.

64. Griggs RC, Moxley RT, Mandell JR, et al: Prednisone in Duchenne dystrophy: A randomized controlled trial defining the time course and dose response. Arch Neurol 48:383, 1991.

65. Amundsen LR, Graves JM: Testing knee extensor muscles of survivors of poliomyelitis. J Hum Muscle Perform 1:25, 1991.

66. Agre JC, Rodriguez AA: Neuromuscular function: Comparison of symptomatic and asymptomatic polio subjects to control subjects. Arch Phys Med Rehabil 71:545, 1990.

67. Munin MC, Jaweed M, Staas WE, et al: Post poliomyelitis muscle weakness: A prospective study of quadriceps strength. Arch Phys Med Rehabil 72:729, 1991.

68. Andersson T, Sidén A: A clinical study of the Guillain-Barré syndrome. Acta Neurol Scand 66:316, 1982.

69. Koller W, Kase S: Muscle strength testing in Parkinson's disease. Eur Neurol 25:130, 1986.

70. Pedersen SW, Öberg B: Dynamic strength in Parkinson's disease. Eur Neurol 33:97, 1993.

71. Pedersen SW, Öberg B, Larsson L-E, Lindval B: Gait analysis, isokinetic muscle strength measurement in patients with Parkinson's disease. Scand J Rehabil Med 29:67, 1997.

72. Corcos DM, Chen C-M, Quinn NP, et al: Strength in Parkinson's disease: Relationship to rate of force generation and clinical status. Ann Neurol 39:79, 1996.

73. Bridgewater KJ, Sharpe MH: Trunk muscle training and early Parkinson's disease. Physiother Theory Pract 13:139, 1997.

74. Bohannon RW, Walsh S: Nature reliability, and predictive value of muscle performance measures in patients with hemiparesis following stroke. Arch Phys Med Rehabil 73:721, 1992.

75. Tsuji I, Nakamura R: The altered time course of tension development during the initiation of fast movement in hemiplegic patients. Tohoku J Exp Med 151:137, 1987.

76. Wierzbicka MM, Wiegner AW, Logigian EL, Young RR: Abnormal most-rapid isometric contractions in patients with Parkinson's disease. J Neurol Neurosurg Psychiatry 54:210, 1991.

77. Bohannon RW, Walsh S: Relationship between isometric torque and velocity of knee extension following stroke with hemiparesis. J Hum Muscle Performance 1:40, 1991.

78. Davies JM, Mayston MJ, Newhan DJ: Electrical and mechanical output of the knee muscles during isometric and isokinetic activity in stroke and healthy adults. Disabil Rehabil 18:83, 1996.

79. Wyke M: Effect of brain lesions on the rapidity of arm movement. Neurology 17:1113, 1967.

80. Baroni A, Benvenuti F, Fantini L, et al: Human ballistic arm abduction movements: Effects of L-dopa treatment in Parkinson's disease. Neurology 34:868, 1984.

81. Godaux E, Koulischer D, Jacquy J: Parkinsonian bradykinesia is due to depression in rate of rise of muscle activity. Ann Neurol 31:93, 1992.

82. Wierzbicka MM, Wiegner AW: Effects of weak antagonist on elbow flexion movements in man. Exp Brain Res 91:509, 1992.

83. Milner-Brown HS, Miller RG: Increased muscular fatigue in patients with neurogenic muscle weakness: Quantification and pathophysiology. Arch Phys Med Rehabil 70:361, 1989.

84. Lenman AJR, Tulley FM, Vrbova G, et al: Muscle fatigue in some neurological disorders. Muscle Nerve 12:938, 1989.

85. Miller RG, Green AT, Moussavi RS, et al: Excessive muscular fatigue in patients with spastic paraparesis. Neurology 40:1271, 1990.

86. Checchia GA, Gionnone F, Miccoli B, et al: Iso-kinetic testing of muscular function and fatigue in patients with multiple sclerosis. Isokinetics Exercise Science 3:101, 1993.

87. Bohannon RW: Relative dynamic muscular endurance of patients with neuromuscular disorders and of healthy matched control subjects. Phys Ther 67:18, 1987.

88. Zelaschi F, Felicetti G: Functional isokinetic parameters in the hemiparetic patient: Training efficacy. Isokinetics Exercise Science 5:25, 1995.

89. Cameron T, Calancie B: Mechanical and fatigue properties of wrist flexor muscles during repetitive contractions after cervical spinal cord injury. Arch Phys Med Rehabil 76:929, 1995.

90. Walker GC, Cardenas DD, Guthrie MR, et al: Fatigue and depression in brain-injured patients correlated with quadriceps strength and endurance. Arch Phys Med Rehabil 72:469, 1991.

91. Sale D: Testing strength and power. In MacDougall JD, Wenger HA, Green HJ (eds): Physiological Testing of the High-Performance Athlete, 2nd ed. Champaign, IL, Human Kinetics, 1991, pp 22–24.

92. Olsen TS: Arm and leg paresis as outcome predictors in stroke rehabiliation. Stroke 21:247, 1990.

93. Friedman PJ: The star cancellation test in acute stroke. Clin Rehabil 6:23, 1992.

94. Friedman PJ, Davis G, Allen B: Semi-quantitative SPECT scanning in acute ischaemic stroke. Scand J Rehabil Med 25:99, 1993.

95. Stone SP, Patel P, Greenwood RJ: Selection of acute stroke patients for treatment of visual neglect. J Neurol Neurosurg Psychiatry 56:463, 1993.

96. Logigian MK, Samuels MA, Falcover J, Zagar R: Clinical exercise trial for stroke patients. Arch Phys Med Rehabil 64:364, 1983.

97. Friedman PJ: Spatial neglect in acute stroke: the line bisection test. Scand J Rehabil Med 22:101, 1990.

98. Abdulwahab SS: Physical disability in patients with hemiparesis. Int J Rehabil Res 19:157, 1996.

99. Segboer SHAM, Terpstra-Lindeman E, Buitenhuis M, Adam JJ: Spastic paresis. I. Relationship between impairment and disability. J Rehabil Sci 6:3, 1993.

100. Lazar RB, Yarkony GM, Ortolano P, et al: Prediction of functional outcome by motor capability after spinal cord injury. Arch Phys Med Rehabil 70:819, 1989.

101. Marino RJ, Huang M, Knight P, et al: Assessing selfcare status in quadriplegia: A comparison of quadriplegia index of function (QIF) and the functional independence measure (FIM). Paraplegia 31:225, 1993.

102. Bohannon RW: Relationship among paretic knee extension strength, maximum weight bearing, and gait speed in patients with stroke. J Stroke Cerebrovasc Dis 1:65, 1991.

103. Nakamura R, Hosokawa T, Tsuji I: Relationship of muscle strength for knee extension to walking capacity in patients with spastic hemiparesis. Tohoku J Exp Med 145:335, 1995.

104. Suzuki K, Nakamura R, Yamada Y, Handa T: Determinants of maximum walking speed in hemiparetic stroke patients. Tohoku J Exp Med 162:337, 1990.

105. Bohannon RW: Knee extension power, velocity, and torque: Relative deficits and relation to walking performance in stroke patients. Clin Rehabil 6:125, 1992.

106. Bohannon RW: Knee extension force measurements are reliable and indicative of walking speed in stroke patients. Int J Rehabil Res 12:193, 1989.

107. Bohannon RW, Andrews AW: Correlation of knee extensor muscle torque and spasticity with gait speed in patients with stroke. Arch Phys Med Rehabil 70:330, 1990.

108. Bohannon RW: Selected determinants of ambulatory capacity in patients with hemiplegia. Clin Rehabil 3:47, 1989.

109. Agre JC, Findley TW, McNally MC, et al: Physical activity in children with myelomeningocele. Arch Phys Med Rehabil 68:372, 1987.

110. Waters RL, Adkins R, Yakura J, Vigil D: Prediction of ambulatory performance based on motor scores derived from standards of the American Spinal Injury Association. Arch Phys Med Rehabil 75:756, 1994.

111. Waters RL, Yakura JS, Adkins R, Barnes G: Determinants of gait performance following spinal cord injury. Arch Phys Med Rehabil 70:811, 1980.

112. Waters RL, Yakura JS, Adkins RH: Gait performance after spinal cord injury. Clin Orthop 288:87, 1993.

113. Perry J, Mulroy SJ, Renwick SE: The relationship of lower extremity strength and gait parameters in patients with post-polio syndrome. Arch Phys Med Rehabil 74:165, 1993.

114. Bohannon RW: Determinants of transfer capacity in patients with hemiparesis. Physiother Can 40:236, 1988.

115. Bohannon RW: Rolling to the nonplegic side: Influence of teaching and limb strength in hemiplegic stroke patients. Clin Rehabil 2:215, 1988.

116. Welch RD, Lobley SJ, O'Sullivan SB, Freed MM: Functional independence in quadriplegia: Critical levels. Arch Phys Med Rehabil 67:235, 1986.

117. Bohannon RW: Determinants of patient gown donning performance soon after stroke. Eur J Phys Med Rehabil 2:70, 1992.

118. Bohannon RW, Walsh S: Association of paretic lower extremity muscle strength and balance with stair climbing ability in patients with stroke. J Stroke Cerebrovasc Dis 1:129, 1991.

119. Tupling SJ, Davis GM, Pierrynowski R, Shepard RJ: Arm strength and impulse generation: Initiation of wheelchair movement by the physically disabled. Ergonomics 29:303, 1986.

120. Shima H: A study of key muscles for wheelchair driving in quadriplegics. J Phys Ther Sci 9:43, 1997.

121. Hesse S, Schauer M, Malezic M, et al: Quantitative analysis of rising from a chair in healthy and hemiparetic subjects. Scand J Rehabil Med 26:161, 1994.

122. Yoshida K, Iwakura H, Inoue F: Motion analysis in the movements of standing up from and sitting down on a chair. Scand J Rehabil Med 15:133, 1983.

123. Engardt M, Olsson E: Body weight-bearing while rising and sitting down in patients with stroke. Scand J Rehabil Med 24:67, 1992.

124. Engardt M, Ribbe T, Olsson E: Vertical ground reaction force feedback to enhance stroke patients' symmetrical body-weight distribution while rising/sitting down. Scand J Rehabil Med 25:41, 1993.

125. Fowler V, Carr J: Auditory feedback: Effects on vertical force production during standing up following stroke. Int J Rehabil Res 19:265, 1996.

126. Engardt M: Long term effects of auditory feedback training on relearned symmetrical body weight distribution in stroke patients. Scand J Rehabil Med 26:65, 1994.

127. Bohannon RW, Larkin PA: Lower extremity weight bearing under various standing conditions in independently ambulatory patients with hemiparesis. Phys Ther 65:1323, 1985.

128. Waldron RM, Bohannon RW: Weight distribution when standing: The influence of a single point cane in patients with stroke. Physiother Pract 5:171, 1989.

129. Caldwell C, MacDonald D, MacNeil K, et al: Symmetry of weight distribution in normals and stroke patients using digital weigh scales. Physiother Pract 2:109, 1986.

130. Arcan M, Brull MA, Najenson T, Solzi P: FGP assessment of postural disorders during the process of rehabilitation. Scand J Rehabil Med 9:165, 1977.

131. Dickstein R, Nissan M, Pillar T, Scheer D: Foot-ground pressure pattern of standing hemiplegic patients. Phys Ther 64:19, 1984.

132. Bohannon RW, Waldron RM: Weightbearing during comfortable stance in patients with stroke: Accuracy and reliability of measurements. Aust J Physiother 37:19, 1991.

133. Bohannon RW, Tinti-Wald D: Accuracy of weightbearing estimation by stroke versus healthy subjects. Percept Motor Skills 72:935, 1991.

134. Goldie P, Evans O, Matyas T: Performance in the stability limits test during rehabilitation following stroke. Gait Posture 4:315, 1996.

135. Turnbull GI, Charteris J, Wall JC: Deficiencies in standing weight shifts by ambulant hemiplegic subjects. Arch Phys Med Rehabil 77:356, 1996.

136. Goldie PA, Matyas TA, Evans OM, et al: Maximum voluntary weightbearing by the affected and unaffected legs in standing following stroke. Clin Biomech 11:333, 1996.

137. Brunt D, Lafferty MJ, McKeon A, et al: Invariant characteristics of gait initiation. Am J Phys Med Rehabil 70:206, 1991.

138. Rogers MW, Pai YC: Dynamic transitions in stance support accompanying leg flexion movements in man. Exp Brain Res 81:398, 1990.

139. Rogers MW, Hedman LD, Pai Y-C: Kinetic analysis of dynamic transitions in stance support accompanying voluntary leg flexion movements in hemiparetic adults. Arch Phys Med Rehabil 74:19, 1993.

140. Von Schroeder HP, Coutts RD, Lyden PD, et al: Gait parameters following stroke: A practical assessment. J Rehabil Res Devel 32:25, 1995.

141. Pai Y-C, Rogers MW, Hedman LD, Hanke TA: Alterations in weight-transfer capabilities in adults with hemiparesis. Phys Ther 74:647, 1994.

142. Perry J, Ireland ML, Gronley J, Hoffer MM: Predictive value of manual muscle testing of gait analysis in normal ankles by dynamic electromyography. Foot Ankle 6:254, 1986.

143. Miyashita M, Matsui H, Miura M: The relation between electrical activity in muscle and speed of walking and running. Medicine and Sport: Biomechanics II 6:192, 1971.

144. Winter DA: Energy generation and absorption at the ankle and knee during fast, natural and slow cadences. Clin Orthop 175:147, 1983.

145. Winter DA, White SC: Cause-effect correlations of variables of gait. In Jonsson B (ed): Biomechanics X—A. Champaign, IL, Human Kinetics, 1987, p 363.

146. Siegler KL, Stanhope SJ, Caldwell GE: Kinematic and kinetic adaptations in the lower limb during stance in gait of unilateral femoral neuropathy patients. Clin Biomech 8:147, 1993.

147. Kramers de Quervain IA, Simon SR, Leurgans S, et al: Gait pattern in the early recovery period after stroke. J Bone Joint Surg 78-A:1506, 1996.

148. Sutherland DH, Cooper L, Daniel D: The role of ankle plantar flexors in normal walking. J Bone Joint Surg 62A:354, 1980.

149. Olney SJ, Griffin MP, Monga TN, McBride ID: Work and power in gait of stroke patients. Arch Phys Med 72:309, 1991.

150. Olney SJ, Griffin MP, McBride ID: Temporal, Kinematic and kinetic variables related to gait speed in subjects with hemiplegia: A regression approach. Phys Ther 74:872, 1994.

151. Hesse SA, Jahnke MT, Schreiner C, Mauritz K-H: Gait symmetry and functional walking performance in hemiparetic patients prior to and after a 4-week rehabilitation programme. Gait Posture 1:166, 1993.

152. Carlsöö S, Dahlöf A-G, Holm J: Kinetic analysis of the gait in patients with hemiparesis and in patients with intermittent claudication. Scand J Rehabil Med 6:166, 1974.

153. Nilsson J, Thorstensson A: Ground reaction forces at different speeds of human walking and running. Acta Physiol Scand 136:217, 1989.

154. Morita S, Yamomoto H, Furuya K: Gait analysis of hemiparetic patients by measurement of ground reaction force. Scand J Rehabil Med 27:37, 1995.

155. Ueno E, Yanagisawa N, Takami M: Gait disorders in Parkinsonism: A study with floor reaction forces and emg. Adv Neurol 60:414, 1993.

156. Lunnen JD, Yack J, LeVeau BF: Relationship between muscle length, muscle activity and torque of the hamstring muscles. Phys Ther 61:190, 1981.

157. Bohannon RW, Reed ML, Gajdosik R: Electrically evoked knee flexion torque increases with increased pelvifemoral angles. Clin Biomech 5:23, 1990.

158. Bohannon W: Decreased isometric knee flexion torque with hip extension in hemiparetic patients. Phys Ther 66:521, 1986.

159. Bohannon RW, Gajdosik RL, LeVeau BF: Relationship of pelvic and thigh motions during unilateral and bilateral hip flexion. Phys Ther 65:1501, 1985.

160. Komi PV: Physiological and biomechanical correlates of muscle function: Effects of muscle structure and stretch-shortening cycle on force and speed. Exerc Sport Sci Rev 12:81, 1984.

161. Svantesson U, Sunnerhagen KS: Stretch-shortening cycle in patients with upper motor neuron lesions due to stroke. Eur J Appl Physiol 75:312, 1997.

162. Wretenberg P, Arborelius UP: Power and work produced in different leg muscle groups when rising from a chair. Eur J Appl Physiol 68:413, 1994.

163. Voss DE, Ionta MK, Myers BJ: Proprioceptive Neuromuscular Facilitation, 3rd ed. Philadelphia, Harper & Row, 1985, pp 293–294.

164. Bohannon RW: Hemiparetic elbow flexion force

production before and after muscle belly tapping. Neurol Report 11:75, 1987.

165. Liberson WT, Holmquest HJ, Scott D, Dow M: Functional electrotherapy: Stimulation of the peroneal nerve synchronized with the swing phase of the gait of hemiplegic patients. Arch Phys Med Rehabil 42:101, 1961.

166. Granat MH, Maxwell DJ, Ferguson ACB, et al: Peroneal stimulator: Evaluation for the correction of spastic drop foot in hemiplegia. Arch Phys Med Rehabil 77:19, 1996.

167. Burridge JH, Taylor PN, Hagan SA, et al: The effects of common peroneal stimulation on the effort and speed of waling a randomized controlled trial with chronic hemiplegic patients. Clin Rehabil 11:201, 1997.

168. Stanič U, Ačimović-Janežič R. Gros N, et al: Multichannel electrical stimulation for correction of hemiplegic gait. Scand J Rehabil Med 10:75, 1978.

169. Faghri PD, Rodgers MM, Glaser RM, et al: The effects of functional electrical stimulation on shoulder subluxation, arm function recovery, and shoulder pain in hemiplegic stroke patients. Arch Phys Med Rehabil 75:73, 1994.

170. Merletti R, Acimovic R, Grobelnik S, Cvilak G: Electrophysiological orthosis for the upper extremity in hemiplegia: Feasibility study. Arch Phys Med Rehabil 56:507, 1975.

171. Bajd T, Kralj A, Turk R: Standing-up of a healthy subject and a paraplegic patient. J Biomech 15:1, 1982.

172. Ewins DJ, Taylor PN, Crook SE, et al: Practical low cost stand/sit system for mid-thoracic paraplegics. J Biomed Eng 10:184, 1988.

173. Jaeger RJ, Yarkony GM, Smith RM: Standing the spinal cord injured patient by electrical stimulation: Refinement of a protocol for clinical use. TEEE Trans Biomed Eng 36:720, 1989.

174. Marsolais EB, Kobetic R: Functional walking in paralyzed patients by means of electrical stimulation. Clin Orthop 175:30, 1983.

175. Bajd T, Kralj A, Turk K, et al: The use of a four-channel electrical stimulator as an ambulatory aid for paraplegic patients. Phys Ther 63:1116, 1983.

176. Petrofsky JS, Heaton H, Phillips CA: Outdoor bicycle for exercise in paraplegics and quadriplegics. J Biomed Eng 5:292, 1983.

177. Bajd T, Štafančič M, Matjacic Z, et al: Improvement in step clearance via calf muscle stimulation. Med Biol Eng Comput 35:113, 1997.

178. Shropshire BM, Broton JG, Cameron TL, Klose KJ: Improved motor function in tetraplegics following neuromuscular stimulation assisted arm ergometry. J Spinal Cord Med 20:49, 1997.

179. Hagbarth KE, Eklund G: The muscle vibrator: A useful tool in neurologic therapeutic work. Scand J Rehabil Med 1:26, 1969.

180. Knutsson E, Lindblom U, Odeen I: Reflex facilitation by muscle vibration in the treatment of spastic hemiparesis. Scand J Rehabil Med 2–3:110, 1970.

181. Matyas TA, Galea MP, Spicer SD: Facilitation of the maximum voluntary contraction in hemiplegia by concomitant cutaneous stimulation. Am J Phys Med 65:125, 1986.

182. Neeman RL, Neeman M: Efficacy of orthokinetic orthotics for post-stroke upper extremity hemiparetic motor dysfunction. Int J Rehabil Res 16:302, 1993.

183. Neeman RL, Neeman HJ, Neeman M: Application of orthokinetic orthoses in habilitation of a person with upper extremity in coordination secondary to spastic quadriplegia due to cerebral palsy. Can J Rehabil 1:145, 1988.

184. Blashy MRM, Fuchs-Neeman RL: Orthokinetics: A new receptor facilitation method. Am J Occup Ther 13:226, 1959.

185. Inaba M, Edberg E, Montgomery J, Gillis MK: Effectiveness of functional training, active exercise, and resistive exercise for patients with hemiplegia. Phys Ther 53:28, 1973.

186. Bütefisch C, Hummelsheim H, Denzler P, Mauritz K-H: Repetitive training of isolated movements improves the outcome of motor rehabilitation of the centrally paretic hand. J Neurol Sci 130:59, 1995.

187. Sharp SA, Brouwer BJ: Isokinetic strength training of the hemiparetic knee: Effects on function and spasticity. Arch Phys Med Rehabil 78:1231, 1997.

188. Engardt M, Knutsson E, Jonsson M, Sternhag M: Dynamic muscle strength training in stroke patients: Effects on knee extension torque electromyographic activity, and motor function. Arch Phys Med Rehabil 76:419, 1995.

189. Knutsson E, Gransberg L, Måartensson A: Facilitation and inhibition of maximal voluntary contractions by the activation of muscle stretch reflexes in patients with spastic paresis. Electroenceph Clin Neurophysiol 70:37P, 1988.

190. MacPhail HEA, Kramer JF: Effect of isokinetic strength-training on functional ability and walking efficiency in adolescents with cerebral palsy. Dev Med Child Neurol 37:763, 1995.

191. Horvat M: Effects of a progressive resistance training program on an individual with spastic cerebral palsy. Am Corr Ther J 41:7, 1987.

192. McCubbin JA, Shasby GB: Effects of isokinetic exercise on adolescents with cerebral palsy. Adapt Phys Act Q 2:56, 1985.

193. Damiano DL, Kelly LE, Vaughn CL: Effects of quadriceps femoris muscle strengthening on crouch gait in children with spastic diplegia. Phys Ther 75:658, 1995.

194. O'Connell DG, Barnhart R: Improvement in wheelchair propulsion in pediatric wheelchair users through resistance training: A pilot study. Arch Phys Med Rehabil 76:368, 1995.

195. Gersten JW: Isometric exercises in the paraplegic and in the patient with weakness of quadriceps and hamstrings. Arch Phys Med Rehabil 42:498, 1961.

196. Davis GM, Shephard RJ: Strength training for wheelchair users. Br J Sports Med 24:25, 1990.

197. McCartney N, Moroz D, Garner SH, McComas AJ: The effects of strength training in patients with selected neuromuscular disorders. Med Sci Sports Exerc 20:362, 1988.

198. DeLorme TL, Schwab RS, Watkins AL: The response of the quadriceps femoris to progressive resistance exercises in poliomyelitic patients. J Bone Joint Surg 30A:834, 1948.

199. Fillyaw MJ, Badger GJ, Goodwin GD, et al: The effects of long-term non-fatiguing resistance exercise in subjects with post-polio syndrome. Orthopedics 14:1253, 1991.

200. Agre JC, Rodriguez AA, Franke TM, et al: Low-intensity, alternate-day exercise improves muscle performance without apparent adverse affect in postpolio patients. Am J Phys Med Rehabil 75:50, 1996.

201. Spector SA, Lemmer JT, Koffman BM, et al: Safety and efficacy of strength training in patients with sporadic inclusion body myositis. Muscle Nerve 20:1242, 1997.

202. Wolf SL, Edwards DI, Shutter LA: Concurrent assessment of muscle activity (CAMA): A procedural approach to assess treatment goals. Phys Ther 66:218, 1986.

203. Bohannon RW: Electromyographic activity of the quadriceps femoris muscles during four activities in stroke rehabilitation. Int J Rehabil Res 13:80, 1990.

204. Augustsson J, Esko A, Thomee R, Svantesson U: Weight training of the thigh muscles using closed versus open kinetic chain exercises: A comparison of performance enhancement. J Orthop Sports Phys Ther 27:3, 1998.

205. Sale DG, Martin JE, Moroz DE: Hypertrophy without increased isometric strength after weight training. Eur J Appl Physiol 64:51, 1992.

206. Behm DG, Sale DG: Intended rather than actual movement velocity determines velocity-specific training response. J Appl Physiol 74:359, 1993.

207. Olney BW, Williams PF, Meneleus MB: Treatment of spastic equinus by aponeurosis lengthening. J Pediatr Orthop 8:422, 1988.

208. Matsuo T, Hara H, Tada S: Selective lengthening of the psoas and rectus femoris and preservation of the iliacus for flexion deformity of the hip in cerebral palsy patients. J Pediatr Orthop 7:690, 1987.

209. Reimers J: Functional changes in the antagonists after lengthening the agonists in cerebral palsy. I. Triceps surae lengthening. Clin Orthop 253:30, 1990.

210. Reimers J: Functional changes in the antagonists after lengthening the agonists in cerebral palsy. II. Quadriceps strength before and after distal hamstring lengthening. Clin Orthop 253:35, 1990.

211. Conine TA, Sullivan T, Mackie T, Goodman M: Effect of serial casting for the prevention of equinus in patients with acute head injury. Arch Phys Med Rehabil 71:310, 1990.

212. Moseley AM: The effect of casting combined with stretching on passive ankle dorsiflexion in adults with traumatic head injuries. Phys Ther 77:240, 1997.

213. Bohannon RW, Larkin PA: Passive ankle dorsiflexion increases in patients after a regimen of tilt table-wedge board standing. Phys Ther 65:1676, 1985.

214. Light KE, Nuzik S, Personius W, Barstrom A: Low-load prolonged stretch vs high-load brief stretch in treating knee contractures. Phys Ther 64:330, 1984.

215. Odéen I: Reduction of muscular hypertonus by long-term muscle stretch. Scand J Rehabil Med 13:93, 1981.

216. Keenan MA: Management of the spastic upper extremity in the neurologically impaired adult. Clin Orthop 233:116, 1988.

217. Petrillo CR, Knoploch S: Phenol block of the tibial nerve for spasticity: A long-term follow-up study. Int Disabil Studies 10:97, 1988.

218. Pierson SH, Katz DI, Tarsy D: Botulinum toxin in the treatment of spasticity: Functional implications and patient selection. Arch Phys Med Rehabil 77:717, 1996.

219. Bhakta BB, Cozens JA, Bamford JM, Chamberlain MA: Use of botulinum toxin in stroke patients with severe upper limb spasticity. J Neurol Neurosurg Psychiatry 61:30, 1996.

220. Reiter F, Danni M, Ceravolo MG, Provinciali L: Disability changes after treatment of upper limb spasticity with botulinum toxin. J Neurol Rehabil 10:47, 1996.

221. Corry IS, Cosgrove AD, Walsh EG, et al: Botulinum toxin A in the hemiplegic upper limb: A double-blind trial. Dev Med Child Neurol 39:185, 1997.

222. Dunne JW, Heye N, Dunne SL: Treatment of chronic limb spasticity with botulinum toxin A. J Neurol Neurosurg Psychiatry 58:232, 1995.

223. Hesse S, Friedrich H, Domasch C, Mauritz K-H: Botulinum toxin therapy for upper limb flexor spasticity: Preliminary results. J Rehabil Sci 5:98, 1992.

224. Féve A, Decq P, Filipetti P, et al: Physiological effects of selective tibial neurotony on lower limb spasticity. J Neurol Neurosurg Psychiatry 63:575, 1997.

225. Steinbok P, Reiner AM, Beauchamp R, et al: A randomized clinical trial to compare selective posterior rhizotomy plus physiotherapy with physiotherapy alone in children with spastic diplegic cerebral palsy. Dev Med Child Neurol 39:178, 1997.

226. Thomas SS, Aiona MD, Buckon CE, Piatt JH: Does gait continue to improve 2 years after selective dorsal rhizotomy? J Pediatr Orthop 17:387, 1997.

227. Levin MF, Hui Chan CWY: Relief of hemiparetic spasticity by TENS is associated with improvement in reflex and voluntary motor functions. Electroenceph Clin Neurophysiol 85:131, 1992.

228. Merletti R, Zelaschi F, Latella D, et al: A control study of muscle force recovery in hemiparetic

patients during treatment with functional electrical stimulation. Scand J Rehabil Med 10:147, 1978.

229. Smith LE: Restoration of volitional limb movement of hemiplegics following patterned functional electrical stimulation. Percept Motor Skills 71:851, 1990.

230. Lagassé PP, Roy M-A: Functional electrical stimulation and the reduction of co-contraction in spastic biceps brachii. Clin Rehabil 3:111, 1989.

231. Winchester P, Montgomery J, Bowman B, Hislop H: Effects of feedback stimulation training and cyclical electrical stimulation on knee extension in hemiparetic patients. Phys Ther 63:1096, 1983.

232. Bowman BR, Baker LL, Waters RL: Positional feedback and electrical stimulation: An automated treatment for the hemiplegic wrist. Arch Phys Med Rehabil 60:497, 1979.

233. Hazlewood ME, Brown JK, Rowe PJ, Salter PM: The use of therapeutic electrical stimulation in the treatment of hemiplegic cerebral palsy. Dev Med Child Neurol 36:661, 1994.

234. Pape KE, Kirsch SE, Galil A, et al: Neuromuscular approach to the motor deficits of cerebral palsy: A pilot study. J Pediatr Orthop 13:628, 1993.

235. Barr FMD, Moffat B, Bayley JIL, Middleton FRI: Evaluation of the effects of functional electrical stimulation on muscle power and spasticity in spinal cord injured patients. Clin Rehabil 3:17, 1989.

236. Rabischong E, Ohanna F: Effects of functional electrical stimulation (FES) on evoked muscular output in paraplegic quadriceps muscle. Paraplegia 30:467, 1992.

237. Farragher D, Kidd GL, Tallis R: Eutrophic electrical stimulation for Bell's Palsy. Clin Rehabil 1:265, 1987.

238. Naeser MA, Alexander MP, Stiassny-Eder D, et al: Acupuncture in the treatment of hand paresis in chronic and acute stroke patients: Improvement observed in all cases. Clin Rehabil 8:127, 1994.

239. Naeser MA, Alexander MP, Stiassny-Eder D, et al: Real versus sham acupuncture in the treatment of paralysis in acute stroke patients: A CT scan lesion site study. J Neurol Rehabil 6:163, 1992.

240. Magnusson M, Johansson K, Johansson BB: Sensory stimulation promotes normalization of postural control after stroke. Stroke 25:1176, 1994.

241. Kjendahl A, Sällström S, Østen PE, et al: A one year follow-up study on the effects of acupuncture in the treatment of stroke patients in the subacute stage: A randomized, controlled study. Clin Rehabil 11:192, 1997.

242. Johansson K, Lindgren I, Widner H, et al: Can sensory stimulation improve the functional outcome in stroke patients? Neurology 43:2189, 1993.

243. Schleenbaker RE, Mainous AG: Electromyographic biofeedback for neuromuscular reeducation in the hemiplegic stroke patient: A meta analysis. Arch Phys Med Rehabil 74:1301, 1993.

244. Glanz M, Klawansky S, Stason W, et al: Biofeedback therapy in post stroke rehabilitation: A meta-analysis of the randomized controlled trials. Arch Phys Med Rehabil 76:508, 1995.

245. Intiso D, Santilli V, Grasso MG, et al: Rehabilitation of walking with electromyographic biofeedback in footdrop after stroke. Stroke 25:1189, 1994.

246. Marciello MA, Herbison GJ, Cohen ME, Schmidt R: Elbow extension using anterior deltoids and upper pectorals in spinal cord-injured subjects. Arch Phys Med Rehabil 76:426, 1995.

247. Bergström EMK, Frankel HL, Galer IAR, et al: Physical ability in relation to anthropometric measurements in persons with complete spinal cord lesion below the sixth cervical segment. Int Rehabil Med 7:51, 1985.

248. Butler PB, Nene AV, Major RE: Biomechanics of transfer from sitting to the standing position in some neuromuscular diseases. Physiotherapy 77:521, 1991.

249. Griffiths RD: Controlling weight in muscle disease to reduce the burden. Physiotherapy 75:190, 1989.

250. Edwards RHT, Round JM, Jackson MJ, et al: Weight reduction in boys with muscular dystrophy. Dev Med Child Neurol 26:384, 1984.

251. Pillar T, Dickstein R, Smolinski Z: Walking reeducation with partial relief of body weight in rehabilitation of patients with locomotor disabilities. J Rehabil Res 28:47, 1991.

252. Visintin M, Barbeau H: The effects of parallel bars, body weight support and speed on the modulation of the locomotor pattern of spastic paretic gait: A preliminary communication. Paraplegia 32:540, 1994.

253. Hesse S, Helm B, Krajnik J, et al: Treadmill training with partial body weight support: Influence of body weight release on the gait of hemiparetic patients. J Neurol Rehabil 11:15, 1997.

254. Hesse S, Bertelt C, Jahnke MT, et al: Treadmill training with partial body weight support compared with physiotherapy in nonambulatory hemiparetic patients. Stroke 26:976, 1995.

255. Hesse S, Bertelt C, Schaffrin A, et al: Restoration of gait in nonambulatory hemiparetic patients by treadmill training with partial body weight support. Arch Phys Med Rehabil 75:1087, 1994.

256. Harrison R, Bulstrode S: Percentage of weightbearing during partial immersion in the hydrotherapy pool. Physiother Pract 3:60, 1987.

257. Harrison R, Hillman M, Bulstrode S: Loading of the lower limb when walking partially immersed implications for clinical practice. Physiotherapy 78:164, 1992.

258. Burdett RG, Habasevich R, Pisciotta J, Simon

SR: Biomechanical comparison of rising from two types of chairs. Phys Ther 65:1177, 1985.

259. Finlay OE, Bayles TB, Rosen C, Milling J: Effects of chair design, age and cognitive status on mobility. Age Ageing 12:329, 1983.

260. Weiner DK, Long R, Hughes MA, et al: When older adults face the chair-rise challenge. J Am Geriatr Soc 41:6, 1993.

261. Arborelius UP, Wretenberg P, Lindberg F: The effects of armrests and high seat heights on lower limb joint load and muscular activity during sitting and rising. Ergonomics 11:1377, 1992.

262. Wretenberg P, Lindberg F, Arborelius UP: Effect of armrests and different ways of using them on hip and knee load during rising. Clin Biomech 8:95, 1993.

263. Wretenberg P, Arborelius UP, Lindberg F: The effects of a pneumatic stool and a one-legged stool or lower limb joint load and muscular activity during sitting and rising. Ergonomics 36:519, 1993.

264. Wretenberg P, Arborelius UP, Weidenhelm L, Lindberg F: Rising from a chair by a spring-loaded flap seat: A biomechanical analysis. Scand J Rehabil Med 25:153, 1993.

265. Thomas L, Fewell E, Walker JM: Energy cost of walking and of wheelchair propulsion by children with myelodysplasia: Comparison with normal children. Dev Med Child Neurol 25:617, 1983.

266. Hawran S, Biering-Sorensen F: The use of long leg calipers for paraplegic patients: A follow-up study of patients discharged 1973–82. Spinal Cord 34:666, 1996.

267. Harburn LK, Spaulding SJ: Muscle activity in spinal cord-injured during wheelchair ambulation. Am J Occup Ther 40:629, 1986.

268. Mulroy SJ, Gronley JK, Newsam CJ, Perry J: Electromyographic activity of shoulder muscles during wheelchair propulsion by paraplegic persons. Arch Phys Med Rehabil 77:187, 1996.

269. Blower P: The advantages of the early use of wheelchairs in the treatment of hemiplegia. Clin Rehabil 2:323, 1988.

270. Blower PW, Carter LC, Sulch DA: Relation between wheelchair propulsion and independent walking in hemiplegic stroke. Stroke 26:606, 1995.

271. Butler C: Effects of powered mobility on self-initiated behaviors of very young children with locomotor disability. Dev Med Child Neurol 28:325, 1986.

272. Butler C: Effects of powered mobility on self-initiated behaviors of very young children with locomotor disability. Dev Med Child Neurol 28:325, 1986.

273. Smith ME, Walton MS, Garraway WM: The use of aids and adaptations in a study of stroke rehabilitation. Health Bull 39:98, 1981.

274. Lu CL, Yu B, Basfored JR, et al: Influences of cane length on the stability of stroke patients. J Rehabil Research Devel 34:91, 1997.

275. Milczarek JJ, Kirby RL, Harrison ER, MacLeod DA: Standard and four-footed canes: Their effect on the standing balance of patients with hemiparesis. Arch Phys Med Rehabil 74:281, 1993.

276. Baxter ML, Allington RO, Koepke GH: Weight distribution variables in the use of crutches and canes. Phys Ther 49:360, 1969.

277. Dickstein R, Abulaffio N, Pillar T: Vertical force loaded on walking canes in hemiparetic patients. Gait Posture 1:113, 1993.

278. Cybulski GR, Jaeger RJ: Standing performance of persons with paraplegia. Arch Phys Med Rehabil 67:103, 1986.

279. Mikelberg R, Reid S: Spinal cord lesions and lower extremity bracing: An overview and follow-up study. Paraplegia 19:379, 1981.

280. Coughlan JK, Robinson CE, Neumarch B, Jackson G: Lower extremity bracing in paraplegia: Follow-up study. Paraplegia 18:25, 1980.

281. Burdette RG, Borello-France D, Blatchly C, Potter C: Gait comparison of subjects with hemiplegia walking unbraced, with ankle-foot orthosis, and with Air-Stirrup brace. Phys Ther 68:1197, 1988.

282. Mojica JAP, Nakamura R, Kobayashi T, et al: Effect of ankle-foot orthosis (AFO) on body sway and walking capacity of hemiparetic stroke patients. Tohoku J Exp Med 156:395, 1988.

283. Isakov E, Mizrahi J, Onna I, Susak Z: The control of genn recurvatum by comgining the Swedish knee-cage and an ankle-foot brace. Disabil Rehabil 14:187, 1992.

284. DeVries J: Evaluation of lower leg orthosis use following cerebro-vascular accident. Int J Rehabil Res 14:239, 1991.

285. Yamamoto S, Miyazaki S, Kubota T: Quantification of the effect of the mechanical property of ankle-foot orthoses on hemiplegic gait. Gait Posture 1:27, 1993.

286. Dieli J, Ayyappa E, Hornbeak S: Effect of dynamic AFOs on three hemiplegic adults. J Prosth Orthot 9:82, 1997.

287. Lehmann JF, Condon SM, Price R, deLateur BJ: Gait abnormalities in hemiplegia: Their correction by ankle-foot orthoses. Arch Phys Med Rehabil 68:763, 1987.

288. Hesse S, Luecke D, Jahnke MT, Mauritz KH: Gait functin in spastic hemiparetic patients walking barefoot, with firm shoes, and with ankle-foot orthosis. Int Rehabil Res 19:133, 1996.

289. Corcoran PJ, Jebsen RH, Brengelmann GL, Simons BC: Effects of plastic and metal leg braces on speed and energy cost of hemiparetic ambulation. Arch Phys Med Rehabil 51:69, 1970.

CHAPTER 8

BIOMECHANICS OF UNPERTURBED STANDING BALANCE

Joseph Mizrahi

THE DYNAMIC NATURE OF BALANCE

Bipedal standing is an unstable position that necessitates a continuous regulation process, involving periodic contractions of muscles in the lower limbs and trunk.[1,2] The direct result of this continuously acting stabilizing system is the existence of body sway in the sagittal, coronal, and transversal planes. The ability to maintain a stable upright position depends on the integrity of the musculoskeletal and neurologic systems. Specifically, the visual,[3] vestibular,[4] and proprioceptive[5] systems play significant roles in controlling human balance. In different pathologies caused by disease or trauma, one or more of these sensitive sources can be damaged, resulting in impaired stability in standing.

Measurement of postural balance has been used in the past to assess stability in bipedal standing and walking. The body situations in which balance ability is needed are, however, diverse: from the easiest ones, in which the body's center of gravity is absolutely within the base of support and in which no motion of the supporting surface takes place (e.g., lying supine), to the most demanding and exacting ones, such as maintaining balance while treading a rope on one leg, or during ice skating. Specifically, standing in the upright position in the absence of external perturbations is a position of fundamental importance. Postural sway tests while standing still are relatively easy to carry out, demanding minimal cooperation and effort from the tested subjects or patients. These tests also provide valuable and reliable information on the mechanisms of unperturbed balance in normal and pathologic conditions. This particularly applies to patients with deficiencies in the locomotor system, such as cerebrovascular accident (CVA) patients, craniocerebral injury (CCI) patients, and amputees wearing their prostheses, as soon as they become able to stand without support.

This chapter discusses the parameters that describe standing balance of able-bodied subjects and of subjects with neuromuscular and skeletal deficiencies. A special emphasis is given to the measurement of the foot–ground reaction forces in standing still. These are easily measurable quantities that provide a natural input to biomechanical models on human standing. At the same time, they can form the basis for the clinical characterization of standing posture in subjects with balance pathologies.

METHODS OF BALANCE MEASUREMENT

UNPERTURBED STANDING TESTS

A commonly used method in the measurement of standing balance deals with the variations of the center of pressure of the vertical foot–ground reaction forces obtained from fixed forceplates.[6–11] In using this method, however, special care should be taken not to confuse the measured trajectory of the center of pressure and that of the body's center of mass.[12] In fact, earlier, Valk-Fai[13] showed the existence of a difference between the center of pressure and center of mass trajectories, and Gurfinkel[6] estimated this difference for various values of the swaying frequency. Later, Shimba[14] proposed a method for the estimation of the trajectory of the body's center of gravity in single-limb stance from the rate of change of the moment of momentum of the whole body, as obtained from forceplate data. This method was later expanded to double-limb stance by Levin and Mizrahi.[15]

Typical trajectories of the center of gravity with respect to the platforms' plane, as reported by Levin[16] for four able-bodied subjects and two subjects with musculoskeletal pathologies, are shown in Figure 8–1. The pathologies included a right below-knee amputation (BKA) and paralysis of the left plantar-flexor muscles. The average position of the center of gravity trajectories is indicated on the surface of the platforms. It can be seen that the average position of the center of gravity trajectories of the able-bodied subjects falls around the separation line between the platforms, outside the contact area between each of the feet and the ground. Conversely, the average position of the center of gravity trajectories of the pathologic subjects is shifted away from the

separation line, toward the direction of the sound leg. These results clearly demonstrate the difference between the trajectory of the center of pressure and that of the center of gravity.

Elaborate methods of measurement of postural sway have included measurement of all the components of the actual reactive foot–ground forces, including those in the tangential plane.[17–20] Additional methods, applied separately or in conjunction with the previously described methods, have included accelerometry of the trunk,[17] goniometry of the ankle joint,[21] and measurement of the motion of various parts of the body by one of the following means: mechanical pen writer,[22] photography,[12] light-emitting diodes,[23] television and light spots,[24] spark microphones,[25] and variable-capacitance sway meter.[26]

A major advantage of measuring the actual re-

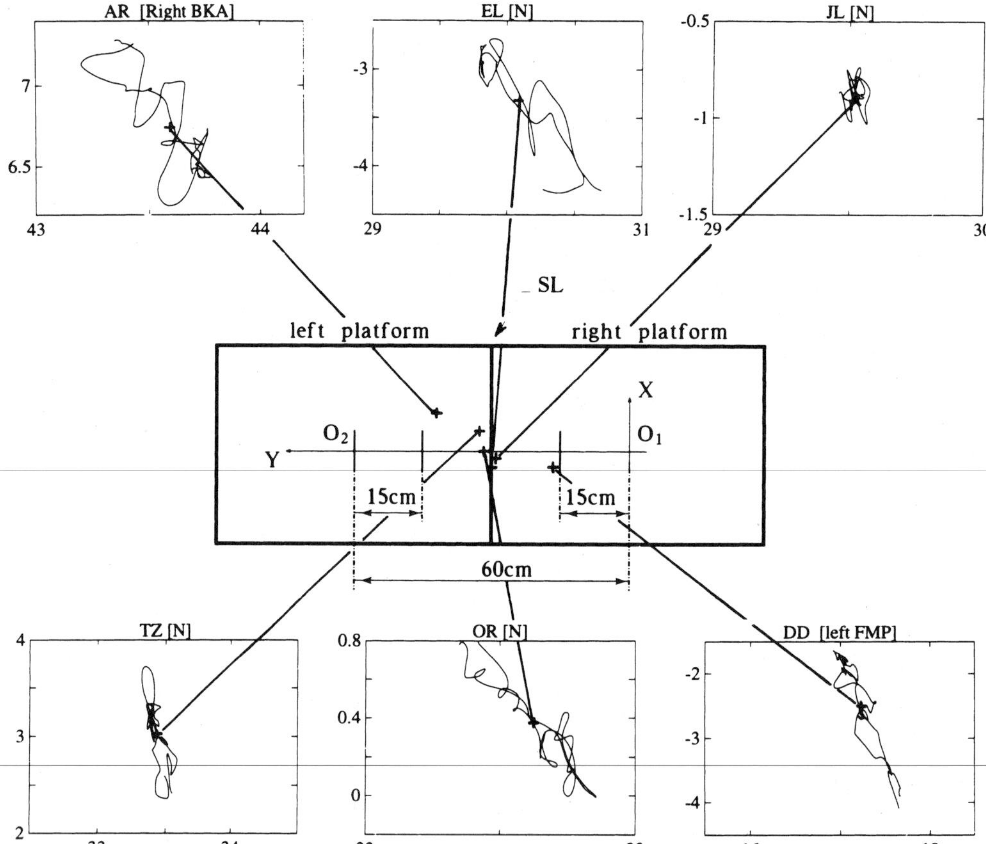

FIGURE 8–1   Typical trajectory of the center of gravity in the transverse plane for four able-bodied subjects (N) and two subjects with pathology: right below-knee amputation (BKA) and paralysis of the left plantar-flexor muscles (FMP). The average position of the center of gravity trajectories is pointed on the surface of the platforms. It is noted that the average positions of the center of gravity trajectories of the able-bodied subjects fall around the separation line (SL) between the platforms. Conversely, the average positions of the center of gravity trajectories of the subjects with pathology are shifted away from the SL, toward the direction of the sound leg. EL, JL, TZ, and OR, normal subjects; AR, below-knee amputee; DD, subject with FMP; O_1, O_2, centers of platform, respectively; X, Y, anteroposterior and mediolateral axes, respectively.

active forces is that the results obtained can be easily related to the acceleration of the center of mass of the body, through the equations of motion. Note, however, that in most of the studies dealing with force measurements, only one force platform was used, thus measuring the sum of the reactive forces, acting on both feet together. The importance of double forceplate measurements was later pointed out in conjunction with both bilateral characterization of the swaying motion and multisegmental modeling of the human body.[15, 27]

TEST PARAMETERS IN UNPERTURBED STANDING

Studies of healthy subjects of different ages have attempted to establish ranges of norms for this population. Variability of the reported results was, however, very large, mainly because of the different methodologies used. An attempt to overcome this problem was made by Kapteyn and colleagues[28] by setting principles for the standardization of postural sway forceplate measurements.

Significant test parameters in postural sway measurements include the following:

Duration of test. The duration of swaying tests ranges in the literature from a few seconds[29] to a few minutes[17, 19, 30]; in most studies, however, the typical duration was within the range of 20 to 80 seconds.[10, 11, 20, 31–33]

Footwear. Differences between swaying tests made with or without shoes were not referred to in most studies on this subject, with the exception of those of Harris and colleagues[10] and Shimba.[20]

Positioning of and spacing between feet. The effect of foot positioning was specifically addressed by Stribley and colleagues,[18] who reported that posture, especially in the mediolateral direction, was more stable with a wide opening between the feet compared with standing with the feet parallel and touching.[31] Similar findings were also reported by Nayak and coauthors[11] and, more recently, by Kirby and associates.[34] Another view is that no restrictions should be made on the foot placement, except that they should be comfortably positioned.[19] The influence of foot positioning and spacing between the feet is especially important when bilateral measurements of postural balance are to be taken.[27]

Visual feedback. The importance of visual feedback in the regulation of posture has been discussed by many investigators, for example, Gantchev and Popov,[35] Hlavacka and Litvinenkova,[36] and Seidel and Brauer.[37] In fact, in most investigations on postural balance, visual feedback was of central interest.[8, 9, 18, 22] It was reported that in the absence of vision, balance becomes less stable.[8, 21] Furthermore, Paulus and colleagues[3] showed that a decrease in visual acuity is usually accompanied by an increase in postural instability.

Other factors. Of special interest were the effects on postural balance stability of factors such as physical fatigue,[29, 38] environment of acoustic noise,[29] anesthetics, drugs and alcohol,[32] the effect of equilibrium lesions,[39–42] the effect of ischemic blocking of the leg,[43] and the effect of other general pathologies.[9, 40, 44–48]

PERTURBED STANDING TESTS

The balance tests described previously were made in unperturbed standing; in some of the more recent reports, dynamic testing conditions were also treated. One method of dynamic testing consists of moving the measuring platform, either linearly or angularly, to create an effect of either unexpected or continuous perturbation.[9, 29, 49–53] Another method of perturbed testing is moving the visual scene in front of the tested subject.[21] In either of these dynamic methods, the role of visual feedback was shown to be much more significant than that found when testing in static conditions.[49, 51]

The relative role of each of the visual, vestibular, and proprioceptive sensors has been described in several studies, using both fixed and sway-referenced supports.[54, 55] Particularly, the relative weighting of the sensors of patients with vestibular deficits using sway-referenced supports and vision was examined.[56, 57] The adaptability and relative contribution of each of the sensors in young children was reported.[58] Fixed and sway-reference supports were also compared in conjunction with chronic low-back dysfunction.[59]

The electrical activity in five lower limb muscles was investigated in dynamic standing balance.[53] The spatial and temporal parameters were measured separately in the sagittal and frontal planes,[60] using an instrumented stabilometer.[61] It was found that the total angular displacement of the tilting platform and its fundamental frequency were strongly correlated. Additionally, spatiotemporal symmetry was shown to indicate subjects' performance and to monitor the learning progress of the dynamic balance tasks.[62]

THE NATURE OF SWAYING MOTION IN STANDING STILL

Swaying motion while standing still has been reported to be periodic, containing waves that follow no recognizable pattern.[17, 63] Although the cycles of this motion are irregular in amplitude and frequency, large low-frequency primary waves are identifiable. Superimposed on these waves are secondary, smaller waves of higher frequencies. The higher-frequency waves were reported to be of greater regularity, with regard to both cycle duration and amplitude. Bizzo and associates[64] determined that the whole frequency range in stabilometry was 0 to 10 Hz. Previous studies[17, 63] reported swaying frequencies exceeding the upper limit of this range. Altogether, three typical frequency groups were identified and reported: (1) above 5 Hz[17, 19, 27, 43, 45, 63]; (2) 0.5 to 5 Hz[6, 13, 14, 19, 20, 27, 29, 63, 65]; (3) below 0.5 Hz.[12, 17, 21, 27, 45] These frequency groups were found in both kinematic (swaying) and dynamic (forceplate data) tests. The existence of the high-frequency group was dissociated from any passive elasticity effects and attributed instead to muscle tremor. According to Thomas and Whitney,[17] this tremor originates from the asynchronous firing of individual motor units, which accompanies all muscular activity.

In most of the previously mentioned investigations, not all the frequency groups were studied. The reason could be either that the investigators have put their emphasis on the more easily detectable frequency group or that, owing to their own methodology, some frequencies simply could not be identified. For example, if the swaying data are sampled at the frequency of 5 Hz,[21] no oscillation frequencies above 2.5 Hz can be detected. On the other hand, a power spectrum analysis of force traces sampled at 50 Hz has demonstrated the above frequency groups: two rather broad ranges of local peaks were detected at the two lower frequencies, that is, about 0.1 and 1 Hz, and a sharp peak was detected at the higher frequency, corresponding to about 7 Hz.[27]

MODELING OF SWAYING MOTION

Relating to modeling of postural sway, the inverted pendulum bisegmental model has gained a significant amount of attention, particularly in the sagittal plane motion. In this motion, the body is considered rigid and hinged above the ankle joint. This representation complies with the conception of using one force platform only for measuring the reactive forces.

In the more simple approach, the restoring components in the system are treated as purely elastic and passive.[6, 66] Later studies have demonstrated that this treatment is erroneous.[17, 19, 24] For one thing, the inverted pendulum representation failed to predict correlations that should emerge from such a model between sway magnitudes and physique variables, such as body height and weight,[19] due to lack of symmetry of the actual body motion around the vertical axis.[21]

Additionally, Thomas and Whitney[17] and Lestienne and colleagues[21] have suggested that postural movements are maintained by continuous muscular action, and not as a simple pendular motion with passive elasticity. Thus, the existence of continuous muscle action with relatively small forces required in the ankle, as well as the other rotating joints, makes it evident that a multisegmental model is more adequate for describing body sway. This suggested modification of the body sway model also sheds light on the regulation mechanism of postural sway, through the detailed action of the leg muscles.

Figure 8–2 illustrates the main muscle groups that are potentially involved in maintaining equilibrium during standing still. Under the assumption of a locked-knee position, the muscle groups shown in the part A of this figure act around the ankle and hip joints. A three-segment model representation of the swaying body in the sagittal plane is presented in part B. In this model, the tibialis anterior and gluteus maximus muscles act as torque generators around the ankle and hip joints, respectively. Note that the more simplistic inverted pendulum model[6, 66] treats the body in terms of two rigid segments, the foot and the remainder above it, with a purely elastic recoil at the ankle-joint level.

Several factors indicate that the mechanism involving the regulatory muscle action may act independently in the left and right legs. These factors are listed as follows:

1. The existence of relative motion between the body segments, which contributes to body corrections,[13] contradicts the previously mentioned bisegmental model. The amplitudes of these compensatory body movements, which are minimized by the influence of visual information,[36] are related to the position of each leg. It was further suggested that the relative and compensatory movements occur in such a way that the ground reaction forces are not predictably invoked.[19]

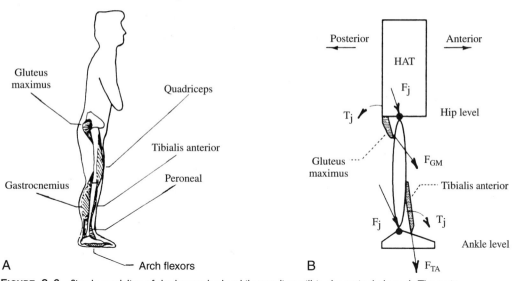

FIGURE 8–2 Simple modeling of the human body while standing still in the sagittal plane. *A,* The main muscle groups involved in maintaining equilibrium during standing with locked knees. *B,* The tibialis anterior and gluteus maximus muscles are shown to act as torque generators around the ankle and hip, respectively, in a three-segment model. Joint forces and torques are denoted as F_j and T_j, respectively, for each joint. Reactive foot–ground forces are not shown. HAT, head and arms and trunk; F_{GM}, force in the gluteus maximus; F_{TA}, force in the tibialis anterior.

2. In addition to the vestibular organs, the mere rotation of the ankles was pointed out as the major source of information of the body's orientation.[29, 50] In comparison to the vestibular organs, ankle rotation, which is based on the stretch and long-loop reflexes of the plantar-flexing posterior muscles,[63] was reported to be more significant in the higher sway frequencies.[50, 67]

3. The source of existence of the high-frequency sway (6 Hz) is associated with muscle tremor,[17] which possibly originates from the asynchronous firing of the individual motor units and which accompanies all muscular activity. This may indicate that each leg acts independently with an individual postural activity pattern.

It is evident that, to relate the externally measured foot–ground reaction forces to the mechanisms of stabilization and posture regulation, data collected from a single force platform on which the subject stands, thus treating the swaying body as a single-supported structure, cannot provide sufficiently detailed information on the individual activity of each of the supporting legs. Such information is essential to understand the mechanism involved in normal postural sway and, even more so, to describe and evaluate postural deficiencies existing in pathologic cases[68, 69] (e.g., center or gravity trajectory; see Fig. 8–1). In particular, if the specific activity of forces on each leg is required, each of the supporting limbs should be represented as a segment. It is obvious that pelvic attachment of the lower limbs requires that each of these limb segments be connected to an upper segment, representing the trunk of the body. The practical implication of a multisegmental model is that measurement of body sway should be made by means of two force platforms, one for each leg, and that the force data obtained from such a system should be used as input values for this model.

A five-segment model of the human body for bipedal standing-still postural sway is shown in Figure 8–3. The reaction forces F_L and F_R are measured bilaterally from both feet, using two force platforms. A block diagram of the iterative calculation procedure[16] for this model is shown in Figure 8–4. Apart from the forceplate data, information of the individual anthropometry of the tested subject is essential. However, a thorough evaluation of the kinematics and dynamics of the model is bounded by the uncertainty of the exact positioning of the joints in space and by the anthropometry of the subject. Consequently, the model is constrained by including a condition that compares model results to actually measured data. The first step in the calculation procedure is the estimation of the trajectory of the center of gravity, as evaluated from forceplate measurements.[15] Kinematics of the segments are then estimated from the center of gravity trajectory, followed by

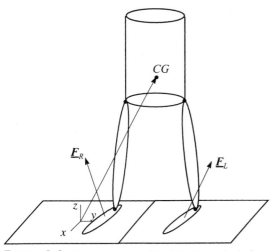

FIGURE 8–3   Five-segment model of the human body for bipedal, standing-still postural sway. The reaction forces $\underline{F}_L$ and $\underline{F}_R$ are measured bilaterally from both feet using two force platforms. CG, center of gravity.

solution of the forces and moments acting on the distal segments of the model by means of inverse dynamics methods. Differences between model and measured forces of the right foot are minimized by readjusting the positioning of the joints and the anthropometric properties of the segments. After minimizing the calculation errors, the iteration procedure of the kinematics and dynamics of the segments is concluded.

BILATERAL MEASUREMENTS OF NATURAL BODY SWAY

It has been argued that in using only one force platform for monitoring postural sway, the lateral forces on both feet are vectorially summed, resulting in a small net lateral force that is within the noise level of the measurements.[27] In using two force platforms, the force components and centers of pressure on each foot can be measured separately. As discussed in the previous section, this is essential if standing sway is to be modeled as a multisegmental model,[70, 71] which accounts for possible asymmetries. The significance of bilateral forceplate measurements in postural sway has been reported for able-bodied populations[27] as well as for populations with neurologic[72–76] or orthopedic[77, 78] pathologies.

It is expected, for example, that in CVA patients, because muscular activity may differ considerably from one side of the body to the other, information on the forces acting on each of the legs in maintaining equilibrium would be of great interest.

METHODOLOGY OF NATURAL SWAY MEASUREMENTS

Bilateral measurements of the natural swaying motion in standing are made by means of two collaterally installed force platforms for the adjacent positioning of the left and right feet during standing. The tested subject is requested to stand still during the test, and the measured quantities include the force components and the coordinates of the center of pressure. A distinction should be made in the vertical and mediolateral directions between the *level* of forces (dc component) and the force *oscillations* around this level (ac component). The force oscillations is the component of interest in studying the dynamics of body sway. A strong correlation was found between the amount of opening between the feet and the level of medi-

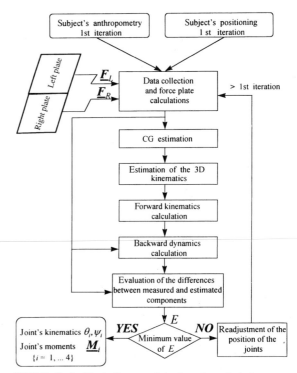

FIGURE 8–4   Block diagram of the iterative calculation procedure of the five-segment model presented in Figure 8–3. The first step is the estimation of the trajectory of the center of gravity (CG), as evaluated from forceplate measurements. Kinematics of the segments are thereafter estimated, from which forces and moments on the distal segments are resolved using inverse dynamics. Differences between model and measured forces are minimized for the right foot by readjusting the positioning of the joints and anthropometric properties of the segments. After minimizing the calculation errors, the iteration procedure of the kinematics and dynamics of the segments is concluded. $\underline{F}_L$, left reaction force; $\underline{F}_R$, right reaction force; E, error of estimation; $\underline{M}_i$, moment about the ith axis.

olateral forces measured, implying that spacing between the feet should be carefully controlled.[27]

The duration of the measuring tests is typically 30 to 60 seconds, of which the central two thirds are considered for data processing. This duration is of the same order of magnitude taken in most previous investigations.[10, 18, 20, 24, 31, 32]

Early works dealing with bilateral measurement of sway were confined to studying weight-bearing imbalance between the legs, that is, through the vertical component of the foot–ground reaction forces. Using foot–ground pressure measurements, a striking asymmetry of 75% in weight bearing between the feet in post-CVA patients was reported.[44] Similar findings were also reported when using two force platforms and when concentrating on the magnitude of the vertical force component only and the coordinate of its center of pressure.[45]

In subsequent studies, bilateral force measurements on the supporting limbs were made to provide a new representation of postural sway, which was implemented to evaluate able-bodied subjects as well as patients suffering from disorders in the musculoskeletal and neurologic systems.[72–78]

Parameters, including frequency amplitude force sequence between the feet, force activity on each foot, and asymmetry, were defined, presented, and compared between the different groups of subjects studied.

DEFINED PARAMETERS

The force traces obtained included a transient, slow oscillation (about 0.1 Hz), above which more rapid oscillations (1 Hz and higher) were superimposed. Tremor oscillations (about 6 Hz) also presented, but with much smaller amplitudes (Fig. 8–5). A procedure was established to measure the peak-to-peak amplitudes of the middle (1 Hz) oscillations and to compute their averages.[27, 77] From these amplitude averages obtained for the anteroposterior, mediolateral, and vertical force components, the following parameters were defined:

1. *Relative sequence of the tangential force vectors* (RSTFV). As a result of body sway, the horizontal component of the foot–ground reaction vector obtained for each leg was found to oscillate periodically and diagonally backward and forward along a given direction. It was also found that the horizontal components of the foot–ground reaction vectors of both feet generally have the same oscillation frequency, although they may appear in various relative sequences.[27, 73, 74] For instance, the anteroposterior force components on both legs can be either concurrent or opposite to each other. The same is true for the mediolateral components. Thus, different configurations may occur, all resulting in time-synchronized diagonal oscillations of the tangential reactive force on both feet. This synchronous appearance discloses the bilateral dynamics of the reactive forces involved in maintaining equilibrium during standing. The RSTFV can be established either by visually inspecting the relative course of the force traces in the time domain or by using the following computerized procedure: The tangential force components in the x and y directions of the two legs are plotted one against the other in different combinations, disclosing the correlations existing between them. From these correlations, the RSTFV can be resolved, as demonstrated in the Poincare plots shown in Figure 8–6. Previous results indicate that the RSTFV has a common pattern in most able-bodied subjects tested.[27] Typical deviations from this pattern are found in defined pathologies, such as in CCI and CVA patients.

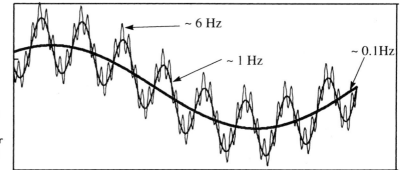

FIGURE 8–5 Schematic demonstration of force oscillations in standing sway. A frequency analysis discloses the existence of three major frequency ranges of about 0.1, 1, and 6 Hz.

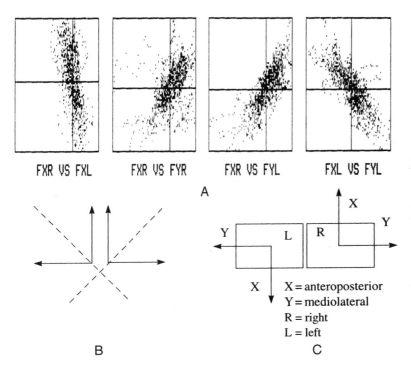

FXR VS FXL   FXR VS FYR   FXR VS FYL   FXL VS FYL

A

B

X = anteroposterior
Y = mediolateral
R = right
L = left

C

FIGURE 8–6 Poincare plots of the force components illustrating the procedure to establish the relative sequence of the tangential force vectors (RSTFV). *A,* The tangential force components in the x and y directions of the two legs plotted against one another in different combinations. *B,* Resolution of the RSTFV from the correlations between the components. *C,* Definition of the axes for the two forceplates used. VS, versus; FX, force in the anteroposterior direction; FY, force in the mediolateral direction; R, right; L, left.

2. *Weight-bearing imbalance* (WBI), in the vertical direction, is defined as follows: WBI = absolute value of vertical force difference between the feet normalized to body weight. Thus, WBI expresses the difference between the average vertical forces supported by each of the legs.

3. *Total sway activity* is defined in the horizontal plane as the added force amplitude averages in the anteroposterior and mediolateral directions (Fig. 8–7). This quantity combines the force activity of both legs and may therefore be directly related to the added muscle activity of both legs and represents the accumulated efforts invested in maintaining standing equilibrium. Note that single-platform measurements would not enable us to obtain such an integrated measure because the measured forces in this case represent the net external force acting on the body.

4. *Asymmetry,* also defined in the horizontal plane, is the subtracted force amplitude averages in the anteroposterior and mediolateral directions (see Fig. 8–7). This quantity is related to the difference in activity existing between both legs, and in the presence of ideal symmetry it should have a zero value. Asymmetry thus indicates the measure in which the force activity required during standing is shared between the two legs.

ESTIMATION OF THE TRAJECTORY OF THE CENTER OF GRAVITY FROM BILATERAL REACTIVE FORCES

An iterative model for the estimation of the center of gravity trajectory by using foot–ground reaction force and center of pressure data was developed.[15] The iterative procedure was used to examine possible effects of the rate of change of angular momentum on the estimated trajectory. It was concluded that the contribution of the time-rate change of the angular momentum is negligible in the iteration procedure of estimating the center of gravity trajectory. The method was illustrated on

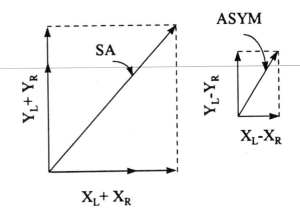

FIGURE 8–7 Vectorial definition of total sway activity (SA) and asymmetry (ASYM).

a group of 11 able-bodied subjects and 2 subjects with musculoskeletal pathologies.

Symmetric standing can be defined in terms of the forces applied by each of the feet or by the location of the average position of the center of gravity trajectory. Under the condition of symmetric positioning of the feet on the forceplates, the separation line between the forceplates can be used as a reference for the average position of the center of gravity trajectory. The latter was found to be considerably displaced from the separation line for the two pathologic subjects, whereby the displacement was found to be significantly large ($P < .005$) compared with that of the able-bodied subjects. Similar results on the effect of pathologic disorders on the shift of the center of gravity trajectory were reported by Snijders and Verduin.[8] Nevertheless, in this study, the data were related to a single forceplate.

A different reported methodology for the prediction of the center of gravity from forceplate measurements during gait is based on a Fourier representation of the acceleration components of the center of gravity, whereby the fundamental harmonic of the Fourier series is one cycle of gait.[79] The problem in applying such a methodology in standing still is the difficulty of identifying one basic harmonic of the standing-still posture sway. As previously mentioned, spectral analysis of forceplate data has in the past identified at least three main frequency ranges.[27]

BALANCE IN ABLE-BODIED SUBJECTS

SUBJECTS TESTED

The postural balance in quiet standing of 23 adult able-bodied subjects (13 men and 10 women) was studied. The average age mass and height were 41 years, 66 kg, and 168 cm, respectively.

FREQUENCIES OF SWAYING MOTION

In all the subjects tested, the force traces corresponding to both feet were synchronous with each other and thus had the same basic frequencies. These frequencies might, however, differ from test to test, as they might in the presence of (as opposed to in the absence of) visual feedback. Although the cycles of the periodic swaying motion are irregular in frequency and amplitude, primary waves are easily identifiable. Superimposed on these waves are secondary smaller waves of higher frequencies. The higher-frequency waves (middle- and high-frequency oscillations) were reported to be of greater regularity with regard to both cycle duration and amplitude.[17, 63] This has also been demonstrated in the power spectrum analysis of the traces.[27]

Average values of the waveform frequencies for all the subjects studied are summarized in Figure 8–8. The orders of magnitude frequencies for the oscillations detected in this study were 6 Hz for the rapid oscillation, 1.2 Hz for the middle oscillation, and 0.1 Hz for the slow oscillation. Because of their regularity, the middle-frequency oscillations (on the order of 1.2 Hz) were the most easily measurable and were, in fact, the only ones referred to by several investigators.[19, 20]

In the literature, the frequency values reported for postural sway vary considerably. Seliktar and colleagues[45] reported on three distinct ranges around the following frequencies: 5, 0.5, and 0.01 Hz. Lakes and associates[32] reported on two frequency bands of 2.9 and 0.56 Hz, and Thomas and Whitney[17] found two frequency components: the high frequency around 10 Hz and the low one

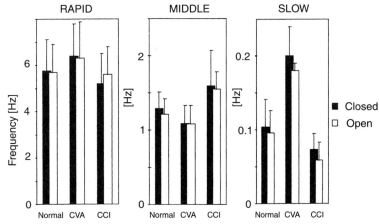

FIGURE 8–8 Average frequencies of oscillations in standing sway in the three major frequency ranges for three population groups: able-bodied (normal), cerebrovascular accident (CVA), and craniocerebral accident (CCI) patients. The vertical bars denote I standard deviation.

around 0.2 Hz. In other studies, however, only one frequency was reported, presumably that which was the most easily measurable or which was judged to be the most significant.

Smith,[63] Thomas and Whitney,[17] and Kapteyn[24] emphasized in their reports the 10-Hz frequency. Other authors[19, 20] focused mainly on the 1-Hz-frequency oscillation. The effect of visual feedback on the waveform frequencies indicates a slight increase in the absence of visual feedback. Particularly, the frequency of the middle oscillation increased by about 7% (from 1.21 to 1.29 Hz) when the visual feedback was eliminated (eyes covered, as compared with eyes open).

RELATIVE SEQUENCE OF THE TANGENTIAL FORCE VECTORS

The recordings obtained indicate that the anteroposterior forces on both feet were always concurrent with each other. The mediolateral forces, however, were in most cases opposite to each other.

The RSTFV on both feet is summarized in Table 8–1. Three vectorial patterns were found in the normal population group tested. The most frequent pattern is shown in the first column and was found in 77% of the cases analyzed. In this pattern, also shown in Figure 8–6, the vectors run synchronously, diverging diagonally from each other in the front side of the body and converging in the rear side of the body. In 18% of the cases analyzed (column 2), the pattern was somewhat similar, except that the intersecting point was shifted toward the front side of the body. It is also noted that the roles of the left and right feet are interchanged in these two patterns. It may be of interest to note that all cases having the second pattern involved women. The least frequent pattern among the healthy subjects tested is shown in column 3 and was noted in only 5% of the

cases analyzed. The vectors in this pattern are concurrent and run somewhat parallel to each other from the left anterior to the right posterior direction of the body.

The vector diagrams presented in Table 8–1 shed light on the force patterns acting on the feet and their relative sequences. Each vector schematically describes the direction of the horizontal reactive force acting on the foot. The synchronous appearance of the vectors, as described separately for each foot, thus discloses the dynamics of the reactive forces involved in maintaining equilibrium during standing. The diagonal patterns, with diverging vectors from the center of the body to the front of the body, were found to be most frequent, indicating that while the anteroposterior forces run concurrently, the mediolateral forces normally run in opposite directions on both feet. Despite the observed different activities on the legs, however, the fact that the tracings on both feet were synchronous with each other tends to indicate that the muscle forces in both legs are controlled by one central source.

AMPLITUDES

Amplitudes of the medium oscillations are expressed separately for the dominant and opposite legs. Average values of the amplitudes for the normal population, expressed in terms of body weight, are given in Figure 8–9. The magnitudes on both legs were comparable. Also, the difference in the presence or absence of visual feedback was not significant.

In the vertical (z) direction, weight-bearing imbalance was 5.4% and 2.1% of body weight, with and without visual feedback, respectively (Fig. 8–10). Oscillations of the vertical forces in the same condition amounted to 1.5% of the body weight. Here, again, the effect of visual feedback was not significant (see Fig. 8–9).

TABLE 8–1 Relative Sequence of the Tangential Force Vectors (RSTFV) on Both Feet*

	1	2	3	4	5	6	7	8
Healthy subjects	77	18.0				5.00		
Subjects with cerebrovascular accident	29.4	1.6	9.7	25.2	5.10	19.2	0.3	0.50
Subjects with craniocerebral injury	62.0		2.9		5.8	5.7	14.7	8.8

*The figures represent percentage occurrence from the recordings obtained for the populations tested.

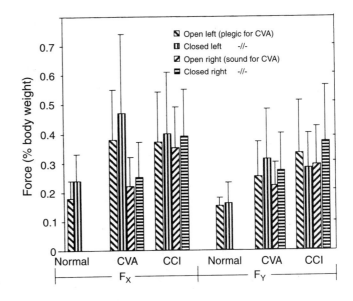

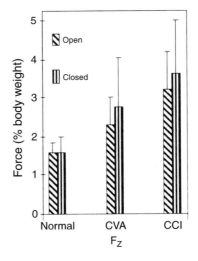

FIGURE 8–9   Average values of forces in standing sway for three population groups: normal, cerebrovascular accident (CVA), and craniocerebral accident (CCI) patients. The forces, expressed in percentage body weight, are presented in three components: anteroposterior (F_X), mediolateral (F_Y), and vertical (F_Z). The vertical bars denote 1 standard deviation.

The values of total sway activity and asymmetry, as defined earlier, are given in Figure 8–11. The total sway activity values were about 0.5% of body weight. Asymmetry values were lower than 0.1% of body weight, indicating that for the normal population, this parameter was negligibly low.

The most common order of magnitude found in the literature for the force amplitudes was about 1 N.[17–19] Shimba[20] reported on different force magnitudes in the various directions measured: 0.5 N in the anteroposterior direction, 0.35 N in the mediolateral direction, and 1.18 N in the vertical direction. Note that these values correspond to the resultant forces acting on both feet together. Our results on the amplitudes of the middle frequency, presented separately for the dominant and the opposite legs, indicate the following:

1. The oscillations of the forces in the tangential plane are approximately 0.2% of body weight, corresponding to about 1.2 N on each leg.
2. The oscillations of the forces in the anteroposterior (x) direction are slightly higher than those in the mediolateral (y) direction.
3. In the vertical (z) direction, the oscillations of the forces were of a much higher amplitude than in the horizontal directions (1.57% of body weight, corresponding to about 9.35 N).
4. Absence of visual feedback has no significant effect on the forces measured, except in the anteroposterior (x) direction, where a slight increase was noticed.

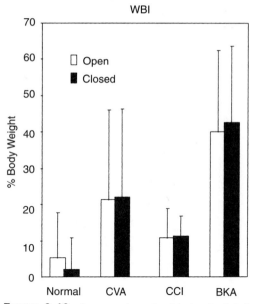

FIGURE 8-10 Average values of weight-bearing imbalance (WBI), expressed in percentage body weight, in standing sway for four population groups: normal, cerebrovascular accident (CVA), craniocerebral accident (CCI), and below-knee amputation (BKA) patients. The vertical bars denote 1 standard deviation.

To compare these results with those found in the literature, vector summations were done and the resultants further evaluated. It was concluded that the results presented by the single-support method are erroneous if the forces on each leg are to be known. The relationship between postural sway and muscular activity around the joint has been discussed in the literature. Thomas and Whitney[17] refer to the high-frequency tremor during sway to criticize the inverted pendulum model, which is based on passive elastic terms only, and to justify the existence of continuous muscular action. Smith[63] states further that the stabilization of the ankle joint during standing is due to two forces: the first originating from the passive tissues resisting dorsiflexion, and the second due to the posterior muscles that are responsible for dorsiflexion of the joint. In this context, the significance of sway activity and asymmetry parameters, as seen in Figure 8-11, is easily understood. Beyond the force magnitudes reported separately for each leg in Figure 8-9, sway activity represents the vector summation of the absolute values of these forces and can therefore be related to the overall muscle activity of both legs. Typical values of sway activity were found to be 3 N, corresponding to 0.5% body weight. Asymmetry is related to the difference in activity existing between both legs, and in the presence of ideal symmetry, this parameter should be zero. Asymmetry in the healthy subjects tested in this study was about 0.4 N (0.07% body weight).

BALANCE IN PATIENTS WITH CEREBROVASCULAR ACCIDENT

PATIENTS TESTED

The postural balance in quiet standing was studied in 16 CVA patients. The average age was 60.9 $\pm$ 10.5 years, and the average time from stroke to

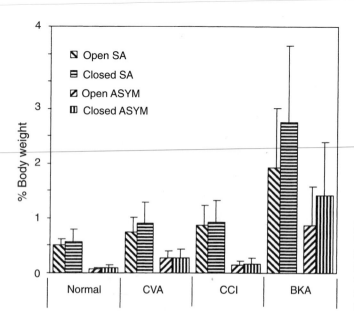

FIGURE 8-11 Average values of total sway activity (SA) and asymmetry (ASYM), expressed in percentage body weight, for four population groups: normal, cerebrovascular accident (CVA), craniocerebral accident (CCI), and below-knee amputation (BKA) patients. The vertical bars denote 1 standard deviation.

first test was 11.8 ±8.6 weeks. Six able-bodied subjects from the group of healthy subjects (average age, 64.6 ±8.1 years) served as controls. Sex and age differences were checked between the patients and the control groups using the chi-square test, and the results showed that no adjustment was required for age or sex.

WAVEFORM FREQUENCIES

Average values of waveform frequencies for the CVA patients are given in Figure 8–8. The average frequencies of the medial and rapid oscillations were in the same range as in the control population. On the other hand, slow oscillations were of a considerably higher frequency in the hemiplegic population. The frequencies tended to be slightly higher in the absence of visual feedback than when visual feedback was present.

RELATIVE SEQUENCE OF THE TANGENTIAL FORCE VECTORS

The RSTFV on both feet is summarized in Table 8–1. Of the various patterns found in the CVA population, the diagonal pattern corresponding to concurrent anteroposterior forces, but opposite to mediolateral forces on both legs (column 1), was found the most frequently, in more than 29% of the tests. Both of the next two common patterns in the CVA population had concurrent mediolateral forces. The anteroposterior components were, however, opposite in one of these patterns (25.2% of the tests, column 4) and concurrent in the second pattern (19.2% of the tests, column 6). Other patterns, with various degrees of occurrence, are shown in Table 8–1. The presence or absence of visual feedback did not affect the RSTFV.

These results show that the patterns in the hemiplegic population are different from those in the control subjects. The most frequent pattern in the control population was found in only 29.4% of the CVA patients. Other patterns, in which the mediolateral and anteroposterior forces are concurrent, were also frequent (see columns 3 to 6 in Table 8–1) and can be considered equivalent. When grouping them together, an occurrence in about 29% of the tests is obtained, approaching the occurrence of the most frequent pattern.

AMPLITUDES

Amplitudes of the medial frequency oscillations are expressed separately for the sound and plegic legs in the hemiplegic patients (see Fig. 8–9). The amplitudes in the hemiplegic group were invari-

ably higher than those found in the control group. The difference between the forces on the sound leg in the hemiplegic population and those on any leg in the control population were statistically significant ($P < .01$) in the mediolateral direction, and even more so in the anteroposterior direction. The force differences between the legs within the hemiplegic population were significant ($P < .01$); however, this was not the case within the control population. It may be seen from Figure 8–9 that absence of visual feedback considerably increased the force amplitudes in the hemiplegic group; however, this increase was not statistically significant. Also, in the vertical (z) direction, amplitudes were higher in the hemiplegic compared with the healthy group for both the weight-bearing imbalance (see Fig. 8–10) and the force oscillations (see Fig. 8–9). The effect of absence of visual feedback was similar in this direction as in the previously described horizontal plane, that is, an increase in amplitude in the hemiplegic population.

Values of total sway activity and asymmetry are given in Figure 8–11. Both parameters had significantly higher values in the hemiplegic group than in the control group ($P < .04$ and $P < .001$, respectively), indicating that the former group requires a higher muscular activity for maintaining postural equilibrium.

It is obvious from the results presented in Figure 8–11 that the sound leg's contribution to this process is much greater than that of the plegic leg. Asymmetry was defined to express the difference in activities between both legs. Although in the control subjects tested, this parameter was very nearly zero, it amounted in the hemiplegic population to 0.27% of the body weight. Absence of visual feedback resulted in an increase in those two parameters. However, the only statistically significant difference was the increase in asymmetry, occurring in the absence of, as opposed to the presence of, visual feedback.

The above results on the amplitudes of the middle frequency, presented separately for the plegic and sound legs in the CVA population, can be summarized as follows:

1. The forces were significantly higher than those of the control group ($P < .01$), amounting to double the value in the anteroposterior component on the sound leg.
2. The force oscillation during sway was higher in the anteroposterior (x) direction than in the mediolateral direction (y) (supporting previous findings[20]). Although in the healthy subjects this difference was

minor, in the hemiplegic group it was considerably higher, especially in the forces on the sound leg.

3. The force magnitudes were always higher in the sound leg than in the plegic leg ($P <$ .01). The most significant difference was found in the anteroposterior (x) directions both with the eyes open and with them closed. The increased force magnitudes on the sound leg in comparison with the plegic leg points to an increased activity of the sound let to compensate for the relative inactivity of the plegic leg, to regain the ability to maintain the standing position. Remember than in the control subjects, no differences were found between the legs.

4. In the vertical (z) direction, the force oscillations were of much higher amplitudes than in the horizontal directions. Both the amplitude oscillations and the weight-bearing imbalance were considerably higher in the hemiplegic compared with the control population.

5. Although absence of visual feedback did not have noticeable effects in the control subjects, it appeared to increase the amplitudes of force oscillations in the hemiplegic group. When comparing the effect of eye closure for both groups separately, the only significant parameter was asymmetry in the normal population. Eye closure did not cause any statistically significant effect in the group of hemiplegics, which may suggest that this population does not extract helpful information from the visual input in the process of maintaining equilibrium during standing. Moreover, because the more significant differences between the groups were obtained with the eyes open rather than closed, it may be concluded that in hemiplegics, visual input may provide conflicting information from the balance point of view.

TIME EFFECT AND LOCOMOTOR OUTCOME

No single parameter or array of parameters of a single dimension—clinical, physiologic, or biomechanical—was found to predict the locomotor outcome of a patient.[75, 76] Nevertheless, some significant findings were reported for the patients with the better locomotor outcome. These included (1) the RSTFV patterns, which became remarkably similar to those of healthy people without hemiplegia; and (2) the total sway activity

and asymmetry values, which tended to be clearly reduced during rehabilitation.

BALANCE IN PATIENTS WITH CRANIOCEREBRAL INJURY

PATIENTS TESTED

Ten CCI patients (9 men and 1 woman), aged 19 to 43 years (28.5 ± 10.3 years), with no previous history of neurologic illness, drug abuse, or alcoholism, took part in the postural balance tests.[74] Eight patients suffered from blunt head injuries due to road accidents, and two patients suffered from penetrating lesions. All the patients were in a coma for at least 24 hours (range, 1 to 20 days; mean, 7.1 ± 4.9 days). Neurobehavioral disturbances were evaluated by previously described methods.[80, 81]

Eleven healthy subjects from the group of normal subjects (average age, 29.9 ± 6.6 years) served as controls. All the subjects included were free from neurologic, orthopedic, vestibular, and visual impairment and had no recent history of skeletal or muscular injury. The two above groups were found to be similar regarding sex and age (t = −0.36; P = .7), therefore requiring no adjustment for these factors.

WAVEFORM FREQUENCIES

Average values of waveform frequencies in the CCI patients are presented in Figure 8–8. The average frequencies of both the low- and high-frequency oscillations were lower in the CCI patients than in the control subjects. In the middle-frequency oscillations, the average was higher in the CCI group. The differences in frequencies between the two population groups, however, were not statistically significant. The effect of visual feedback on the oscillation frequencies tended to be altogether minor in the CCI patients, as it was also for the control subjects.

RELATIVE SEQUENCE OF THE TANGENTIAL FORCE VECTORS

The RSTFV on both feet is summarized in Table 8–1. The most frequent pattern was the diagonal pattern corresponding to concurrent anteroposterior (x) forces but opposite mediolateral (y) forces on both legs (62%). The next most common pattern in the CCI group consisted of opposite forces in both the anteroposterior and mediolateral directions on the two legs in relation to each other (8.8 + 14.7 = 23.5%; see columns 7 and 8 in Table

8–1). None of the control subjects exhibited this pattern. The pattern corresponding to concurrent forces in both the anteroposterior and mediolateral directions on the two legs had an occurrence of 2.9 + 5.7 = 8.6% in the CCI patients (see columns 3 and 6 in Table 8–1). The least frequent pattern in the CCI group, with concurrent mediolateral but opposite anteroposterior forces, is shown in column 5. Presence or absence of visual feedback or of a curtain drawn between the patient and site of measurement did not affect the RSTFV found for any patient.

AMPLITUDES

Our results on the amplitudes of the middle frequency are presented in Figure 8–9 and indicate the following:

1. The forces were significantly higher in the CCI patients than in the control subjects (P < .05), amounting to double the value.
2. The force oscillation during sway was higher in the anteroposterior (x) direction than in the mediolateral direction (y), supporting previous findings.[20]
3. The differences between left and right legs within each of the two groups tested were not statistically significant. The high asymmetry values obtained for the CCI patients (see Fig. 8–11) indicate, however, that within this group, at the individual level, differences are found between the forces on both legs.
4. The force oscillations were much higher in the vertical (z) direction than in the horizontal directions. Both the amplitude oscillations (see Fig. 8–9) and the weight-bearing imbalance (see Fig. 8–10) were considerably higher in the CCI group than in the control group.
5. Absence of visual feedback caused no noticeable effects.

Values of the sway activity parameter were significantly higher in the CCI population studied than in control subjects (P < .02), indicating that the former group requires a higher muscular activity for maintaining postural equilibrium. Asymmetry amounted in the CCI population to 0.15% body weight, nearly double the value for the control subjects.

CORRELATION BETWEEN MECHANICAL AND CLINICAL PARAMETERS

An attempt to grade the patients according to ascending magnitude of neurologic deficits dis-closed that their sway disturbances, as revealed by the magnitudes of total sway activity and asymmetry, tended to be related to the severity of neurobehavioral disturbances,[74] the correlation coefficients being 0.97 and 0.60, respectively, for sway activity and asymmetry.

BALANCE IN PATIENTS WITH BELOW-KNEE AMPUTATION

THE QUESTION OF PROPRIOCEPTIVE DEFICIT

Published results about the standing stability in people who have had amputations are controversial. An increased postural sway in people with above-knee and below-knee amputations was demonstrated.[82] On the other hand, it has been stated that sway in people with below-knee amputation is comparable to that of a matched control group.[83] Additional questions about standing stability of BKA patients relate to the effects of visual feedback and of compensation and adaptation on improved stability in these subjects. It has been assumed that in subjects with BKA, unlike in able-bodied subjects, when the visual and vestibular systems are intact, the main cause for insecure standing is a quantitative decrease in proprioceptive inflow due to the loss of foot and leg muscles. The proprioexteroceptive information is transmitted by different receptors localized in the skin, subcutis, joint capsule, ligaments, tendons, and muscles.

Intense responses to afferent inputs arising within the environment are mediated primarily by exteroceptive inputs.[5] Muscular responses resulting from proprioceptive inputs are mild. Therefore, the muscle spindles, which are highly sensitive proprioceptors, evoke the stretch reflex and a muscular response even after small disturbances. As a result, postural instabilities should increase only when inputs from muscle spindle afferents are eliminated. Nevertheless, published results regarding the relationship between visual inflow and postural stability are still controversial. As far as we know, no investigations have been performed to test whether lower limb amputation results in proprioceptive deficit. In fact, it has been found that amputation above the knee affects postural sway only when the subject's eyes are closed.[82] Surprisingly, it has also been found that the postural sway of people with BKA was significantly greater than it was for people with above-knee amputations when the patients' eyes were either open or closed. Bilateral measurements were thus undertaken to address these questions.

SUBJECTS

Eleven men who had BKA, with an average age of 64.8 ± 9.2 years (range, 49 to 80 years), were included in this study. The level of amputation was below the left knee in seven men and below the right knee in four men. In all patients, amputation was performed because of gangrene secondary to diabetes mellitus. Nine able-bodied men from the group of control subjects (mean age, 65.6 ± 8.6 years) served as controls. Patients or subjects with partial blindness, neurologic problems, or any disease known to affect equilibrium were excluded from the study. To establish integrity of equilibrium in the test subjects, a preliminary Romberg test[82] was conducted. Those who failed to maintain equilibrium during the test were excluded from the study.

Subjects with BKA were tested after exercising with their new prostheses. The first test was done 1 to 2 days after the subjects with BKA received their prostheses. They were tested again 3 to 4 weeks later on completion of their prosthetic rehabilitation program.

AMPLITUDES OF SWAY

Values of sway activity, asymmetry, and weight-bearing imbalance (WBI) (expressed in percentage of body weight) obtained in subjects with BKA are shown in Figures 8–10 and 8–11. All three quantities were substantially higher in the BKA patients than in control subjects: 3.8-, 13.1-, and 3.84-fold higher for sway activity, asymmetry, and WBI, respectively. The differences were statistically significant. Results for the second testing period for the subjects with BKA indicate that improvement was achieved in all three parameters. In the second test, performed on completion of the prosthetic rehabilitation program, there was a reduction in sway activity, asymmetry, and WBI by 11%, 28%, and 16%, respectively. There was a significant reduction for sway activity with eyes open ($P = .01$) and for WBI with eyes closed ($P = .027$). When visual feedback was present, there was a significant decrease in asymmetry in the subjects with BKA, both in the early and in the late testing periods. Total sway activity decreased in the late testing period only.

There was no significant improvement in WBI in either group when the test was performed with eyes open or closed. Comparison between results obtained by subtracting values for closed eyes from values for open eyes indicates that the differences obtained in the early test and the late test were not significant. It may be assumed, in those cases in which no significant differences were found between closed eyes and open eyes when comparing subjects with BKA with the able-bodied controls, that the influence (or lack of influence) of vision is similar in both groups tested. To address the issue of the role of proprioception deficit in subjects with BKA, the differences obtained from tests of subjects in both groups with closed eyes and open eyes were compared. These results show that the differences were significantly higher in subjects with BKA for the sway activity and asymmetry parameters in the late testing period. The difference was less pronounced for sway activity in subjects with BKA in the early testing period. These differences have no effect on WBI. Therefore, the obvious difference in values obtained from tests of subjects with BKA with eyes open and eyes closed indicates that they are less stable and less secure, probably owing to proprioceptive deficit. This is further emphasized by the fact that the differences remain in people with BKA throughout rehabilitation.

It has also been demonstrated that in people who have recently experienced BKA, there is a continuous process of compensation and adaptation to the new situation of a partial limb loss. In fact, with prosthesis use for 3 to 4 weeks, significant improvement was seen in sway activity (eyes open) and WBI (with eyes closed). Other parameters also improved, but to a lesser extent.

In conclusion, subjects with BKA were found to be significantly less stable than able-bodied people during standing. Deficits in proprioceptive inflow due to limb amputation contribute even more to this difference. There is a process of habituation and compensation achieved by means of prosthetic training and use. Future studies on subjects with BKA should be conducted to test the effects of longer periods of prosthetic use.

INFLUENCE OF PROSTHESIS ALIGNMENT ON STANDING BALANCE

Alignment of a prosthesis is established by the relative geometric position and orientation of the various prosthetic components, such as the socket, shaft, joints, and foot. Optimal alignment is a crucial factor for the successful rehabilitation of the amputee. No less important are the quality of the fit of the socket, quality of suspension, mass properties of the prosthesis, and cosmesis.[84–87]

Several investigators have attempted to establish the optimal range of alignment for the BKA patient, through subjective impression of several prosthetists and direct feedback from the patient.[88] Other approaches to investigate the effect of changing prosthetic alignment on gait have included indices of symmetry between limbs.[89, 90] It was shown that maximum symmetry of kinematic parameters does not always correspond to a subjectively determined optimal alignment. Therefore, gait symmetry should not be the only goal of the clinician when aligning a prosthesis.

The standing BKA patient adapts to the prosthesis alignment through accommodation by the contralateral limb. Therefore, use of unilateral measurement techniques[91, 92] has the disadvantage of not considering interaction of the contralateral limb, and monitoring of both limbs simultaneously is essential to determine the combined effect of alignment on standing balance.

Two relevant questions thus arise: (1) What are the foot–ground force patterns obtained by BKA patients when standing while the prosthesis is optimally aligned? (2) Do changes in prosthesis alignment influence the bilateral foot–ground force patterns and the standing sway activity?

To address these questions, the following bilateral sway measurements were made.

Subjects and Tests

We assessed three volunteers, one woman and two men, with traumatic BKA. The sides of amputation for the three subjects respectively were right, left, and right: ages 45, 30, and 52 years; masses 75, 78, and 90 kg; heights 1.62, 1.80, and 1.80 meters; and time from amputation 15, 19, and 25 years. All were excellent walkers who used their prostheses on a regular basis and were conducting an active normal family life.

The test was conducted while the subject was wearing his or her regular prosthesis. All subjects used a modular patellar-tendon–bearing prosthesis with belt suspension and a solid ankle-cushioned heel foot. Because the subjects were excellent walkers and were satisfied with their prostheses, the existing prosthesis alignment in each of the three amputees tested was considered optimal and was therefore taken as the reference position.

The optimal alignment was changed by tilting the pylon in the anterior, posterior, medial, and lateral directions. The maximal tilt in each direction, obtained by maneuvering the coupler, was 9 degrees.

Results

The results indicate that the anteroposterior force differences between the amputated and contralateral limbs were found to be highly significant in all alignment positions. The measured mediolateral force did not differ significantly.

For each leg and each alignment position, the anteroposterior and mediolateral forces were also compared with those in the optimal position. In the amputated limb, the anteroposterior and mediolateral forces in varus tilting and the anteroposterior force in valgus tilting were significantly higher than in the optimal position. In the contralateral limb, no significant differences were found between the optimal and other alignments. A possible explanation is that an inert prosthesis is incapable of compensating for the missing function of the joints of an anatomic foot and ankle. This imposes on the musculature of the contralateral limb an additional balancing activity in the anteroposterior direction. This increased level of activity of the contralateral limb prevails in the optimal alignment as well as in the modified alignments in the anteroposterior direction. The amputated limb activity increased significantly, however, in the anteroposterior and mediolateral directions when the prosthesis was tilted into varus and in the anteroposterior direction only when tilted into valgus.

Sway activity obtained with optimally aligned prostheses was compared with sway activity in the different measured alignments. Changing the prosthesis alignment did not significantly influence the sway activity during standing. Asymmetry and WBI were also verified; neither differed significantly between the optimal and the other tested alignment configurations, except for asymmetry in the valgus tilting, which was significantly higher in this position. It can therefore be concluded that the standing, well-trained BKA patient is able to adapt to drastic alignment changes while preserving a well-balanced position.

SUMMARY

Postural sway is the result of the minute movements of the different body segments while standing still. Forceplate measurements are only one expression of this phenomenon; they can, however, be very significant if properly made. Measurement of postural sway, as reported in the literature, has for many years been based on monitoring the variations of the center of pressure of both feet together when standing on one force platform. Most of the sway studies erroneously interpreted the trajectory of the center of pressure to reflect the trajectory of the center of mass of the body. In our work, we have corrected this misconception in the following two respects: (1) we measure the actual *forces* between foot and ground, rather than their center of pressure; and (2) we make our measurements bilaterally, that is, in each leg separately.

Normal posture by nature has some systematization, although intricate, allowing quantification and delineation of possible patterns of associated postural adjustments. In patients with orthopedic or neurologic disorders, motor and sensory deficits may influence the resulting swaying mechanisms and balance outcome. Although some of these features are difficult to assess and quantify accurately, however, common standing patterns can often be identified in the different groups of patients. The possibility of characterizing the swaying features of the various pathologies is of major importance for both diagnostic and follow-up purposes.

Acknowledgment: This study was supported by the Segal Foundation, Tel Aviv, Israel.

References

1. Basmajian JV: Muscles Alive: Their Functions Revealed by Electromyography. Baltimore, Williams & Wilkins, 1962.
2. Winter DA: A.B.C. of Balance During Standing and Walking. Waterloo, Ontario, Canada, Waterloo Biomechanics, 1995.
3. Paulus WM, Straube A, Brandt T: Visual stabilization of posture: Physiological stimulus characteristics and clinical aspects. Brain 107:1143–1163, 1984.
4. McClure JA: Vertigo and imbalance in the elderly. J Otolaryngol 15:248–252, 1985.
5. Evarts EV: Sherrington's concept of proprioception. Trends Neurosci 4:44–46, 1981.
6. Gurfinkel EV: Physical foundations of oscillography. Agressologie 14C:9–13, 1973.
7. Hirashawa Y: Study of human standing ability. Agressologie 14C:37–43, 1973.
8. Snijders CJ, Verduin M: Stabilograph, an accurate instrument for sciences interested in postural equilibrium. Agressologie 14C:15–20, 1973.
9. Herman R, MacEwen GD: Idiopathic scoliosis: A visuo-vestibular disorder of the central nervous system? *In* Zorab PA (ed): Sixth Symposium on Scoliosis. New York, Academic Press, 1980, p 61.
10. Harris GF, Knox TA, Larson SJ, et al: A method for the display of balance platform center of pressure data. J Biomech 15:741–745, 1982.
11. Nayak VSL, Gabell A, Simons MA, Isaacs B: Measurement of gait and balance in the elderly. J Am Geriatrics Soc 30:516–520, 1982.
12. Koozekanani SH, Stockwell CW, McGhee RB, Firoozmand F: On the role of dynamic models in quantitative posturography. IEEE Trans Biomed Eng 27:605–609, 1980.
13. Valk-Fai T: Analysis of the dynamical behaviour of the body whilst "standing still." Agressologie 14C:21–25, 1973.
14. Shimba T: An estimation of center of gravity from force platform. J Biomech 17:53–60, 1984.
15. Levin O, Mizrahi J: An iterative model for estimation of the trajectory of center of gravity

16. from bilateral reactive force measurements in standing sway. Gait Posture 4:89–99, 1996.
16. Levin O: Dynamic parameters in human standing posture. M.Sc. Thesis, Technion, Israel Institute of Technology, Haifa, Israel, March 1994.
17. Thomas DP, Whitney RJ: Postural movements during normal standing in man. J Anat (London) 93:524–539, 1959.
18. Stribley RF, Albers JW, Tourtellotte WW, Cockrell JL: A quantitative study of stance in normal subjects. Arch Phys Med Rehabil 55:74–80, 1974.
19. Soames RW, Atha J: The validity of physique-based inverted pendulum models of postural sway behaviour. Ann Human Biol 7:145–153, 1980.
20. Shimba T: Ground reaction forces during human standing. Eng Med 12:177–182, 1983.
21. Lestienne F, Soechting J, Berthoz A: Postural readjustments induced by linear motion of visual scenes. Exp Brain Res 28:363–384, 1977.
22. Walsh EG: Standing man, slow rhythmic tilt, importance of vision. Agressologie 14C:79–85, 1973.
23. Pollak VA, Wyss UP: A simple and inexpensive technique for the measurement of head sway. J Biomech 16:349–350, 1983.
24. Kapteyn TS: Afterthought about the physics and mechanics of the postural sway. Agressologie 14C:27–35, 1973.
25. Gueguen G, Leroux J: Identification d'un modele representant les deplacements du centre de gravite de l'homme. Agressologie 14C:73–77, 1973.
26. Lee DN, Lishman JR: Visual proprioceptive control of stance. J Hum Movement Stud 1:87–95, 1975.
27. Mizrahi J, Susak Z: Bi-lateral reactive forces patterns in postural sway activity of normal subjects. Biol Cybernet 60:297–305, 1989.
28. Kapteyn TS, Bles W, Njiokiktjien ChJ, et al: Standardization in platform stabilometry being a part of posturography. Aggressologie 24C:321–326, 1983.
29. Era P, Heikkinen E: Postural sway during standing and unexpected disturbance of balance in random samples of men of different ages. J Gerontol 40:287–295, 1985.
30. Kataoka J, Sakamoto K, Hara T, Hayami A: Principal component analysis of spontaneous physical movements in sustained standing posture of children. J Hum Ergol 10:61–71, 1981.
31. Yamomoto T: Changes in postural sway related to age. J Phys Fitness Jpn 28:249–256, 1979.
32. Lakes RS, Korttila K, Eltoft D, et al: Instrumented force platform for postural sway studies. IEEE Trans Biomed Eng 28:725–729, 1981.
33. Hashizume K, Ito H, Marruyama H, et al: Age-related changes of stability in standing posture. Jpn J Geriatr 23:85–92, 1986.
34. Kirby RL, Price NA, MacLeod DA: The influence of foot position on standing balance. J Biomech 20:423–427, 1987.
35. Gantchev G, Popov: Quantitative evaluation of induced body oscillations in man. Agressologie 14C:91–94, 1973.

36. Hlavacka F, Litvinenkova V: First derivative of the shabilogram and posture control in visual feedback conditions in man. Agressologie 14C:45–49, 1973.

37. Seidel H, Brauer D: Effects of visual information, conscious control and low-frequency whole-body vibration on postural sway. Agressologie 20C:189–190, 1979.

38. Yamamoto T: Changes in postural sway related to fatigue. J Phys Fitness Jpn 28:18–24, 1979.

39. Tokita T, Miyata H, Matsuoka T, et al: Correlation analysis of the body sway in standing posture. Agressologie 17B:7–14, 1975.

40. Hufschmidt A, Dichgans J, Mauritz KH, Hufschmidt M: Some methods and parameters of body sway quantification and their neurological applications. Arch Psychiat Nervenkr 228:135–150, 1980.

41. Nashner LM, Black OF, Wall C III: Adaptation to altered support and visual conditions during stance: Patients with vestibular deficits. J Neurosci 2:536–544, 1981.

42. Black OF, Wall C III, Nashner LM: Effects of visual and support surface orientation references upon postural control in vestibular deficient subjects. Acta Otolaryngol 95:199–210, 1983.

43. Dietz V, Mauritz KH, Dichgans J: Body oscillations in balancing due to segmental stretch reflex activity. Exp Brain Res 40:89–95, 1980.

44. Arcan M, Brull MA, Najenson T, Solzi P: FGP assessment of postural disorders during the process of rehabilitation. Scand J Rehabil Med 9:165–168, 1977.

45. Seliktar R, Susak Z, Najenson T, Solzi P: Dynamic features of standing and their correlation with neurological disorders. Scand J Rehabil Med 10:59–64, 1978.

46. Taguchi K: Spectral analysis of the movement of the center of gravity in vertiginous and ataxic patients. Agressologie 19B:69–72, 1978.

47. Mauritz KH, Dichgans J, Hufschmidt A: Quantitative analysis of stance in late cortical cerebellar atrophy of the anterior lobe and other forms of cerebellar ataxia. Brain 102:461–468, 1979.

48. Dichgans, Mauritz KH, Allum JHJ, Brandt Th: Postural sway in normals and atactic patients: Analysis of the stabilizing and destabilizing effects of vision. Agressologie 17C:15–24, 1976.

49. Bles W, DeWit G: Study of the effects of optic stimuli on standing. Agressologie 17C:1–5, 1976.

50. Nashner LM: Adapting reflexes controlling the human posture. Exp Brain Res 26:59–72, 1976.

51. Soechting JF, Berthoz A: Dynamic role of vision in the control of posture in man. Exp Brain Res 37:551–561, 1979.

52. Vidal PP, Berthoz A, Millanvoye M: Difference between eye closure and visual stabilization in the control of posture in man. Aviation Space Environ Med 53:166–170, 1982.

53. Dvir Z, Trousil T: EMG study of several lower limb muscles during maintenance of dynamic balance in the frontal plane. Agressologie 23:71–73, 1982.

54. Booth JB, Stockwell CW: A method for evaluating vestibular control of posture. Otolaryngology 86:93–97, 1978.

55. Ishida A, Imai S, Fukuoka Y: Analysis of the posture control system under fixed and sway-referenced support conditions. IEEE Trans Biomed Eng 44:331–336, 1997.

56. Nashner LM, Block FO, Wall C: Adaptation to altered support and visual conditions during stance: Patients with vestibular deficits. J Neurosci 2:536–544, 1982.

57. Allum JHJ, Pfaltz CR: Visual and vestibular contributions to pitch sway stabilization in the ankle muscles of normals and patients with bilateral peripheral vestibular deficits. Exp Brain Res 58:82–94, 1985.

58. Forssberg H, Nashner LM: Ontogenetic development of postural control in man: Adaptation to altered support and visual conditions during stance. J Neurosci 2:545–552, 1982.

59. Dvir Z, Daniel-Atrakci R, Mirovski Y: The effect of frontal loading on static and dynamic balance reactions in patients with chronic low back dysfunction. Basic Applied Myol 7:91–96, 1997.

60. Dvir Z, Trousil T: A multiple parameter study of dynamic balance in the frontal and sagittal planes. Agressologie 22:129–134, 1981.

61. Dvir Z, Trousil T: Instrumented stabilometer for dynamic balance studies. Med Biol Eng Comput 20:19–22, 1982.

62. Trousil T, Dvir Z: Dynamic balance: A learning strategy. Hum Movement Sci 2:211–218, 1983.

63. Smith JW: The forces operating at the human ankle joint during standing. J Anat (London) 91:545–564, 1957.

64. Bizzo G, Guillet N, Patat A, Gagey PM: Specifications for building a vertical force platform designed for clinical stabilometry. Med Biol Eng Comput 23:474–476, 1985.

65. Kodde L, Caberg HB, Mol JMF, Massen CH: An application of mathematical models in posturography. J Biomed Eng 4:44–48, 1982.

66. Magnusson M, Johannson R: Characteristic parameters of anterior-posterior body sway in normal subjects. In Amblard B, Berthoz A, Clarac F (eds): Posture and Gait: Development, Adaptation and Modulation. Excerpta Medica International Congress Series 812. Amsterdam, Elsevier, 1988, p 177.

67. Nashner LM: A model describing vestibular detection of body sway motion. Acta Otolaryngol 72:429–436, 1971.

68. Nashner LM: Analysis of movement control in man using the movable platform. Adv Neurol 39:607–619, 1983.

69. Nashner LM, Shumway-Cook A, Marin O: Stance posture control in select groups of children with cerebral palsy: Deficits in sensory organization and muscular coordination. Exp Brain Res 49:393–409, 1983.

70. Fioretti S, Leo T, Maurizi M, et al: Functional evaluation of multiple sclerosis patients at an early stage. *In* Woollacott M, Horak F (eds): Posture and Gait: Control Mechanisms, vol 2. XIth International Symposium of the Society for Postural and Gait Research. Portland, OR, University of Oregon Books, 1992, p 63.

71. Fioretti S, Leo T, Maurizi M, Pieroni R: A CAMA system for the functional evaluation of posture maintenance. *In* Woollacott M, Horak F (eds): Posture and Gait: Control Mechanisms, vol 2. XIth International Symposium of the Society for Postural and Gait Research. Portland, OR, University of Oregon Books, 1992 p 67.

72. Mizrahi J, Najenson T, Nissel R: Asymmetry and total activity analysis of postural sway option in cerebral vascular accident patients. Proc 14th Int Conf on Med and Biol Eng Espoo, Finland. Med Biol Eng Comput 23(Suppl 1):418–419, 1985.

73. Mizrahi J, Solzi P, Ring H, Nisell R: Postural stability in stroke patients: Vectorial expression of asymmetry, sway-activity and relative sequence of reactive forces. Med Biol Eng Comput 27:181–190, 1989.

74. Mizrahi J, Groswasser Z, Susak Z, Reider-Groswasser I: Standing posture of craniocerebral injured patients: Bi-lateral reactive force pattern. Clin Phys Physiol Meas 10:25–37, 1989.

75. Ring H, Mizrahi J: Bilateral postural sway in stroke patients: New parameters for assessing and predicting locomotor outcome. J Neurol Rehabil 5:175–179, 1991.

76. Ring H, Mizrahi J: Biomechanical sway parameters in the evaluation of stroke patients. Neurorehabilitation 2:27–35, 1992.

77. Isakov E, Mizrahi J, Ring H, et al: Standing sway and weight bearing distribution in people with below-knee amputations. Arch Phys Med Rehabil 73:174–178, 1992.

78. Isakov E, Mizrahi J, Susak Z, et al: Influence of prosthesis alignment on the standing balance of below-knee amputees. Clin Biomech 9:258–262, 1994.

79. Crowe A, Schiereck P, deBoer R, Keessen W: Characterization of gait of young adult females by means of body center of mass oscillations derived from ground reaction forces. Gait Posture 1:61–68, 1993.

80. Stern B, Stern FM: Neuropsychological outcome during late stage of recovery from brain injury: A proposal. Scand J Rehabil Med Suppl 12:27–30, 1985.

81. Stern JM, Melamed S, Silbey S, et al: Behavioral disturbances as an expression of severity of cerebral damage. Scand J Rehabil Med Suppl 12:36–41, 1985.

82. Fernie GR, Holling PJ: Postural sway in amputees and normal subjects. J Bone Joint Surg (Am) 60:895–898, 1978.

83. Vittas D, Larsin TK, Jansen EC: Body sway in below-knee amputees. Prosthet Orthot Int 10:139–141, 1986.

84. Porter D, Roberts VC: A review of gait assessment in the lower limb amputee. 2. Kinetic and metabolic analysis. Clin Rehabil 3:157–168, 1989.

85. Nissen SJ, Newman WP: Factors influencing reintegration to normal living after amputation. Arch Phys Med Rehabil 73:548–551, 1992.

86. Burgess EM: Amputations. Surg Clin North Am 63:749–770, 1983.

87. Skinner HB, Effeney DJ: Gait analysis in amputees. Am J Phys Med 64:82–89, 1985.

88. Zahedi MS, Spence WD, Solomonidis SE, Paul JP: Alignment of lower limb prostheses. J Rehabil Res Dev 23:2–19, 1986.

89. Hannah RE, Morrison JB, Chapman AE: Prostheses alignment: Effect on gait of persons with below-knee amputations. Arch Phys Med Rehabil 65:159–162, 1984.

90. Andres RO, Stimmel SK: Prosthetic alignment effects on gait symmetry: A case study. Clin Biomech 5:88–96, 1990.

91. Jones D, Paul J: Analysis of variability in pylon transducer signals. Prosthet Orthot 2:35–50, 1973.

92. Wilson AB Jr, Pritham C, Cook T: Force-line visualisation system. Prosthet Orthot 3:85–87, 1979.

CHAPTER 9

BIOMECHANICS OF MANUAL THERAPY

Michael Lee, Julianna Gál, and Walter Herzog

Manipulative procedures have been used for hundreds, perhaps thousands, of years.[1] This century, especially since World War II, detailed descriptions of the techniques have been published, and the training of practitioners of manual therapy has become increasingly formalized. Despite the recent formal codification of the procedures involved, there has been little attempt to develop a comprehensive analysis of the mechanics of manual therapy techniques using realistic assumptions about the nature of joint movements. A complete mechanical analysis would describe the physical effects on all relevant tissues, would take into account the effects of tissue abnormalities associated with disease or trauma, and could be validated by experimental data. Further, the consequences of variations in therapeutic technique would be considered, to allow prediction of the treatment methods most likely to produce the desired outcome. Such an analysis has not yet been presented. Certain elements of the manual therapy process have been examined, but the development of a complete analysis requires research in many areas.

There are two main classes of manual techniques, categorized on the basis of the rate of strain and number of loading phases. One class is commonly known as *manipulation*. In a manipulation, the manual force is usually delivered using a single high-speed thrust. The other class of techniques is often referred to as *mobilization* and is associated with relatively slow loading rates, ranging from almost static loading to cyclic loading at rates as high as 5 to 6 Hz. Mobilization, however, is generally performed at less than 2 Hz, and in the case of higher frequencies (5 Hz), the amplitude of oscillation is probably quite small, so that the tissue strain rates are small compared

with manipulation. In addition to the loads being applied slowly, mobilizations are distinguished by a large number of loading cycles and a much longer duration of loading than manipulations. In this chapter, the two classes of techniques are treated separately.

Although the term *manual therapy* strictly applies to any therapy delivered with the practitioner's hands, the use of the term in this chapter is confined to that group of procedures in which there is an attempt to focus the treatment directly on the joints—either the joints of the vertebral column or the peripheral joints. The objective of this chapter is to review the current state of knowledge of the mechanics of manual therapy techniques. This information is potentially valuable for practitioners who are attempting to understand the possible mechanisms involved in manual therapy and to develop theories that may optimize the use of manual techniques.

JOINT MOVEMENTS AND LOADS: DESCRIPTION AND QUANTIFICATION

Because we are considering a therapy that is directed at joints, we need to be able to describe the mechanical effects of the therapy on joints. This description process essentially involves two elements. First, we need to describe the joint kinematics—the movements that occur between the bones that form the target joint and any other joints that may be of interest. Second, we need to describe the joint dynamics—the forces and moments applied to the bones involved and acting across the joints of interest, and their role in causing joint movements.

KINEMATICS

Movement Produced by the Clinician: "Physiologic" and "Accessory" Movements

In manual therapy, the clinician applies a moment, tending to produce rotation at a joint, or a force, tending to translate one bone relative to another. The rotational movements, simulating the movements produced by the patient's muscles, are known as *physiologic movements.* Isolated translation between bones cannot normally be produced by the patient through voluntary activation of muscles, and these movements are often known as *accessory movements.* The degree to which a manual therapy procedure produces physiologic or accessory movements is not necessarily evident, especially when spinal joints are involved. Although the clinician may be attempting to produce a pure accessory translation between two bones, some rotation may also be produced. Similarly, the clinician's attempt to produce a physiologic movement may not produce the same pattern of rotation and translation that would result from activation of the patient's own muscles.

Joint and Bone Structures

A typical synovial joint can be characterized as shown in Figure 9–1. There is one concave and one convex joint surface, but the radius of curvature is not constant along the joint surface and not exactly the same on the concave and convex surfaces. For any given joint position, a point, such as point C, at the center of the arc that forms the convex joint surface at the point of contact, can be located. Because the joint surface does not form a perfect circle, the point C will be in a different location for each different point of contact.

The size and shape of the bones that compose the joint are important variables for the clinician. Part of the manual therapy process often involves the application of moments to one bone. These moments may be required to stabilize one bone to prevent movement or to produce rotation of a bone. The long bones allow forces to be applied at two points some distance apart, allowing a large moment to be applied. In contrast, smaller bones, such as the vertebrae and the bones of the foot and wrist, are most likely to be subject to manual force application that can be represented as acting through a single point. In the latter case, variation in the amount of joint rotation can be produced by altering the point of application and orientation of the applied manual force in relation to the other forces applied to the bone by tissues, such as ligaments, disk, and joint cartilage, that are in contact with the bone.

Body Segment Movements and Joint Surface Movements

The relationship between bone movements and joint surface movements may be of interest to the clinician who believes that there is a limitation of relative movement between the joint surfaces that is amenable to manual therapy treatment procedures. Consider again the typical joint shown in Figure 9–1. Let us first examine the case of an idealized version of this joint, in which the two joint surfaces have the same constant radius forming circular arcs around the same center, C. Imagine that the ligaments, joint capsule, and muscles hold the surfaces in close contact. Physiologic movement of either bone will occur in a pattern that involves rotation of *all points* on the moving bone around the center of the joint surface arc, C. Hence, if a given joint conforms to this ideal structure, the bone movements, including joint surface movements, can be predicted from the structure. Each point on the bone, including the joint surface, would move in a circular path around the joint center, C. As rotation occurs, the joint surfaces slide past each other, the "gliding" movement described by Kaltenborn.[2] It can be noted that in this ideal case, the amount of linear movement (glide) between the two joint surfaces at the interface is $s = r\theta$, where θ is the angular movement between the bones (measured in radians), and r is the radius from the surface to point C, the center of the radius of curvature. The hip joint is perhaps the joint that conforms most with this ideal morphology in three dimensions,[3] while the elbow joint is a joint with a two-dimensional profile that is close to ideal.[4]

In the case of a nonideal joint, with two joint surfaces that do not have the same radius and are not held in close congruence, "rolling" of one joint surface on another may occur. Pure rolling

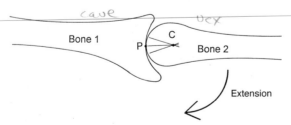

FIGURE 9–1 Typical joint, showing point P, the point of contact between the two joint surfaces; point C, the center of the arc describing the bone 2 joint surface at the point of contact; and the direction that is arbitrarily designated extension.

may occur when there is no gliding between the joint surfaces at the point of contact, but in most cases, rolling and gliding occur together. The relative amounts and directions of the rolling and gliding determine the amount and direction of movement of the point of contact between the two bones. Rolling that would move the point of contact in one direction can be combined with gliding that would move the point of contact in the opposite direction, to maintain the contact point in one location.

Description of Joint Movements

One of the major aims of a manual therapy technique is to produce joint movements; that is, an attempt is made to produce relative movement between two bones. In many cases, the two bones are readily identifiable, and the success of the technique can thus be partly measured by describing the relative motion between the two bones. In the next two sections, methods of describing physiologic and accessory movement will be given that can be used for this purpose.

In some cases, there are more than just two bones whose relative movement must be described. For example, the kinematic outcome of manual therapy techniques in the foot may be given by describing the relative motion between the tibia and the calcaneus, between the talus and the calcaneus, between the talus and the first metatarsal, or between many other bone pairs. There may not be just a single anatomic joint between the bones whose relative movements are of interest. The spine presents a similar situation. When we apply a manual force to a vertebra, we are usually interested in relative movement in at least two intervertebral joints, proximal and distal to the target vertebra, as well as between other bones. Therefore, the complete description of the movement response may involve multiple applications of the methods described next.

Methods Used for Describing Physiologic Movements

Because normal voluntary joint movements predominantly involve rotations of one body segment relative to another, the most appropriate method for describing those movements is a method that focuses on the rotation. Rotational movements are best defined by describing the *helical axis of motion* (HAM) for the motion. This method is capable of giving a full three-dimensional description of the movement of the segment. The key element of the description process is the defining of the helical axis itself. The axis is an imaginary line in

space, around which the moving body segment rotates (Fig. 9–2). Because of the irregularity of human joints, the axis is almost never exactly perpendicular to a cardinal plane, such as the sagittal plane. Further, the axis does not usually stay fixed in space during an entire movement through the available range of motion. Fully describing a physiologic movement pattern involves giving the location of the axis at as many points in the movement as practical. It is possible that during a physiologic movement, there is also a small amount of translation along the axis of motion. For example, if a person produced knee flexion in a sitting position, this translation would correspond to translation in an approximately mediolateral direction. Obviously, in normal joints, this along-axis translation would be small, but its presence in abnormal amounts may be a sensitive indicator of certain injuries.

In some situations, the HAM is simplified by representing it as a single point, with the implicit assumption that the axis is perpendicular to the plane on which the point is located. This point, known as a *center of rotation,* can be a valid way of representing the movement, provided the HAM really is perpendicular to the plane concerned, and provided there is negligible movement of the body segment out of the plane (along the axis).

If we perform a manual therapy technique that involves a passive physiologic movement, we can use the HAM to describe the way the joint moves in response to that technique. The HAM data for this movement could be compared with the HAM data for both voluntary active movements and passive physiologic movements performed on subjects with no abnormalities, to establish the degree of normality of the passive physiologic movement.

An alternative approach to movement description is to divide the total movement into *main* and *coupled* movements, where a main movement is one that occurs in the direction of the externally applied force (or moment) delivered by the clinician. The vertebra's movement in response to the clinician's force is influenced by the restraints offered by the connecting tissues. Many different tissue forces are applied to a vertebra, as well as the clinician's force, and the vertebral movement may therefore take place with components of movement in any direction. Movements that occur concomitantly with the main movement, but in directions other than that of the clinician's force, are known as coupled movements. As shown in Figure 9–3, there can be translations in three directions (1, 2, 3; the directions of the x, y, and z axes) and rotations in three directions (4, 5, 6; about lines parallel to these three axes). Hence, there are six possible movement components. In

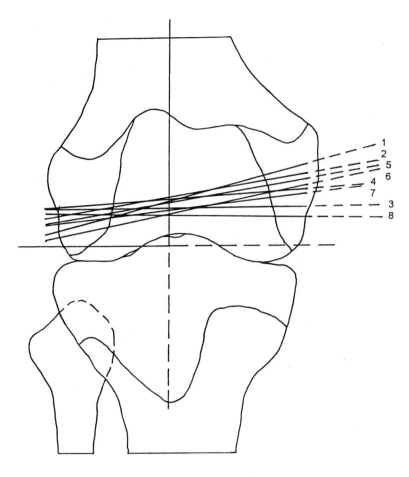

FIGURE 9–2 Helical axes of motion corresponding to eight steps of knee flexion from 0 to 109 degrees, shown in an anteroposterior view of axes projected onto the frontal plane. (Adapted from Huiskes R, van Dijk R, de Lange A, et al: Kinematics of the human knee joint. *In* Berme N, Engin AE, Correia da Silva KM [eds]: Biomechanics of Normal and Pathological Human Articulating Joints. Dordrecht, The Netherlands, Martinus Nijhoff, with kind permission of Wolters Kluwer Academic Publishers, 1985, p 165.)

other words, in addition to the main movement, there can be five coupled movement components. For a complete movement description, just as the HAM components must be given for as many small steps as practical throughout the movement, use of the main and coupled movement approach requires that the amount of these main and coupled movements be given for each small portion of the total range of movement.

Methods Used for Describing Accessory Movements

In contrast to physiologic movements, the aim of performing accessory movements is usually to produce translations of the body segment involved. Therefore, if we are to describe the resulting movements, there must be an emphasis on translation, although some rotation may also occur. In the HAM method, translation along the axis is explicitly described, whereas translation in a direction perpendicular to the axis is accommodated by movement of the axis location in time. For example, if a cylinder is rolling along a table, then the HAM that describes this movement is instantaneously located along the line of contact between the cylinder and the table. In an end view of the cylinder, the HAM is seen as a point at the bottom of the cylinder. The movement of the cylinder means that some time later, the HAM has moved parallel to its original position, to a new line of contact between the cylinder and the table. The direction of movement from the initial HAM to the final HAM is perpendicular to the axis. Therefore, if an accessory movement in which there is a mixture of rotation and translation is produced, the movement can be adequately described using the HAM approach.

If we are primarily interested in translations, however, we may wish to choose an approach that focuses more on translation. If the manual therapy technique involves a force applied in a particular direction, then the variable in which we are probably most interested is the amount of translation in the direction of the applied force. Therefore, it is most common to describe the movement response by partitioning into main and coupled movements. The sizes of the coupled displacements may be expressed in absolute terms or as a proportion of the main displacement. In a clinical context, the

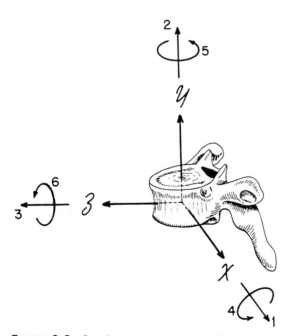

FIGURE 9-3 Coordinate system located at the center of the vertebral body, showing the six possible movements in relation to the x, y, and z axes. (From Panjabi MM, Brand RA, White AA: Three-dimensional flexibility and stiffness properties of the human thoracic spine. J Biomech 9:185, 1976, with permission from Elsevier Science.)

main displacement is usually assessed manually, often while assuming that the coupled displacements are negligible.

KINETICS

Joint Loads During Manual Therapy

Ideally, the clinician would like to know the loads experienced by each relevant anatomic structure as a result of the manual force being applied. In practice, the net force and net moment acting across a joint may be more readily estimated, using the techniques of inverse dynamics. Alternatively, direct measurement of tissue forces[5] and strains[6] is possible, and tissue loads can also be predicted using theoretical models.[7] The loads applied by the clinician can be measured by interposing a transducer between the hands and the patient's skin,[8] or they may be estimated by placing either the clinician or the patient on a forceplate to measure the ground reaction force.[9]

Mechanical Behavior of Joints

The mechanical behavior of a joint is commonly characterized by describing the relationship between an applied force (or moment) and the main

movement, and perhaps coupled movements. For example, a flexion torque may be applied to an elbow joint, and the joint's response can be characterized by showing the variation of flexion angle with applied torque. For anteroposterior accessory movement at the shoulder, the joint's response is characterized by the relationship between the applied anteroposterior force and the anteroposterior movement of the head of the humerus. In clinical practice, the clinician attempts to feel only the main movement, but laboratory studies[10] have described the variation of coupled movements as well as the main movement.

This approach can be applied to both physiologic and accessory movements. The joint mechanical behavior can be measured, or in clinical practice, the clinician performs a manual evaluation. When a manual assessment is performed, the documented joint behavior is often called a *movement diagram*[11] (Fig. 9-4). The movement diagram shows the clinician's perception of the amount of movement as a proportion of the perceived range of available movement, in relation to the resistance to movement, presumably the force opposing the clinician's applied force. In a movement diagram, the movement concerned is the absolute movement of the point at which the clinician's load is applied over the target bone.

To understand the clinical significance of the movement diagram more fully, however, we would also need to know the relationship between the target bone movement and the movement of other relevant bones. For example, in the case of the anteroposterior movement at the shoulder, we might like to know how much of the anteroposter-

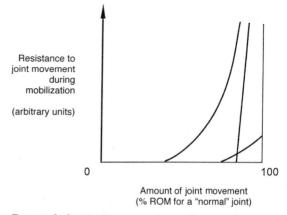

FIGURE 9-4 The "movement diagram" is the clinician's perception of the variation of resistance with displacement (with displacement expressed as a proportion of the normal range of motion [ROM]). Maitland[11] has stated that the perceived pattern of resistance could take a number of forms, including curves such as the three curves shown.

ior movement is occurring at the joint of primary interest, the glenohumeral joint. We may also like to know the amount of movement of the scapula in relation to the rib cage and movement at the acromioclavicular joint. It is an implicit assumption of many manual therapy techniques that a substantial contribution to the absolute movement of the target bone comes from the joint that is of primary interest, but for most joints, there have been no studies of this issue.

THE MANUAL THERAPY PROCESS

The aim of manual therapy treatment is usually to relieve pain; however, there is said to be a link between lack of joint mobility and joint pain.[12] Also, some patients describe problems that appear to be primarily due to joint hypomobility in one or more directions. Therefore, many clinicians use treatments aimed at increasing the mobility of joints.

The manual therapy intervention can be quantified in terms of the mechanical input to the patient or in terms of the outcome of the treatment. In traditional medical language, the nature of the treatment input can be described as the *dose*. The manual therapy dose can largely be measured in mechanical variables, but the treatment outcome measures often include measures of pain and other symptoms as well as physical measures. In this chapter, only mechanical outcome measures that are assessed by manual application of force to a joint are considered. Other types of outcome measurement tools, such as pain scales or range-of-motion measures, may be valid as indicators of the patient's status but are outside the scope of this chapter.

POSSIBLE METHODS FOR MEASURING DOSE

A number of approaches have been suggested for quantifying the dose involved in manual therapy.

Force

The variation of applied manual force with time during the manual therapy procedure is one of the most commonly measured mechanical dosage characteristics. The area under the curve showing applied force versus time is the impulse applied by the manual force.[8] The impulse may be a more important variable than the magnitude of the force alone. The instantaneous or short-term average *rate of change of force* can also be computed to describe the behavior of the applied manual force.[12] The maximum value of the applied force

is a commonly quoted variable,[13] whereas the amplitude of force variation[14] is relevant to cyclic loading conditions, as occur during mobilization. During both cyclic and single-thrust loading cases, there is often a base level of force that is applied before the main manual therapy force.[8] The magnitude of this base level of force is also of interest.

Displacement

The amount of relative displacement (linear and angular) between the bones that make up the target joint is a variable in which clinicians are likely to be interested. Manual therapy is often directed at increasing the amount of relative displacement at a joint. Therefore, the joint kinematic behavior during the manual therapy intervention, as detailed previously, can be used as a measure of the mechanical input to the joint.

Energy

The energy transferred to the joint can be calculated as the area under the force–displacement curve during loading. During unloading, much of this energy is returned to the clinician, with the energy returned being the area under the unloading curve. Because, in the case of biologic materials, the unloading curve follows a different (lower) path than the loading curve, there is a net transfer of energy into the tissues. The amount of energy transferred is equal to the area between the loading and unloading curves.[15]

Sounds

It has been observed that when manual forces are applied to joints, a clicking noise sometimes arises from the joint. This noise is more commonly associated with high-speed manipulation than is the case when forces are applied slowly. Some practitioners regard the occurrence of the click as a criterion for the "success" of the manipulation. A discussion of the possible causes and significance of the click is given later in the section on manipulation.

OUTCOME EVALUATION BY MANUAL TECHNIQUES

Many manual therapists use manual methods to evaluate the force–displacement or torque–angle characteristics of a joint, as described previously. These characteristics are assessed before and after the treatment to indicate the effect of the manual treatment on the mechanical behavior of the joint. One method of describing the manual findings is to represent the perceived variation of resistance (force or torque) on a movement diagram.[11] The accuracy of such subjective representations has not been evaluated. An alternative is to use clinical jargon to express the nature of the mechanical behavior, often without unambiguously defining those terms. For example, the range of joint movement has been divided into movement up to the "first stop" and movement between the "first stop" and the "final stop," without defining these terms.[2] The mechanical behavior in the latter part of the movement between the first stop and the final stop, the "end-feel" of the joint, has been described in terms such as "soft," "firm," and "hard." It has also been implied that a relationship exists between the type of end-feel and the tissue that prevents further movement.[2] As pointed out by Riddle,[16] there are few data to support the idea that there is a consistent relationship between the tissue that limits movement and the nature of the end-feel. Further, the terms soft, firm, and hard are subjective and cannot be unambiguously translated into measurable parameters. Therefore, in this chapter, we consider only methods and descriptive terms that can be understood as measurable physical variables.

MOBILIZATION

There has been little systematic study of the response of joints to mobilization. Those data that are available are mostly experimental results referring to the lumbar spine. In the future, similar experimental methods could be applied to peripheral joints to allow an analysis of the effects of relevant variables to be quantified. By examining the current lumbar spine data, together with information about the mechanical behavior of joints and isolated tissues, however, some principles may be established that could, to some extent, be applied to joints that have not yet been studied.

MOBILIZATION DOSE: THE APPLIED MANUAL FORCE

The manual force is usually applied with a magnitude and pattern that is varied in a graded manner and dependent on the patient's problems and the aims of treatment.[11, 17] The force applied during mobilization has been measured in a number of studies, all involving the spine. The forces have been measured during mobilization of healthy subjects,[9, 18, 19] patients with low back pain,[20] and physical models of patients.[21]

Perhaps the most commonly recorded parameter related to force has been the maximum value,

which depends on the "
land[11] defined a series
in terms of the location
the range of motion of
land's definitions, a g
small-amplitude moveme
range; a grade II mobiliz
movement that occurs in
does not involve signific
mobilizations are perform
tude and do involve sig
grade IV mobilizations are
ments performed near the
Different clinicians show
of the levels of force c
grades,[9] probably because   inter-
pretation of concepts such as "significant resistance" and "end of range."

Performing a Maitland[11] grade II mobilization of the L3 vertebra, a group of experienced physical therapists applied an average maximum vertical component of force of 33.3 N. Using a similar measurement method, and also applying grade II mobilization, Matyas and Bach[9] found that the peak forces when mobilizing four thoracic vertebrae varied from 7.6 N to 87.1 N among a group of seven specialist manual therapists. They found high variability in peak applied force among the clinicians tested.[9] In another study using the L3 vertebra,[14] the average maximum force applied to a group of 18 healthy subjects by an experienced physical therapist performing grade IV mobilization was 92.5 N. Threlkeld,[19] using two experi-

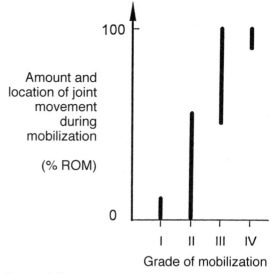

FIGURE 9–5   The grades of mobilization for mobilization of a normal joint with a "hard end-feel." The amount of movement is expressed as a proportion of the total range of motion (ROM). (Data from Maitland.[11])

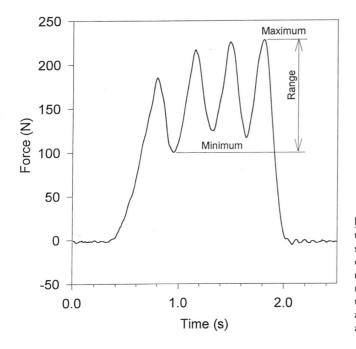

FIGURE 9-6 Force-time graph for mobilization of the L4 vertebra during assessment of stiffness of a subject lying prone. The range is defined as the difference between the maximum force and the minimum force during a set of oscillations. The magnitude of the applied force shown is the sum of the two major components: the vertical component and the horizontal component. (Data from Viner and associates.[45])

enced physical therapists to mobilize the mid-thoracic spine, found peak vertical forces of 140 and 206 N in grade I, and 232 and 500 N in grade IV. Simmonds and colleagues[21] performed an investigation that used a physical model of the spine based on a spring. In part of the experiment, a spring with a stiffness of 22.2 N/mm was used to produce stiffness similar to a high level of lumbar posteroanterior stiffness.[22] Ten physical therapists applied average maximum forces of 58 N, 86 N, 116 N, and 108 N during mobilization at grades I, II, III and IV, respectively, according to the Maitland[11] grading system.[21] All these studies found that there is high variability among clinicians and that peak mobilizing forces ranged from 10 N to 500 N depending on joint location, patient, clinician, and grade of mobilization.

Different grades of mobilization are used for different purposes, with relatively large forces being used in cases in which the clinician is attempting to produce increased movement at a joint, whereas smaller forces are often used when pain is the primary problem.[19] The relationship between applied manual force and particular tissue forces has not been established for any spinal or peripheral joints. Although it would be expected that greater applied forces would produce greater tissue forces, the pattern of load sharing among the tissues would be expected to vary with the level of applied load, owing to the nonuniformity among tissues and nonlinearity of the tissue behavior.[23]

The amplitude of the applied manual force dur-

ing cyclic loading has been reported much less frequently than the magnitude of the peak force. We can define the *range* of forces as the difference between the maximum force and the minimum force during oscillations (Fig. 9-6). Threlkeld[19] reported an average range of about 39% of the peak force in grade I thoracic mobilization, and 27% of the peak force in grade IV. Petty[14] found a mean range of about 10% of the peak force for a grade IV mobilization at L3. Maitland[11] described the different grades of mobilization movement as having either a small or large amplitude (grades I and IV have small amplitude, grades II and III have large amplitude), but the rationale for using a particular amplitude of force is not clear. One factor may be the desire to keep the amount of soft tissue stretch at a level that is beyond the toe region, the region corresponding to low loads and strains (Fig. 9-7). It has been argued that if the load is at a level beyond the toe region, microfailure is more likely to occur.[19] As previously stated, however, the relationship between applied force and the tension within each resisting tissue is unknown.

The frequency of the mobilizing force varies among individual clinicians[19] and, within one assessment session, may be varied by a clinician to alter his or her perception of the nature of the resistance to movement.[11] In a small number of cases, the mobilizing frequency has been measured, and frequencies in the range of 1.5 to 5.5 Hz have been observed.[14, 19] Greater frequency of loading is associated with increased stiffness of

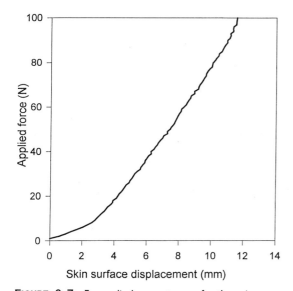

FIGURE 9–7 Force–displacement curve for thoracic posteroanterior loading showing a nonlinear region below an applied load of about 20 N.

the overall response (see later) and may also be linked to more localized movement,[24] although this hypothesized relationship has not yet been proved.

The dose of mobilization therapy could also be measured by reference to the amount of displacement produced, energy transferred to the patient, or whether clicking sounds were released. For mobilization, however, these methods do not appear to have been used.

PATIENT RESPONSES TO MOBILIZATION FORCES

Bone Movements in Peripheral Joint Mobilization

There have been few published studies of the mechanical behavior of peripheral joints of living subjects during actual or simulated mobilization procedures. The investigations that have been performed have not involved detailed kinematic analysis. Most peripheral joint mobilization procedures performed involve accessory movements, with the clinician almost always attempting to produce translations at the joint surface. Questions to be answered by a kinematic analysis would include the following: What joint surface movements are produced during the mobilization? How do the movements produced during mobilization compare with the movements that occur during active movement? Does the "fixed" bone (stabilized by the clinician or the patient) actually remain stationary? If an aim of the mobilization is

to produce one of the components of joint surface movement without the presence of the other movements (e.g., translation without the main rotation), a kinematic analysis is needed to examine whether this objective is being met.

Movements of Vertebrae

The movements of the many vertebrae involved in spinal mobilization are potentially more complex than bone movements during peripheral mobilization, in which only two bones are usually involved. A major issue to be considered is how the various vertebrae move when the mobilizing force is applied to one point on a single target vertebra. The behavior of the most commonly studied region, the lumbar spine, can be seen in terms of principles that are also applicable to other parts of the spine, although their application to a particular region must take into account the special characteristics of that region.

One of the first to study the vertebral movements arising from manual force applied to the lumbar spine was Ward (cited in Lee and Moseley,[25] p. 155). Ward reported a single case study of the application of a static 100-N force to the L3 spinous process. Qualitative comparison of lateral-view radiographs made in the unloaded and loaded cases showed that the force produced a general increase in lumbar extension. The individual intervertebral movements were small. In a subsequent experimental investigation,[24] cyclic loading at 0.5 and 1.0 Hz in the vertical direction was applied over the L3 spinous process. Measurement of skin surface movements showed that at both frequencies, there was a measurable response as far away as T8. Another study of L3 mobilization, using a slower mobilization frequency, found that pelvic anterior rotation also occurred. There were about 2 degrees of pelvic anterior rotation for every 100 N of applied L3 force.[26]

An approach that allows more detailed description of the vertebral movements is to use a mathematical model to predict the response to the manual force. Such a model was used by Lee and associates[27, 28] to simulate posteroanterior forces being applied to the lumbar spinous processes, as occurs during mobilization. A validation study found that the model behaved in a way that was reasonably representative of an average healthy subject.[27] The model predicted that the intervertebral rotation and translation at each joint were small—generally less than 1 degree or 1 mm per 100 N of applied force (Fig. 9–8).

Figure 9–8 shows that the greatest degree of extension was predicted to occur in the joints adjacent to the target bone, with the joints above

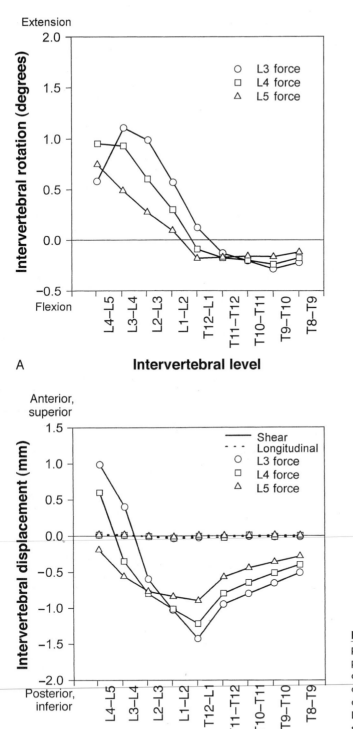

A

B

FIGURE 9–8 Predicted response to 100-N posteroanterior force applied to the spinous process of the L3, L4, or L5 vertebra. A, Angular displacement in the sagittal plane. B, Linear displacement in the shear and longitudinal directions. (From Lee M, Kelly DW, Steven GP: Lumbar spine manual therapy: Effect of choice of target vertebra. In Proceedings of the First Australian Biomechanics Conference, Sydney, 1996, p 104.)

and below the target bone showing similarly sized rotations. Shear displacements were predicted to be maximal around the thoracolumbar junction and to be small in the joints adjacent to the target

vertebra. The model predicted that lumbar mobilization is not a localized technique. Many joints move concomitantly, in contradistinction to the textbook image of isolated intervertebral movements at joints immediately cephalic and caudal to the target vertebra.[11, 29]

Because lumbar mobilization produces movement at many joints and deformation of a number of anatomic structures,[11] the total amount of movement of the skin surface where the clinician applies the force can be quite large, on the order of 10 mm of displacement under 100 N of applied force.[30] The relation between the joint mechanical properties of interest to the practitioner and the total movement under the practitioner's hands is not clear. For lumbar spine mobilization, it has been implied that intervertebral shear displacements are the major focus and that these movements are reflected in the movement felt by the clinician during mobilization.[11, 29] Although modeling studies indicate that the intervertebral shear displacements are likely to be less than 10% of the total posteroanterior movement,[28] it is possible that the intervertebral joint properties could have a palpable influence on the overall movement.

The general patterns of movement described previously for lumbar spine mobilization may also apply similarly to other spinal regions, although kinematic studies have not yet been performed. The movements occurring in the thoracic spine are likely to reflect the additional constraints offered by the rib cage, whereas the cervical spine movements are influenced by the high segmental mobility and the variable degree of constraint provided over its length. The manner in which the patient's head is supported on the treatment couch may be an important variable.

Tissue Loads

The loads sustained by various anatomic elements during mobilization are important determinants of the effects on the tissues.[19] In relation to spinal mobilization, there is little direct evidence about the load distributions. Lee and Evans[7] used a simple model of the lumbar spine to predict the pattern of posteroanterior shear force and extension moment variation under an L4 posteroanterior manual force of 150 N. They predicted anterior shear loads of about 120 N at joints caudal to the point of loading and posterior shear loads of about 30 N at cephalic joints, with extension moments of 2 N m and 6.5 N m at L5–S1 and L4–L5, respectively, and varying from 5 N m at L1–L2 to 8 N m at L3–L4 at lumbar joints cephalic to the target vertebra. The extent of simplifying assumptions and the lack of validation studies mean that these predictions may not be good indicators of the true load distribution.

Tissue Resistance to Mobilization

Another important aspect of spinal mobilization dynamics is the pattern of resistance to the mobilizing force, as perceived by the clinician. Because the manual force is applied slowly, the clinician is able to perceive the nature of the mechanical response. This response is thought to be indicative of the mechanical behavior of relevant spinal joints, although there are few data to support this assumption. The pattern of resistance, shown as a movement diagram, gives the relationship between applied manual force and body surface displacement. Throughout this chapter, the gradient of this force–displacement curve is described as the stiffness of the mobilization movement. In the terminology of Latash and Zatsiorsky,[31] this could be described as the apparent quasi-stiffness because the physical nature of the resistive forces is not known, and it is not measured at equilibrium. It should be emphasized that the movement stiffness, measured in this way, cannot necessarily be directly related to purely elastic behavior and the storage of elastic potential energy.

The force–displacement curves have been found to have two phases.[24, 30] The first phase is a region in which the stiffness (the gradient of the force–displacement relation) begins at a low level and then increases rapidly, producing a nonlinear response. The nonlinear region continues up to about 20 to 30 N and is followed by a linear region.[24, 30] A number of investigations have found this region to be linear in the range 30 to 100 N,[24, 30] but a recent case study found that when a large range of forces was considered (about 250 N), there was observable nonlinearity[32] (Fig. 9–9). There was found to be a modest stiffening of the movement with increasing force, so that if a large range of forces was considered, the force–displacement relationship would need to be represented by a nonlinear function, such as a parabola. Because most investigations have employed a moderate range of forces (less than 100 N), the region above 30 N has been satisfactorily represented as linear and has been fitted with a straight-line relationship between force and displacement. In such cases, the entire force–displacement relationship has been characterized by the length of the toe region up to 30 N (D30) and the slope of the subsequent linear region (stiffness coefficient K).[33] Average values of K for normal young subjects have been found to be about 15 N/mm for L3 loads, with the normal values ranging from about 8 to 29 N/mm.[22, 30, 34]

Factors Associated With an Alteration in Lumbar Mobilization Stiffness

Many manual therapists believe that one sign of joint disease or dysfunction is the presence of

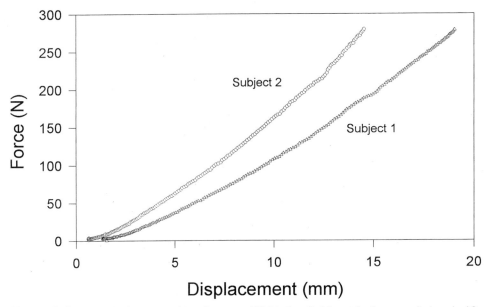

FIGURE 9–9   Force–displacement relationship up to 275 N of applied force, for forces applied to the L3 vertebra at 0.5 Hz. Data for two subjects are shown. (From Lee M, Latimer J, Maher C: Normal response to large postero-anterior lumbar loads: A case study approach. J Manipulative Physiol Ther 20:369, 1997.)

altered stiffness during manual assessment using mobilization procedures. As described previously, it is likely that many tissues contribute to the movement felt by the clinician during mobilization. The lumbar spine can be seen as a flexible, segmented complex that is suspended between two supporting structures: the pelvis and the rib cage.[35] A conceptual model of this structure is given in Figure 9–10. The posteroanterior movement of the target vertebra is produced by many intervertebral movements. Further, the deformation of the rib cage and movement of the pelvis also contribute to the total displacement. Referring to the conceptual model in Figure 9–10, the displacement through space of a lumbar vertebra under a manual load, A, is partly dependent on the intervertebral joint stiffness at nearby intervertebral joints. Flexible intervertebral joints allow greater movement of the target vertebra in relation to its neighbors. The degree to which the mobilization stiffness is affected by the stiffness of any single intervertebral joint is unknown. A number of factors that are associated with significant increases in stiffness during lumbar mobilization have been identified.

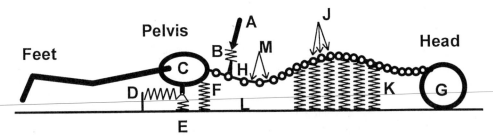

FIGURE 9–10   Simple schematic model of application of manual force to spine (not to scale). The head (G), pelvis (C), and vertebrae (such as J) can be considered rigid bodies. The spine may be represented as a stiff segmented beam comprising the vertebrae and the interconnecting tissues (M). The spine is supported by the head, by a series of springs (K, representing the rib cage), and by the pelvis. The pelvis in turn is supported by springs restraining vertical (E) and horizontal (D) movement and a spring that resists pelvic rotation around the axis (F). The manual force (A) is applied through a spring representing the dorsal soft tissues (B) to the spinous process (H), and the patient lies on a bed (L). (Modified from Lee M, Steven GP, Crosbie J, et al: Variations in posteroanterior stiffness in the thoraco-lumbar spine: Preliminary observations and proposed mechanisms. Phys Ther 78:1277, 1998. With permission of the American Physical Therapy Association.)

Muscle Activity

One factor that has the potential to have a large influence on the stiffness during lumbar mobilization is the degree of activity of lumbar muscles. When a person with no low-back pain lies in a relaxed prone position, it is normal for there to be no activity of the lumbar extensors.[36, 37] It has been reported that patients with low-back pain do have variable amounts of muscle activity present when lying in a position that is used for manual therapy,[36] although much information on the presence of muscle activity is based on unsubstantiated clinical observation. When healthy subjects maximally activated their spinal extensors, with the pelvis and thorax restrained, there was a 350% increase in mean posteroanterior stiffness at L3 during mobilization at 0.7 Hz.[34]

It has also been found that spinal extensor activation at levels below maximum produces increases in posteroanterior stiffness that are nearly proportional to the level of activation of the lumbar erector spinae.[38] A hypothesized mechanism for this effect relates to the orientation of the major lumbar extensors, the erector spinae group.[34] It has been noted that the erector spinae pass posteroinferiorly from their origin on the lumbar vertebrae to their insertion on the pelvis, so that their action produces a posterior shear force on the lumbar vertebrae.[39] Therefore, because posteroanterior mobilization produces anterior movement of the lumbar vertebrae relative to the pelvis, the activated erector spinae tend to oppose this movement. Mobilization tends to stretch these muscles, and their stiffness is nearly proportional to the level of activation,[40] thus producing mobilization stiffness that depends on the level of muscle activation. The question remains open about whether patients with low-back pain might have increased stiffness during mobilization as a result of this mechanism or whether the actual levels of activation are too low to produce a significant effect. In this regard, it should be noted that patients with low-back pain were found to have 8% higher posteroanterior stiffness than when they had little or no pain.[33]

Mobilization Frequency

Mobilization is usually performed at frequencies of up to 3 to 5 Hz. In isolated tissues, resistance to stretch increases as the rate of stretch increases.[41] During lumbar mobilization, this stiffening effect is also apparent. The posteroanterior stiffness has been observed to increase by an average of about 25% when the frequency of mobilization changes from very slow loading to 0.5 Hz.[22] Smaller average increases in stiffness are observed when changing frequency from 0.5 to 1 Hz.[24] The stiffness of the posteroanterior responses observed by Lee and Liversidge[22] under very slow loading were highly correlated with the stiffness values observed at 0.5 Hz, with correlation coefficients of 0.82 at L3, 0.91 at L4, and 0.97 at L5. The tissues that are the source of this increasing stiffness with increasing frequency are not known because many tissues contribute to the stiffness felt by the clinician, and all show properties that depend on strain rate.[22]

Location of Target Bone

Within the spine, the location of the target vertebra is an important variable in determining the stiffness during mobilization.[22] There are a number of possible reasons for this, but it has been proposed that the proximity of the target vertebra to the relatively rigid pelvis is a major factor.[22]

As indicated in the conceptual model of Figure 9–10, deformation of the rib cage and displacement of the pelvis can allow movements of the entire lumbar spine, adding to intervertebral movements within the lumbar spine to produce the total movement of the target vertebra. Imagine that the lumbar spine is a rigid beam connected between two flexible supports, so that no intervertebral movement occurs. A load is applied at various points along the beam. It can be shown that if the flexibility of the two supports is different, the movement at the point of loading would be greatest when the load was applied at the more flexible support. The movement would be least under a load applied at the stiffer support. For loads applied along the beam at points between the supports, the movement would be intermediate between the values at the two ends, with the movement increasing as the load moved from the stiff support toward the flexible support.

In the human body, the rib cage would be expected to provide a less rigid support to the lumbar spine than would the pelvis, owing to the relative flexibility of the ribs and costal cartilages. If the target vertebra is close to the relatively rigid support of the pelvis, then the posteroanterior displacement of the target vertebra would be expected to be less. Hence, the posteroanterior mobilization stiffness would be greater. Consequently, the lumbar posteroanterior stiffness could decrease as the point of load application moves away from the sacrum toward the rib cage, as has been observed.[22, 42] This simple model is not directly applicable to the spine because the lumbar spine itself is not rigid. Hence, the actual variation of posteroanterior movement would depend on the intervertebral joint stiffness as well as on the stiffness of the supports.

Another possible factor that could be involved in the variation of posteroanterior stiffness between target vertebrae is the orientation of the mobilizing force. The mobilizing force tends to be oriented in a direction that takes into account the sagittal lumbar curve,[42] and hence the force direction changes in association with change of the target vertebra. Altering the force direction results in application of different components of load to the intervertebral joints. For example, a more caudally applied force at lower lumbar levels is associated with a relatively higher longitudinal component of force and changes the moment of force at many intervertebral joints. Changing the direction of applied force also changes the moment of force around the center of pressure through which the pelvis is supported by the treatment bed and thus may alter the amount of pelvic rotation. These factors could account for some changes in stiffness due to change in force direction per se.

Some support for this hypothesis comes from a modeling study. Lee and colleagues[27] predicted that at the lower lumbar levels, where the mobilizing force is inclined somewhat caudad, a change in direction involving a more caudad inclination would result in greater stiffness. Hence, the change in force direction alone with change in the target vertebra may be responsible for some increase in stiffness. Another possibility is that higher posteroanterior stiffness at inferior levels reflects a greater stiffness of the more caudal intervertebral joints. It is unclear to what extent this factor might account for the systematic changes in posteroanterior stiffness that have been observed[22] because the lumbosacral joint stiffness appears to be lower than at superior joints under anteroposterior and posteroanterior shear but higher under flexion and extension moments.[43]

Degree of Lordosis

The sagittal curve of the lumbar spine varies among patients and, during therapy, can be altered by the clinician by adjusting the treatment couch or by placing pillows under parts of the patient. One experiment has been conducted in which the lordosis was increased by upwardly tilting the upper trunk while maintaining the position of the pelvis and lower limbs. The more lordotic posture produced in this way was found to be associated with greater posteroanterior stiffness.[25] It is unclear whether it was the increase in lordosis per se that was responsible for this change in stiffness because a number of other variables were

changed. For example, both the angle between the applied force and the target vertebra, and the pressure distribution on the anterior body surface may have changed concomitantly with the degree of lordosis.

Mobilizing Force Magnitude

The magnitude of mobilizing force varies with the grade of mobilization.[11] As mentioned previously (see Fig. 9–9), the gradient of the force–displacement relation, the movement stiffness, depends to some extent on the level of applied force. A case study has shown that the linear phase of the force–displacement response may actually be nonlinear if a large range of forces is considered.[32] Further, depending on the grade of mobilization, some clinicians apply only small forces that may involve responses in the nonlinear region below 30 N.[9, 21] Therefore, in some cases of mobilization in which the applied force is below 30 N, or if the range of forces is large, the mobilization stiffness is dependent on the level of applied force. In such cases, the overall stiffness coefficient gives an indication of the patient's response, but a more appropriate approach to evaluation of stiffness could be used. First, a nonlinear function such as a parabola could be fitted to the data, allowing the tangent stiffness to be calculated at any given point on the force–displacement relation. Parabolas have been successfully fitted to the nonlinear region below 20 N[24] as well as to the region between 30 and 275 N,[32] although there has been no documented attempt to fit a single nonlinear function to the entire force–displacement relationship. A second approach could be to represent the force–displacement relationship as piecewise linear. That is, the force–displacement relationship could be broken into a number of segments, each of which can be reasonably fitted with a straight line. If such an approach is taken with the data for subject 2 in Figure 9–9, the variation in stiffness is more readily apparent (Table 9–1).

The latter method of analysis would be appropriate if it was known that a particular interval of force with a linear force–displacement relationship was the focus of the mobilization. If stiffness coefficients are to be compared between patients or between occasions, it is necessary to use the same range of forces in each case.

Breathing

During inspiration, the lumbar spine moves in an anteroposterior direction. Therefore, there is potential for breathing to produce artefacts as well as to produce real changes in the posteroanterior

TABLE 9–1   **Calculated Stiffness Coefficients for Force Intervals in the Force–Displacement Relationship for Subject 2***

FORCE INTERVAL (N)	STIFFNESS COEFFICIENT (N/MM)
0–10	6.8
10–30	13.8
30–100	17.5
100–170	21.5
170–240	23.4

*See Figure 9–9.
Data from Lee M, Latimer J, Maher C: Normal response to large postero-anterior lumbar loads—a case study approach. J Manip Physiol Ther 20:369, 1997

stiffness when evaluation of the mechanical behavior of the spine is attempted. One investigation found that, when measuring the posteroanterior stiffness of healthy subjects at L3 during 0.5-Hz mobilization, posteroanterior stiffness was lower when associated with breath-holding at the end of a normal expiration than when the stiffness was measured during breathing.[44] This result can probably be explained by the subjects' timing of their breathing so that inspiration tended to coincide with the loading phase of the mobilization, thus increasing the stiffness as a result of the action of the inspiratory muscles. Clinicians attempting to evaluate stiffness during mobilization need to be aware of the possible influence of this variable.

Skin-Fold Thickness and Body Mass Index

It has been observed that both skin-fold thickness (measured over the anterior superior iliac spine) and body mass index (mass divided by height squared) are significant predictors of the lumbar posteroanterior stiffness in the linear region during mobilization, accounting for up to half of the variance in the stiffness at lower lumbar levels.[45] People with small skin-fold thickness or a low body mass index tend to have greater stiffness. At least two mechanisms are likely to be responsible for this relationship. The skin and subcutaneous fat overlying the target bone are compressed by the mobilizing force. Because of the nonlinear behavior of these tissues,[46] most of the compression takes place at relatively low loads. Nonetheless, beyond the toe region, some compression of these compliant superficial soft tissues occurs, providing greater displacement under the clinician's hands than would otherwise take place. If there is a large initial thickness of the superficial tissues, there are relatively larger amounts of soft tissue compression and hence more overall displacement.

A similar mechanism may also operate on the anterior surface of the patient to produce direct effects on stiffness. The thickness of the anterior skin and subcutaneous fat may be important in providing a compliant element that allows movement of the bony elements, giving additional displacement under the clinician's hands. For example, more anterior soft tissue might allow more pelvic rotation and hence may increase the target bone displacement and reduce the posteroanterior stiffness. A model study suggested that the mobilization stiffness would be very sensitive to the manner in which the pelvis was constrained, which is likely to be related to the mechanical properties of the anterior soft tissues.[27] The constraint provided by the anterior soft tissues is likely to be applied in at least two ways: to resist both anterior displacement and anterior rotation of the pelvis. Greater thickness of anterior superficial soft tissues tends to be associated with lower constraints to pelvic movements and hence low mobilization stiffness.[27] Although recent observations[45] have demonstrated a strong negative correlation between soft tissue thickness and lower lumbar posteroanterior stiffness, the hypothesized mechanisms to produce this relationship remain unconfirmed.

Treatment Couch Padding

Through a mechanism similar to that described for skin compression, the thickness and compliance of the padded surface of the treatment couch on which the patient is lying can affect the stiffness felt by the clinician during mobilization.[47] A standard treatment couch gives lumbar posteroanterior stiffness values that are on average 19.2% lower than those perceived if the patient is assessed on an unpadded surface,[47] although the change in stiffness with the addition of padding varies substantially among subjects.

Other Variables

Many other variables may have an influence on the characteristics of the responses to mobilization, including diurnal variation in tissue behavior, various pathologic processes within and outside the spine, postural variation among patients, and physiologic range of joint movement. However, there is currently no direct evidence to link these factors with the response to mobilization.

There is some evidence that the posteroanterior movement response is similar in the thoracic spine,[48, 49] and it is likely that the factors that increase the posteroanterior stiffness in the lumbar spine are also applicable in the thoracic region.

Few data, however, are available to support this suggestion, and there is even less information about the responses in the cervical spine.

RESISTANCE TO MOBILIZATION AT PERIPHERAL JOINTS

A number of tests of joint responses have been made to applied moments to establish the normal pattern of resistance to physiologic movements. Such responses may indicate the general pattern of resistance to mobilizations that employ physiologic movements, even though the data were obtained without any specific attempt to simulate the loading pattern of mobilization. The general nature of the responses of peripheral joints to physiologic moments is shown in a typical curve for the hip joint in Figure 9–11. The response is characterized by a region with minimal resistance close to the neutral position and by a gradual, nonlinear increase in resisting moment toward the end of range of motion.[50]

This characteristic pattern of responses can also be seen in the behavior of other joints, including the knee, shoulder, and ankle,[10] although some aspects of the response vary depending on the joint and the direction of movement. For example, for shoulder movements in most directions, there is a large amount of movement with low resistance close to the neutral position, whereas ankle flexion and extension may not show any substantial resistance-free zone.[10]

Mobilization using accessory movements is more common than using physiologic movements, but little information is available about the pattern of resistance. The only joint that has been studied to any great extent appears to be the knee. The anteroposterior force–displacement relationship at the tibiofemoral joint has been studied because of its demonstrated relationship to cruciate ligament integrity.[51] In the normal tibiofemoral joint, the anteroposterior force–displacement relationship shows only a small zone of low-resistance movement, but this zone enlarges when there is loss of restraints at the joint (Fig. 9–12). A similar pattern of normal resistance in the intact joint has been demonstrated for the humeral anteroposterior movement.[52] Logically, this pattern also applies to most other peripheral joints because the structures around the joint are intended to allow movements that are controlled by muscles (physiologic movements) but to prevent movements that cannot be controlled by the muscles (accessory movements).

Factors associated with an increase in stiffness of accessory movements are likely to be similar to those established for the spine, as explained previously. In particular, the degree of activity in muscles crossing the joint; the thickness of superficial soft tissue; the frequency of mobilization; the location, direction, and magnitude of applied force; and the degree of restraint offered by the treatment couch could be all expected to affect the pattern of the patient's response.

MANIPULATION

Treatment with manipulation is commonly used for disorders involving the spine. Although most often associated with the chiropractic profession,

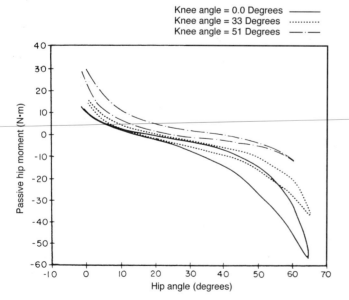

Knee angle = 0.0 Degrees ——————
Knee angle = 33 Degrees ············
Knee angle = 51 Degrees ——·——

FIGURE 9–11 Pattern of resistance of the hip joint to flexion moments. The flexion direction is positive. One subject's loading and unloading curves for knee flexion angles of 0, 33, and 51 degrees are shown. (From Yoon YS, Mansour JM: The passive elastic moment at the hip. J Biomech 15:905, 1982, with permission of Elsevier Science.)

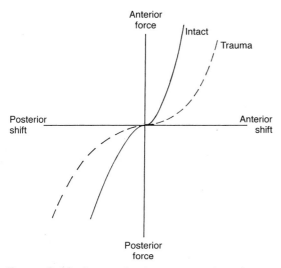

FIGURE 9–12 Pattern of resistance to anterior and posterior forces at the knee in cases of intact ligaments and after trauma has occurred. (From Huiskes R, van Dijk R, de Lange A, et al: Kinematics of the human knee joint. *In* Berme N, Engin AE, Correia da Silva KM [eds]: Biomechanics of Normal and Pathological Human Articulating Joints. Dordrecht, The Netherlands, Martinus Nijhoff, with kind permission of Wolters Kluwer Academic Publishers, 1985, p 165.)

spinal manipulative therapy (SMT) is also used by groups of physical therapists and other practitioners. In particular, the site-specific, short-lever, high-velocity, low-amplitude spinal adjustment is the most commonly used manipulative technique. This method of SMT involves the rapid application of a thrustlike force to the vertebral processes (spinal, transverse, or mamillary), the iliac and ischial spines, or the mastoid, in a specific direction.[53, 54]

Clinicians typically administer SMT in response to a number of problematic scenarios, as indicated primarily by manual diagnoses (palpation) and radiography. In summary, these diagnostic scenarios include vertebral malposition (a vertebra does not appear to be in the correct orientation or location; that is, it is a question of static positioning or alignment); abnormal vertebral motion (a vertebra does not appear to be moving in the correct way; that is, it is a question of dynamic range of motion or direction of motion); abnormal joint play or end-feel (a purely subjective determination of passive motion, elasticity or "give" in a joint within its physiologic range); soft tissue abnormalities (palpable changes in paraspinal soft tissue, such as tenderness, muscle spasm, and trigger points); and muscle contraction or imbalance (palpable spinal contracture in synergistic or opposing muscle groups).[53]

Despite the considerable success of SMT in alleviating pain and restoring functionality,[53, 55–61] the mechanisms (mechanical, physiologic, psychological, or combinations thereof) by which SMT continues to achieve the observed beneficial results are, as yet, unknown. Because SMT is clearly a mechanical procedure, several groups of researchers have endeavored to implement a biomechanical approach in an attempt to understand and characterize the application and efficacy of SMT.

Biomechanically speaking, the clinician delivers a force of specific magnitude, direction, and time-history to a specific location on the patient. As such, the clinician is free to alter only a finite number of variables with respect to the delivery of a manual treatment. The text that follows summarizes the salient features of the current knowledge base regarding the biomechanics of SMT from the perspective of the external observer (e.g., the clinician or scientist).

FORCE MAGNITUDES AND TIME HISTORIES

The earliest attempts at measuring the forces exerted by clinicians during SMT were made by Adams and Wood.[62, 63] By using a "treatment simulator," they were able to characterize the force-time–histories exerted by clinicians of varying levels of experience, during mock sacroiliac treatment sessions. Although it was recognized that treatment simulations are of limited use for the understanding of the mechanics of true clinician–patient interactions, the results that they obtained were important in their clear demonstration of the variable nature of SMT. Later, Triano and Schultz[64] used an inverse dynamics approach to estimate indirectly the forces exerted by clinicians onto the cervical spines of subjects. Despite the fact that this approach requires the quantification of accelerations of body segments and is thus susceptible to errors when high-velocity, low-amplitude movements are involved, their results represent the first attempt at quantifying the mechanics at the clinician–patient interface.

By innovative use of a pressure pad, originally designed for measuring foot and insole pressure (EMED Inc., Munich, Germany), Hessel and colleagues[8] were the first to measure directly the forces exerted by clinicians onto patients during SMT. They clearly showed the distinctive nature of the treatment: the preload force, in which the clinician aims to move the targeted vertebral body through to the end-point of its physiologic range of movement; the treatment thrust; and a termination of clinician–patient contact, wherein the externally applied forces ultimately drop to zero (sometimes referred to as *resolution*; Fig. 9–13).

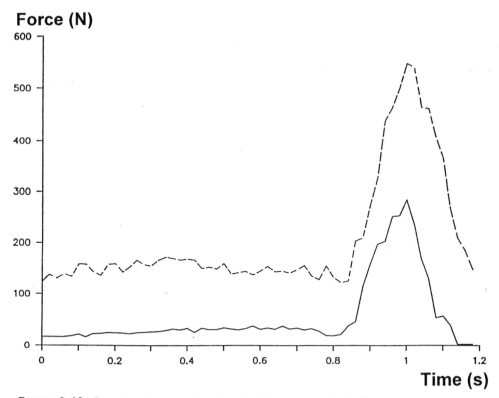

Force (N)

Time (s)

FIGURE 9-13   Force-time–histories of spinal manipulative therapy using the Thompson technique on the sacroiliac joint of a single subject. The solid line and dashed line represent chiropractor 1 and chiropractor 2, respectively. (Adapted from Hessel BW, Herzog W, Conway PJ, McEwen MC. Experimental measurement of the force exerted during spinal manipulation using the Thompson technique. J Manipulative Physiol Ther 13[8]:448–453, 1990.)

Since the study by Hessel and colleagues,[8] several studies employing the same pressure pad system have been conducted (Table 9–2). Comparisons of data among the various studies involving homologous vertebral sites show that, in general, preload and peak forces and treatment times tend to overlap in widely ranging bands. This suggests that there may be considerable variation among clinicians treating the same patient (as illustrated in Fig. 9–13) and within a particular clinician's approach to treating similarly diagnosed patients (Fig. 9–14).

Specifically, SMTs delivered to the cervical region were done faster and used lower peak forces than SMTs delivered to the thoracic or sacroiliac regions, as illustrated in Figure 9–15. Preloads were often so small that they were virtually imperceptible by the pressure pad. Thus, experienced clinicians appear to be able to judge, through direct manual contact, the amount of force required to achieve the desired result. The more compliant joints of the cervical region require less force than the more massive and stiffer joints of either the thoracic or sacroiliac region.

To what extent, however, could this mechanism of manual feedback be expected to be capable of transducing changes in joint stiffness during the rapid application of the treatment thrusts? Herzog and associates[65] investigated the relationships among the preload forces, the peak forces, and the rates at which those peak forces were achieved during SMTs to the cervical, thoracic, and sacroiliac regions of the spine of a large subject pool. They found, as illustrated in Figure 9–16, that a significant variation in the peak forces achieved during SMT could be explained by the magnitudes of the corresponding preload forces applied. As such, they suggested that perhaps it was during the preload phase of the SMT that the clinician was interpreting most of the manual feedback associated with the physiologic and mechanical condition of a particular joint, when the time frame was slow enough that changes in applied force or contact area could be made. Because it appeared that the change from preload to peak thrusting force was effectively brought about by a preprogrammed movement, they concluded that controlling the preload force precisely could be an easy

TABLE 9–2 Summary of Selected Force–Time Characteristics of Spinal Manipulative Therapy

Study	Site	Treatment Technique	Measurement Technique	Preload Force Mean (N)	Preload Force Range (N)	Peak Force Mean (N)	Peak Force Range (N)	Treatment Time Mean (ms)	Treatment Time Range (ms)	Time to Peak Mean (ms)	Time to Peak Range (ms)
Wood & Adams, 1984[63]	SI	Thompson technique	Simulator			257 ± 76R 254 ± 82L			175–547		
Hessel et al, 1990[8]	SI	Thompson technique	EMED pressure pad		20–180		250–450 220–550	271 (1) 280 (2)	200–420		
Herzog et al, 1993[67]	SI	Thompson technique	EMED pressure pad	88 ± 78		328 ± 78					
Herzog et al, 1993[67]	T4	Posterior to anterior, hypothenar	EMED pressure pad	139 ± 46		399 ± 119				150 ± 77	
Triano & Schultz, 1990[64]	C	R, L rotate	Force plate inv. dynamics			123 R 111 L			200–300		
Kawchuk et al, 1992[85]	C1, C2	Toggle technique	EMED pressure pad	2 ± 2	0–11	118 ± 16	99–140	102 ± 15	90–120	48 ± 15	30–65
Kawchuk et al, 1993[68]	C1, C2	Lateral break	EMED pressure pad	40 ± 5		102 ± 7				87 ± 3	
Kawchuk et al, 1993[68]	C1, C2	Gonstead technique	EMED pressure pad	25 ± 7		110 ± 6				92 ± 5	
Kawchuk et al, 1993[68]	C1, C2	Rotation technique	EMED pressure pad	29 ± 4		41 ± 5				79 ± 4	

Force (N)

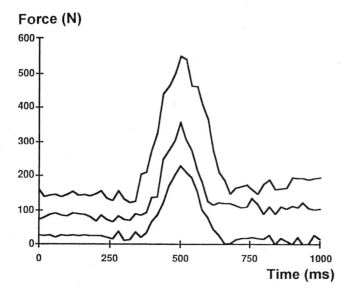

FIGURE 9–14 Selected force-time–histories of spinal manipulative therapy on the thoracic spine (T4). Treatments were performed by one physician on three different patients. Treatments were performed in a posteroanterior direction using a reinforced hypothenar contact on the left transverse process of T4. (Adapted from Herzog W, Conway PJ, Kawchuk GN, et al: Forces exerted during spinal manipulative therapy. Spine 18:1206, 1993.)

method of potentially controlling the ultimate magnitude of the peak thrusting force.

In a study aimed at investigating the effects of preload and initial positioning of the head on the subsequent movements of the head and thorax during two distinct methods of cervical SMT, Triano and Schultz[66] came to a similar conclusion: that clinicians can successfully modify their application of procedures to control the amplitude and direction of body segment displacements that arise during SMT. They concluded that this was an

important clinical skill, particularly with respect to minimizing potentially dangerous manipulative outcomes to which the cervical vertebrae are most susceptible.

FORCE DIRECTIONS

The discussions of force magnitudes thus far have been referring only to the forces directed perpendicularly to the measuring surface. For example, the pressure pad used by Herzog and coworkers[67]

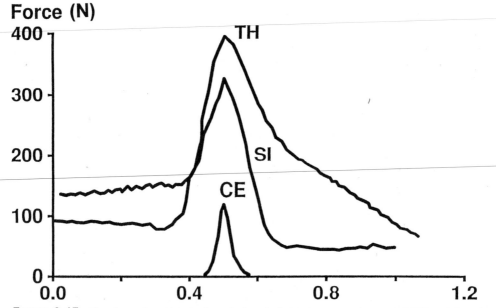

FIGURE 9–15 Mean force-time–histories for spinal manipulative therapy on the cervical (CE) and thoracic (TH) spine and the sacroiliac joint (SI). (Adapted from Herzog W, Conway PJ, Kawchuk GN, et al: Forces exerted during spinal manipulative therapy. Spine 180:1206, 1993.)

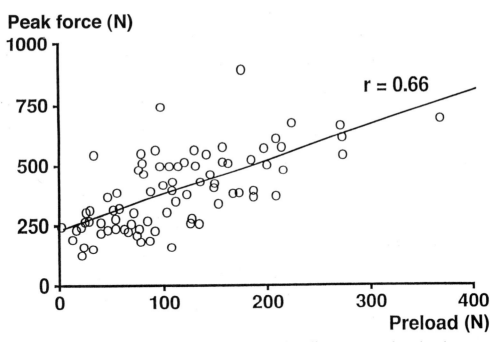

FIGURE 9–16   Correlation between preload force and peak force for treatments performed on the sacroiliac joint. (Adapted from Herzog W, Kawchuk GN, Conway PJ: Relationship between preload and peak spinal manipulative treatments. J Neuromusculoskeletal Syst 1:52, 1993. Reprinted by permission of Journal of the Neuromuscular Skeletal System, Data Trace Publishing Company.)

was oriented in such a way as to record the posterior-to-anterior forces delivered during SMTs to the left transverse process of T4. Even though this particular technique of force delivery appeared to be distinctly unidirectional, it is entirely possible that force vectors other than those measured by the pressure pad may play an important role in the outcome of a successful SMT. In an effort to characterize more specifically the force-time–histories of several different types of cervical SMT, Kawchuk and associates[68] readily acknowledged the likelihood of underestimating the shear or laterally directed forces, particularly in rotatory-type techniques. The development and implementation of a "three-dimensional" force measurement device would be useful in determining the specific force components associated with the variety of available SMT techniques and would be invaluable in the teaching of prospective clinicians.

MULTIPLE SUCCESSIVE SMT

Insofar as a clinician is able to differentiate a successful SMT from an unsuccessful one, the option may be taken to repeat the treatment immediately. Kawchuk and associates[68] asked the participating clinicians to identify whether SMTs that they had administered were satisfactory or unsatisfactory. When allowed to repeat a treatment immediately (within 1 or 2 seconds), clinicians consistently delivered the second "satisfactory" treatment faster and to a higher peak force.

Similarly, Conway and colleagues[69] noted that during an investigation aimed at exploring the cracking sounds often acknowledged to be an indication of a successful SMT, the participating clinician chose to follow a noncracking treatment immediately with another SMT. The force-time profile of the second SMT (which did result in a cracking sound) differed from the first attempt in that it (again) was delivered more rapidly and to a higher peak force. Thus, it would appear that while a clinician is not likely capable of changing the course of a treatment thrust once it has begun, he or she is quite adept at effectively perceiving the mechanical response of the patient and, if necessary, repeating the treatment with correspondingly altered mechanical input, ultimately to achieve the desired goal.

CRACKING SOUNDS

The audible cracking sound that so often accompanies SMT is likely one of the most universally and clearly perceived mechanical responses of the patient. Varying levels of significance have been ascribed to this sound, ranging from absolute unimportance to absolute necessity, for successful manipulative treatment.[70]

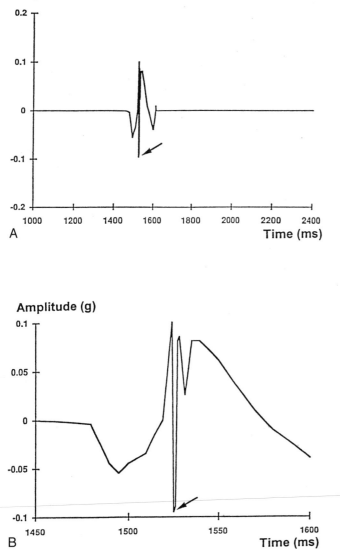

Amplitude (g)

A

Time (ms)

Amplitude (g)

B

Time (ms)

FIGURE 9-17 Acceleration versus time signal for posteroanterior spinal manipulative therapy at T4, which caused cavitation. The graphs depicted in *A* and *B* are identical, except for the time scale on the horizontal axis. (Adapted from Herzog W, Zhang Y, Conway P, et al: Cavitation sounds during spinal manipulative treatments. J Manipulative Physiol Ther 16:523, 1993.)

Investigations aimed at understanding the physical mechanisms of articular sounds were traditionally conducted using metacarpophalangeal (MCP) joints.[71] In his review, Sandoz[70] pointed out some of the features of MCP joint-cracking sounds, namely that they were associated with the appearance of radiolucent spaces on x-ray film and that an MCP joint could not produce a cracking sound a second time until a minimum refractory period had elapsed. More recently, Meal and Scott[72] have shown that when the finger is subjected to increasing tensile forces, an audible cracking sound is associated with a significant reduction in the resistive tension across the MCP joint. Further, by using microphones, they showed that the cracking sounds of the MCP joint are similar to the cracking sounds associated with cervical spine manipulation.

Herzog and colleagues[73] showed that by taping a uniaxial accelerometer to the skin, the vibrations associated with the joint crack during SMT could be measured directly. Figure 9-17 illustrates the vibrations recorded for a typical posteroanterior SMT to T4. The lower-frequency triphasic wave represents the vibration associated with the manipulative thrust. Superimposed on this lower-frequency wave is the higher-frequency vibration of the cracking sound. When a crack was not heard, the corresponding higher-frequency acceleration wave was absent. Later, Conway and associates (unpublished data, 1998) were able to confirm that the higher-frequency accelerometric signals indeed corresponded to cracking sounds recorded by highly sensitive microphones. Herzog, Conway, and their colleagues[73] concluded not only that the cracking sound associated with SMT was clearly perceived by clinicians but also that it was a vibration phenomenon distinct from the manipulation itself, warranting further study.

Conway and associates[69] conducted a study aimed at determining what specific force-time variables were responsible for triggering the cracking sound during SMT. By combining the use of a pressure-sensitive pad with uniaxial accelerometry, both the posteroanterior forces and accelerations were synchronously recorded for a series of manipulative treatments to a current patient pool. In 8 of the 10 trials, the cracking sound and corresponding higher-frequency vibration occurred just before the peak manipulative force, as shown in Figure 9–18. In the remaining 2 trials, the crack occurred just after peak thrusting force had been achieved. During one test, an SMT that did not result in an audible crack was followed almost immediately by a second SMT that did produce a crack. The second SMT was applied more rapidly and to a greater peak force than the initial thrust. In considering all of their data pertaining to the preloads, peak forces, rates at which peak thrusts were delivered, and impulses

of the treatments, they were unable to attribute the cracking phenomenon to a single force-time variable. They suggested that a complex interaction of a number of these variables was responsible for eliciting the cracking response and that unraveling the hierarchy of the potentially important influences would require a more systematic investigation. Interestingly, in a more recent investigation, Reggars and Pollard[74] showed that the cracking sound associated with cervical rotatory SMT was recorded significantly more often on the ipsilateral side of the rotation movement, that is, opposite to the side of the thrust. Their study, and in fact all of the studies previously mentioned in which joint cavitation had been recorded by external sound-vibration methodologies, suffers from the inability to identify precisely which joint had cracked.

Although the joint crack has been demonstrated to be a physical phenomenon that is intimately associated with SMT, its mechanistic importance in general and its importance to the success of SMT specifically has only recently been investigated and challenged. Traditionally, the audible cracking sound has been thought to be the result of cavitation in the spinal facet joints. The proposed sequence of events first involves an increase in synovial joint space (or volume). The concomitant

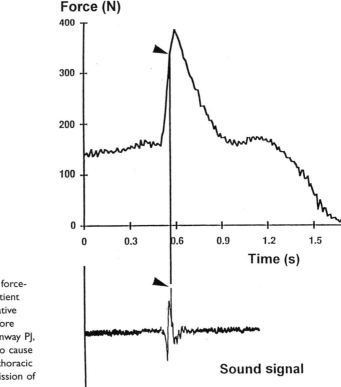

FIGURE 9–18 Representative example of force-time and cavitation-time signals from one patient subjected to posteroanterior spinal manipulative therapy at T4. Here, cavitation occurred before peak force was achieved. (Adapted from Conway PJ, Herzog W, Zhang Y, et al: Forces required to cause cavitation during spinal manipulation of the thoracic spine. Clin Biomech 8:210, 1993, with permission of Elsevier Science.)

reduction in synovial joint pressure allows gases to come out of the synovial fluid, in the form of a bubble. At the same time, fluid flows into the area of low pressure, causing the gas bubble to collapse. The energy that is released when the bubble collapses is perceived as the audible crack.[70] Brodeur[75] offered an alternative mechanism for the cracking sound. He suggested that the reduction in synovial joint pressure would cause the capsular ligaments to invaginate and that the cracking sound was caused by the snapping back of the capsular ligaments away from the synovial interface. Although neither of these explanations for the origins of synovial joint cracking sounds has been conclusively demonstrated, both rely on considerable deformation of the joint capsule.

REFLEX MUSCLE CONTRACTION

Deformation of the synovial joint capsule appears to be at the heart of many hypotheses for the mechanisms by which SMT reduces back pain and restores functionality. It is thought, for example, that interarticular adhesions may be broken or that entrapped synovial folds may be released during manipulative treatments and that these could lead to enhanced intervertebral mobility. Moreover, it has been speculated that articular facet mechanoreceptors and muscle spindles may be suitably stimulated during SMT, thereby causing reflex inhibition of spastic muscles in the treatment area. This increase in sensory input is also thought to reduce the transmission of nociceptive activity, resulting in a decrease in perceived pain.[76–78]

Brodeur[75] suggested that the cavitation process provided a simple means for initiating a reflex activation of muscles in the area of treatment application and that without the cavitation process, it would be difficult to generate the forces in the appropriate tissues without causing muscular damage. Thus, although it appeared that reflex muscle contraction could be an important aspect of a successful SMT, it was not clear how the reflex contractions observed were elicited and what role, if any, was played by spinal joint cavitation during the manipulative process.

Herzog and colleagues[79] conducted a pilot investigation aimed at solving this particular problem: Was joint cavitation a prerequisite for the onset of muscle reflex activity? A pressure-sensitive pad was used to record the posteroanterior force-time–history of two distinct types of manipulation: the rapid SMT as described earlier, and a slowly increasing type of force in which peak magnitudes were achieved several thousands of milliseconds after the initiation of the manipulation, compared with 30 to 200 ms for the normal rapid SMT (see Table 9–2). A uniaxial accelerometer was taped to the skin over the spinous process of the target vertebra to record the cavitation sounds. Finally, the electromyographic (EMG) activity of back muscles just opposite to the area of treatment was recorded using a pair of standard silver–silver chloride bipolar surface electrodes. For the "fast" SMTs, the investigators consistently observed a significant EMG independent of any record of a cavitation response. In contrast, the slowly applied forces were never accompanied by an EMG response, even when a cavitation sound was clearly perceived by the clinician and recorded by the accelerometer. It appeared that the audible crack did not (by itself) evoke muscle activation or a joint proprioceptive reflex response, as had been speculated in the literature.

Suter and coworkers[80] conducted a similar but larger study, which included more EMG and manipulation sites and a larger pool of asymptomatic subjects. Fast and slow manipulations were administered to T3, T6, and T9, and electrode pairs were positioned over the back muscles just opposite the three preselected locations. Additionally, a fourth electrode pair was positioned laterally over the posterior inferior serratus muscle. Their results showed that reflex muscle contraction was observed only during the regular fast SMTs, about 50 to 200 ms after the onset of the thrusting force. These bursts of EMG activity would typically last for about 120 ms, well beyond the time at which peak force was observed, but clearly disappearing before the manipulative forces dropped back to preload levels. These bursts were observed not only in the back musculature directly opposite to the site of each fast treatment but also in the most lateral electrode pair. By considering the timing of the onset of each EMG response, the duration of each response, and the fact that the response was consistently observed at all four electrode locations, these authors concluded that the most likely origin of the observed muscle activity was associated with the excitation of type II articular mechanoreceptors, located in the articular joint capsules of the vertebrae. The ideas proposed by Brodeur[75] concerning the relationship between joint cavitation and muscle reflexes, and the protective nature thereof, were not supported by these new experimental data.[81] Thus, the clinical significance of the manipulative joint crack remains somewhat of a mystery.

MOVEMENTS OF VERTEBRAE

The assumption that vertebrae move relative to one another during SMT has virtually become manipulative therapy dogma. Certainly, with respect to the diagnostic scenarios introduced at the beginning of this section, manipulative therapy is thought to be most efficacious for the improvement or elimination of vertebral pathomechanics, that is, for the restoration of normal vertebral position and normal intervertebral mobility.[53, 82, 83] Yet despite its implicit importance, few investigations have specifically addressed the problem of quantifying the relative movements of vertebral bodies during SMT. Indeed, the few studies that do exist have been primarily concerned with quantifying spinal deformation during the mobilization type of manipulative therapy and were thus considered earlier in this chapter.

As previously described (see Table 9–2), SMT thrusting forces are typically applied rapidly. As such, the subsequent vertebral movements could be expected to be equally rapid. This would preclude the use of bone imaging techniques such as radiography, fluoroscopy, and magnetic resonance imaging, which are useful when studying static situations or when movements take place slowly. Thus, by using an invasive approach with unembalmed post–rigor mortis human cadavers and high-speed cinematography (Fig. 9–19), Gal and associates[84] were able to investigate whether significant relative movements occurred between vertebrae subjected to SMT.

Bone pins were embedded in T10, T11, and T12 to project into the sagittal and transverse plane. Posteroanterior SMTs were delivered to T10, T11, and T12 by a clinician using a reinforced hypothenar contact. The posteroanterior forces were recorded using the pressure pad system previously described, to ensure that the ma-

nipulative thrusts were as similar to genuine clinician–patient force-time–histories as possible. Two electronically synchronized high-speed cine cameras were used to record the movements of the embedded bone pins. This allowed for the calculation of posteroanterior translation, lateral translation, axial rotation, and sagittal rotation of T10, T11, and T12 when the SMT was executed at each of those vertebral sites (Fig. 9–20).

In general, significant relative movements tended to be small and target specific, such that during an SMT to T10, for example, statistically significant relative movements were observed between T10 and T11 but not between T11 and T12. When it is remembered that during the preload phase of each SMT, the clinician endeavors to move the target vertebra through its physiologic range of motion, the mean relative translations and rotations observed by Gal and associates[84] of about 0.4 to 1.1 mm, and 0.2 to 1.6 degrees, respectively, take on new significance. Relative sagittal rotation was particularly interesting in that it appeared that SMT consistently evoked a hyperextension response between T10, T11, and T12, regardless of which vertebral body was the target of the manipulation (Fig. 9–21). Moreover, the hyperextended condition of T11–T12 persisted even as the thrusting forces returned to their preload levels.

Although this latter observation tends to support the hypothesis that SMT may result in realignment of vertebrae from unfavorable positions to more favorable ones, the duration of this hyperextension remains unknown. It appeared that successive manipulations tended to evoke similar magnitudes and directions of absolute translations and rota-

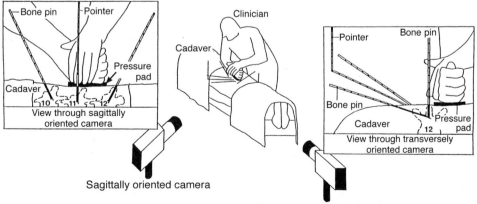

FIGURE 9–19   The experimental setup used by Gal and colleagues[84] to record the movements of vertebrae during posteroanterior spinal manipulative therapy to T10, T11, or T12 of unembalmed post–rigor mortis cadavers. (Adapted from Gal JM, Herzog W, Kawchuk GN, et al: Movements of vertebrae during manipulative thrusts to unembalmed human cadavers. J Manipulative Physiol Ther 20:30, 1997.)

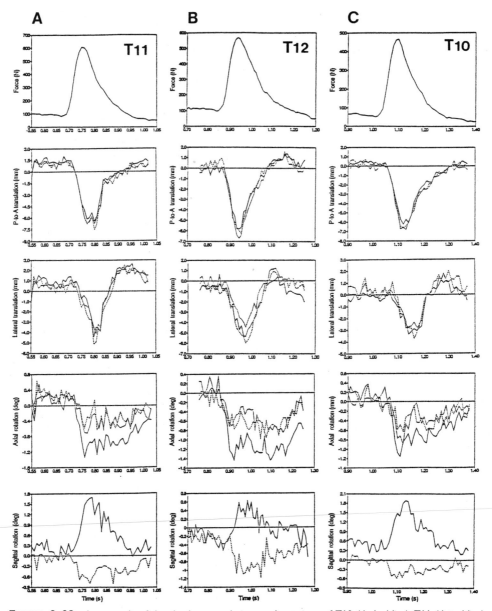

FIGURE 9–20 An example of the absolute translations and rotations of T10 *(dashed line)*, T11 *(dotted line)*, and T12 *(solid line)* for one posteroanterior spinal manipulative therapy to T11 *(A)*, T12 *(B)*, and T10 *(C)* of an unembalmed post–rigor mortis cadaver. (Adapted from Gal JM, Herzog W, Kawchuk GN, et al: Movements of vertebrae during manipulative thrusts to unembalmed human cadavers. J Manipulative Physiol Ther 20:30, 1997.)

tions, which suggests that any cumulative effects of multiple manipulations (separated by about 10 minutes each) on the mechanics of the cadaveric spines were minimal. Thus, it was concluded that the realignment of vertebrae after SMTs was perhaps a short-term observation. Nonetheless, this study was the first to confirm the long-suspected notion that vertebrae do indeed move relative to one another during SMT, even after the vertebrae had been forced to the end ranges of physiologic movement by the applied preload forces. A fully three-dimensional analysis of all six degrees of freedom, using a larger number of unembalmed cadavers, was suggested as the next logical step in attempting to clarify the relationships between the externally applied thrusting forces and the

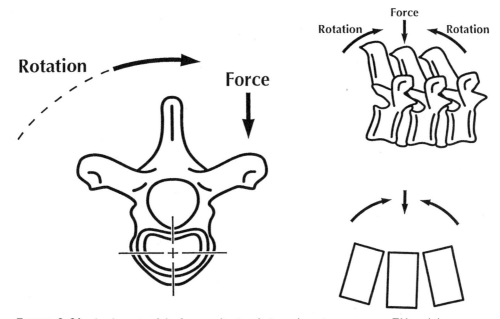

FIGURE 9–21   A schematic of the force application during a thoracic treatment to T11, and the corresponding rotation of the target vertebra around its longitudinal axis (axial rotation, *left*) and the vertebrae immediately adjacent to the target vertebra around their transverse axes (sagittal rotation, *right*). (Adapted from Herzog W: Mechanical, physiologic, and neuromuscular considerations of chiropractic treatments. *In* Advances in Chiropractic, vol 3. St Louis, Mosby–Year Book, 1996, p 269.)

observed relative movement patterns of vertebrae during SMT.

CONCLUSIONS

To understand the possible mechanisms of action of both manipulation and mobilization techniques, we need to understand the kinematics and kinetics of the procedures. Clinicians need to know the movement patterns of the bones to which the manual force is applied, including the relative movements at the joint surfaces and between other key points on the bones as well as the loads that are applied through manual therapy to particular tissues. The major advances in manual therapy biomechanics during the past 10 years have largely been in three areas.

First, there has been substantial progress in describing the applied manual force and its variation with time during a single dose of treatment. This type of information is useful for the training of manual therapy practitioners and also contributes to the understanding of how the techniques might work. For example, a "successful" treatment can be characterized in terms of its force-time behavior, so that practitioners being trained in manual therapy can be taught to apply similar levels of force. It is also possible that aspects of manual

treatment can be optimized using a process that involves measurement of the force-time–history of the treatment procedure and correlating aspects of this with the resulting clinical outcome.

The second major area of progress has been in the description of movements of the target bones, largely during manual therapy of the spine. During some types of both SMT and spinal mobilization, the intervertebral movements have been estimated. The situations that have been studied are somewhat limited at this stage, but there is clear evidence that a major component of the movement response to posteroanterior force techniques is localized intervertebral extension. The sensitivity of the movement responses to variations in technique or differences between patients has not been well studied. In addition, the question of whether the movements produced by the manual therapy have a desirable effect in patients with spinal pain has not yet been explored.

The third aspect of manual therapy biomechanics that has been examined recently is related mostly to mobilization. Practitioners who use this form of therapy may use their perception of the displacement that occurs in response to the manual force to attempt to evaluate the stiffness of the movement response. Recent research has established that certain variables have systematic effects on the stiffness of the spinal mobilization movements. Although many of these variables are of clinical interest, the mechanisms that are involved in determining the resistance to spinal mobilization are not known. Therefore, the interpretation of variations in the stiffness of the mobilization response is somewhat obscure at this stage. In particular, we do not know the degree to which the response reflects the behavior of any one intervertebral joint.

Manual therapy continues to alleviate pain and restore musculoskeletal functionality. Mechanistic descriptions of precisely how this beneficial effect is accomplished remain elusive. We are confident, however, that substantial progress will be made in this area of research using technologies that will allow for more accurate quantification of, and ultimately the prediction of, the changes in the internal mechanics of the patient.

Acknowledgment: Drs. Julianna Gál and Walter Herzog would like to acknowledge the support of the College of Chiropractors of Alberta, the Chiropractic Foundation for Spinal Research, and the Killam Foundation.

References

1. Schiotz EH, Cyriax J: Manipulation Past and Present. London, William Heinemann Medical Books, 1975.
2. Kaltenborn FM: Mobilization of the Extremity Joints. Oslo, Olaf Norlis Bokhandel Universitetsgaten, 1980.
3. Singleton MC, LeVeau BF: The hip joint: Structure, stability, and stress, a review. Phys Ther 55:957, 1975.
4. London JT: Kinematics of the elbow. J Bone Joint Surg 63-A:529, 1981.
5. Vleeming A, Pool-Goudzwaard AL, Hammudoghlu D, et al: The function of the long dorsal sacroiliac ligament: Its implication for understanding low back pain. Spine 21:556, 1996.
6. Buttermann GR, Janevic JT, Lewis JL: Description and application of instrumented staples for measuring in vivo bone strain. J Biomech 27:1087, 1994.
7. Lee R, Evans J: Towards a better understanding of spinal posteroanterior mobilisation. Physiotherapy 80:68, 1994.
8. Hessel BW, Herzog W, Conway PJ, McEwen MC: Experimental measurement of the force exerted during spinal manipulation using the Thompson technique. J Manip Physiol Ther 13(8):448–453, 1990.
9. Matyas TA, Bach TM: The reliability of selected techniques in clinical arthrometrics. Aust J Physiother 31:175, 1985.
10. Engin AE: Passive and active resistive force characteristics in major human joints. *In* Berme N, Engin AE, Correia da Silva KM (eds): Biomechanics of Normal and Pathological Human Articulating Joints. Dordrecht, Martinus Nijhoff Publishers, 1985, p 137.
11. Maitland GD: Vertebral Manipulation, 5th ed. London, Butterworths, 1986.
12. Twomey LT: A rationale for the treatment of back pain and joint pain by manual therapy. Phys Ther 72:885, 1992.
13. Herzog W, Nigg BM, Read LJ: Quantifying the effects of spinal manipulations on gait using patients with low back pain. J Manip Physiol Ther 11:151, 1988.
14. Petty NJ: The effect of posteroanterior mobilisation on sagittal mobility of the lumbar spine. Man Ther 1:25, 1995.
15. Loebl WY: The assessment of mobility of metacarpophalangeal joints. Rheum Phys Med 11:365, 1972.
16. Riddle DL: Measurement of accessory motion: Critical issues and related concepts. Phys Ther 72:865, 1992.
17. Kaltenborn FM: Orthopedic manual therapy for physical therapists. Nordic system: OMT Kaltenborn-Evjenth concept. J Manual Manip Ther 1:47, 1993.
18. Lee M, Moseley A, Refshauge K: Effect of feedback on learning a vertebral joint mobilization skill. Phys Ther 70:97, 1990.
19. Threlkeld J: The effects of manual therapy on connective tissue. Phys Ther 72:893, 1992.
20. Goodsell M, Lee M: The effect of spinal mobilisation on pain and range of motion in patients with low back pain. *In* Proceedings of 12th International Congress of World Confederation for Physical Therapy. Washington, DC, 1995, p 945.
21. Simmonds M, Kumar S, Lechelt E: Use of a spinal model to quantify the forces and motion that occur during therapists' tests of spinal motion. Phys Ther 75:212, 1995.
22. Lee M, Liversidge K: Posteroanterior stiffness at three locations in the lumbar spine. J Manip Physiol Ther 17:511, 1994.
23. Lee M: Dynamics of the Human Body, 4th ed. Sydney, Zygal, 1997.
24. Lee M, Svensson NL: Effect of frequency on response of the spine to lumbar posteroanterior forces. J Manip Physiol Ther 16:439, 1993.
25. Lee M, Moseley A: Dynamics of the Human Body, 2nd ed. Sydney, Zygal, 1991.
26. Lee M, Lau T, Lau H: Sagittal plane rotation of the pelvis during lumbar posteroanterior loading. J Manip Physiol Ther 17:149, 1994.
27. Lee M, Kelly DW, Steven GP: A model of spine, ribcage and pelvic responses to a specific lumbar manipulative force in relaxed subjects. J Biomech 28:1403, 1995.
28. Lee M, Kelly DW, Steven GP: Lumbar spine manual therapy: Effect of choice of target vertebra. *In* Proceedings of the First Australian Biomechanics Conference. The University of Sydney, Sydney, 1996, p 104.
29. Paris SV: Mobilization of the spine. Phys Ther 59:988, 1979.

30. Lee M, Svensson NL: Measurement of stiffness during simulated spinal physiotherapy. Clin Phys Physiol Meas 11:201, 1990.

31. Latash ML, Zatsiorsky VM: Joint stiffness: Myth or reality? Hum Movement Sci 12:653, 1993.

32. Lee M, Latimer J, Maher C: Normal response to large postero-anterior lumbar loads—a case study approach. J Manip Physiol Ther 20:369, 1997.

33. Latimer J, Lee M, Adams R, et al: An investigation of the relationship between low back pain and lumbar posteroanterior stiffness. J Manip Physiol Ther 19:587, 1996.

34. Lee M, Esler M-A, Mildren J, et al: Effect of extensor muscle activation on response to lumbar posteroanterior forces. Clin Biomech 8:115, 1993.

35. Lee M, Steven GP, Crosbie J, et al: Variations in posteroanterior stiffness in the thoraco-lumbar spine: Preliminary observations and proposed mechanisms. Phys Ther 78:1277, 1998.

36. Shirley D, Lee M: A preliminary investigation of the relationship between lumbar postero-anterior mobility and low back pain. J Manual Manip Ther 1:22, 1993.

37. Pauly JE: An EMG analysis of certain movements and exercises. I. Some deep muscles of the back. Anat Rec 155:223, 1966.

38. Shirley D, Lee M: Muscle activity as a possible contributing factor to lumbar posteroanterior stiffness. p. 145 In Proceedings of the 9th Biennial Conference of the Manipulative Physiotherapists Association of Australia, Manipulative Physiotherapists Association of Australia, Gold Coast, 1995.

39. Bogduk N, Twomey LT: Clinical anatomy of the lumbar spine, 2nd ed. Melbourne, Churchill Livingstone, 1991.

40. Crisco JJ, Panjabi MM: Postural biomechanical stability and gross muscular architecture in the spine. In Winters JM, Woo SL-Y, eds: Multiple Muscle Systems: Biomechanics and Movement Organization. New York, Springer-Verlag, 1990, p 438.

41. Fung YC: Biomechanics: Mechanical properties of living tissues, 2nd ed. New York, Springer-Verlag, 1993.

42. Viner A, Lee M: Direction of manual force applied during assessment of stiffness in the lumbosacral spine. J Manip Physiol Ther 18:441, 1995.

43. McGlashen KM, Miller JAA, Schultz AB, et al: Load displacement behavior of the human lumbosacral joint. J Orthop Res 5:488, 1987.

44. Beaumont A, McCrum C, Lee M: The effects of tidal breathing and breath-holding on the postero-anterior stiffness of the lumbar spine. Proceedings of the 7th Biennial Conference of the Manipulative Physiotherapists Association of Australia, 1991, p 244.

45. Viner A, Lee M, Adams R: Postero-anterior stiffness in the lumbosacral spine: The relationship of stiffness between adjacent vertebral levels. Spine 22:2724, 1997.

46. Bader DL, Bowker P: Mechanical characteristics of skin and underlying tissues in vivo. Biomaterials 4:305, 1983.

47. Latimer J, Holland M, Lee M, et al: Plinth padding and measures of posteroanterior lumbar stiffness. J Manip Physiol Ther 20:315, 1997.

48. Lee M, Latimer J, Maher C: Manipulation: Investigation of a proposed mechanism. Clin Biomech 8:302, 1993.

49. Panjabi MM, Brand RA, White AA: Three-dimensional flexibility and stiffness properties of the human thoracic spine. J Biomech 9:185, 1976.

50. Yoon YS, Mansour JM: The passive elastic moment at the hip. J Biomech 15:905, 1982.

51. Huiskes R, van Dijk R, de Lange A, et al: Kinematics of the Human Knee Joint. In Berme N, Engin AE, Correia da Silva KM (eds): Biomechanics of Normal and Pathological Human Articulating Joints. Dordrecht, Martinus Nijhoff Publishers, 1985.

52. Lee M: Assessment of the glenohumeral joint through passive accessory movements. In Current Concepts in the Management of Shoulder Region Dysfunction. Sydney, Manipulative Therapists Association of Australia, 1988, p 41.

53. Haldeman S: Spinal manipulative therapy: A status report. Clin Orthop Rel Res 179:62, 1983.

54. Buerger AA: A non-redundant taxonomy of spinal manipulative techniques suitable for physiologic explanation. Man Med 1:54, 1984.

55. Greenland S, Reisbord LS, Haldeman S, Buerger AA: Controlled clinical trials of manipulation: A review and a proposal. J Occup Med 22:670, 1980.

56. Deyo RA: Conservative therapy for low back pain. JAMA 250:1057, 1983.

57. Herzog W: Biomechanical studies of spinal manipulative therapy. J Can Chiropract Assoc 35:156, 1991.

58. Boline PD, Kassek K, Bonfort G, Nelson C: Spinal manipulation vs. amitriptyline for the treatment of chronic tension-type headaches: A randomized clinical trial. J Manip Physiol Ther 18:148, 1995.

59. Dabbs V, Lauretti WJ: A risk assessment of cervical manipulation vs. NSAIDs for the treatment of neck pain. J Manip Physiol Ther 18:530, 1995.

60. Nilsson N, Christensen HW, Hartvigsen J: Lasting changes in passive range of motion after spinal manipulation: A randomized blind controlled trial. J Manip Physiol Ther 19(3):165–168, 1996.

61. Vernon H: Spinal manipulation for chronic low back pain: A review of the evidence. J Can Chiropract Assoc 40:180, 1996.

62. Adams A, Wood J: Comparison of forces used in selected adjustments of the low back: A preliminary study. The Research Forum. Palmer College of Chiropractic. 1:5, 1984.

63. Wood J, Adams A: Forces used in selected chiropractic adjustments of the low back: A preliminary study. The Research Forum. Palmer College of Chiropractic. 1:16, 1984.

64. Triano JJ, Schultz AB: Cervical spine

manipulation: Applied loads, motions and myoelectric responses. Proceedings of the 14th Annual Meeting of the American Society of Biomechanics, Miami, vol 14. 1990, p 187.

65. Herzog W, Kawchuk GN, Conway PJ: Relationship between preload and peak forces during spinal manipulative treatments. J Neuromusculoskeletal Sys 1:52, 1993.

66. Triano JJ, Schultz AB: Motions of the head and thorax during neck manipulations. J Manip Physiol Ther 17:573, 1994.

67. Herzog W, Conway PJ, Kawchuk GN, et al: Forces exerted during spinal manipulative therapy. Spine 18:1206, 1993.

68. Kawchuk GN, Herzog W: Biomechanical characterization (fingerprinting) of five novel methods of cervical spine manipulation. J Manip Physiol Ther 16:573, 1993.

69. Conway PJ, Herzog W, Zhang Y, et al: Forces required to cause cavitation during spinal manipulation of the thoracic spine. Clin Biomech 8:210, 1993.

70. Sandoz R: The significance of the manipulative crack and of other articular noises. Ann Swiss Chiropract Assoc 4:47, 1969.

71. Roston JB, Haines RW: Cracking in the metacarpophalangeal joint. J Anat 81:165, 1947.

72. Meal GM, Scott RA: Analysis of the joint crack by simultaneous recording of sound and tension. J Manip Physiol Ther 9:189, 1986.

73. Herzog W, Zhang Y, Conway P, et al: Cavitation sounds during spinal manipulative treatments. J Manip Physiol Ther 16:523, 1993.

74. Reggars JW, Pollard HP: Analysis of zygapophyseal joint cracking during chiropractic manipulation. J Manip Physiol Ther 18:65, 1995.

75. Brodeur R: The audible release associated with joint manipulation. J Manip Physiol Ther 18:155, 1995.

76. Raftis K, Warfield CA: Spinal manipulations for back pain. Hosp Pract 15:89, 1989.

77. Zusman M: Spinal manipulative therapy: Review of some proposed mechanisms, and a new hypothesis. Aust J Physiother 32:89, 1986.

78. Gillette RG: A speculative argument for the coactivation of diverse somatic receptor populations by forceful chiropractic adjustments: A review of the neurophysiological literature. Man Med 3:1, 1987.

79. Herzog W, Conway PJ, Zhang Y, et al: Reflex responses associated with manipulative treatments on the thoracic spine: A pilot study. J Manip Physiol Ther 18:233, 1995.

80. Suter E, Herzog W, Conway PJ, et al: Reflex response associated with manipulative treatment of the thoracic spine. J Neuromusculoskeletal Sys 2:124, 1994.

81. Herzog W: On sounds and reflexes. J Manip Physiol Ther 19:216, 1996.

82. Cassidy JD, Potter GE: Motion examination of the lumbar spine. J Manip Physiol Ther 2:151, 1979.

83. Carrick FR: Treatment of pathomechanics of the lumbar spine by manipulation. J Manip Physiol Ther 4:173, 1981.

84. Gal JM, Herzog W, Kawchuk GN, et al: Movements of vertebrae during manipulative thrusts to unembalmed human cadavers. J Manip Physiol Ther 20:30, 1997.

85. Kawchuk GN, Herzog W, Hasler EM: Forces generated during spinal manipulative therapy of the cervical spine: A pilot study. J Manip Physiol Ther 15:275, 1992.

CHAPTER 10

LOWER LIMB ORTHOTICS

John Stallard

Historically considered a last resort, to be used only when all else fails, orthoses have in recent years become a more respected treatment option for many conditions. Orthoses have increasingly seen as having the potential to provide a positive contribution to the rehabilitation of severely handicapped patients, and orthotists are now commonly included in the clinical team. Many enlightened practitioners[1, 2] advocate therapy regimens in which the elements of surgery, physical therapy, and orthotics are integrated at the beginning of treatment to ensure the optimum functional outcome for the patient. An understanding of the potential of orthotics to contribute to the well-being of a patient is therefore an important part of the armory of skills for modern clinicians, whatever their discipline.

Confusion about the role of orthotics does still exist. It is therefore necessary to have a clear understanding of its scope. Being a comparatively modern profession, there are still a number of definitions that are applied. Two of these give a good indication of the role of the orthotist and the scope of orthotics:

"An external device designed to apply or remove forces to or from the body with the object of supporting, correcting or for an anatomical deformity or weakness, however caused. It may be applied with the additional object of assisting, allowing or restricting movement of the body" (UK DHSS definition).

"An externally applied device used to modify the structural or functional characteristics of the neuro-muscular-skeletal system" (International Standards Organisation definition).

There is a wide range of orthotic devices, and they are given a variety of names. This can cause great confusion because local custom frequently determines the description of an orthosis, which often is named for the person who is alleged to have pioneered the design. To overcome this potentially troubling problem, the American Academy of Orthopaedic Surgeons proposed that orthoses should be defined by the joints of the body they cross. Thus, a long-leg caliper is described as a knee-ankle-foot orthosis (KAFO). A knee brace is called a knee orthosis (KO), a wrist splint a wrist-hand orthosis (WHO), a below-knee brace an ankle-foot orthosis (AFO), and so on. This system has now been widely adopted and is accepted as an International Standard (ISO 8549–3:1989 E/F: Prosthetics and orthotics–Vocabulary–Part 3: Terms relating to external orthoses). The adoption of this system is becoming ever more common, and this has certainly been a boost to international exchange of information, which in turn is fostering an improvement in treatment in most countries.

There are surprisingly few standards governing the design and manufacture of orthotic devices. This is more a reflection of the paucity of data on the loading applied to these devices than of the lack of need for such documents. In prosthetics (external artificial limbs), international cooperation has led to funding for research to establish performance specifications for lower limb devices, and an ISO Standard[3] has recently been published. The loads on orthoses are much less easily defined, and the research to establish an equivalent standard would therefore be considerably more expensive. This has inhibited the financing of work that is accepted as being as necessary as that achieved in the field of prosthetics. Initiatives are being pursued, and it is hoped that international collaboration will one day make performance specifications available to professionals working in the field of orthotics.

To make the most of an orthosis, it is important to understand the principles on which it works and the potential benefits it can provide for the patient receiving rehabilitation care. This means that, ideally, not only must the function of an orthosis and the objective of the forces it applies or resists be appreciated, but also the long-term outcome for the patient should be identified. In a young profession such as orthotics, there is not yet a wealth of research data establishing long-term outcomes for particular treatments. However, the scientific background is growing rapidly, and clinical research is commonly regarded as a necessary requirement to underpin new developments. Consequently, it is now possible to establish evidence of efficacy for some orthoses, and it should be expected that this body of information will grow exponentially as the professions allied to medicine increasingly turn their attention to the need to produce proven findings.

The contributions that orthotics can make to the treatment of patients fall under a number of headings. Although there is no formally adopted system of clinical categorization of orthoses, a commonly adopted practice is to group them according to the area of the body they are intended to treat. This logical approach is a convenient means of structuring an examination of the subject. Lower limb orthoses perform a wide range of functions, almost all of them related to ambulation for handicapped patients. Because all lower limb devices have biomechanical principles that are related to the functional requirements, an essential starting point is a knowledge of the fundamentals of walking.

THE WALKING CYCLE

Lower limb orthoses are prescribed mainly to treat walking disorders. The degree of handicap and the commensurate complexity of the biomechanical solution can vary from the simple to the highly complex. Successful treatment clearly demands an accurate evaluation of the problems faced by the patient, so that the appropriate biomechanics to ensure the most effective outcome can be achieved. Analysis of handicapped gait is enhanced by an understanding of normal gait. It permits a sharper focus on the problem areas and a better grasp of the mechanical controls that must be applied to achieve the most practical outcome for an individual patient.

Normal ambulation is an effective compromise that enables people to function in a wide range of conditions. It is generally observed while subjects are walking on a flat surface that allows good grip, but it adapts well to slopes, rough ground, and different amounts of friction. Gait has evolved to minimize energy expenditure, consistent with maintaining its inherent flexibility, to permit adaptation to different conditions. To achieve overall efficiency, the normal gait cycle is arranged to minimize excursions of the general body center of gravity. Other mechanisms of normal gait are invoked to smooth impact loads by absorbing energy (e.g., in muscles and tendons), some of which can be recovered later in the gait cycle.

It can be seen, therefore, that walking consists of complex and sophisticated interactions of a number of simultaneous mechanisms that demand a high degree of control. Whenever neurologic control mechanisms are compromised, gait inevitably increases in difficulty and decreases in efficiency. The greater the degree of the control deficit, the more extensive the handicap. Lower limb orthoses can compensate for lack of subtle neuromuscular control through the use of cruder, pure mechanical controls. Although these have the capacity to permit ambulation, this inevitably has a lower efficiency than normal walking[4] because these orthoses do not permit the subtle interplay of finely controlled biomechanics.

It is a great advantage in identifying the most appropriate mechanical controls for handicapped gait to have a knowledge of the normal gait cycle. The normal gait cycle (Fig. 10–1) is generally considered to have six distinct major events (on both sides), as follows:

1. Heel-strike
2. Foot-flat
3. Mid-stance
4. Heel-off
5. Toe-off
6. Mid-swing

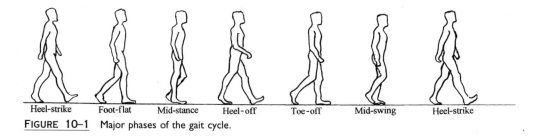

| Heel-strike | Foot-flat | Mid-stance | Heel-off | Toe-off | Mid-swing | Heel-strike |

FIGURE 10–1   Major phases of the gait cycle.

This cycle repeats with heel-strike. The temporal relationships between these events lead to recognizable phases of the gait cycle and have an important influence on performance. In the sagittal plane, viewed from the right side of the body, these relationships are as follows:

Heel-strike to foot-flat. At right heel-strike the leg is in front of the trunk, with the hip at its maximum degree of flexion (while walking), the knee slightly flexed, and the ankle in the neutral position. Immediately after the heel contacts the ground, the ankle joint absorbs energy by plantar-flexing under eccentric muscle control until the foot is flat on the ground, while the knee flexes slightly and the hip maintains its flexed position. This phase takes about 10% of the cycle and is also known as the *ankle rocker.*

Mid-stance. In this phase of the cycle, the foot remains flat on the ground as the rest of the body progresses forward over the ankle joint, which moves progressively from plantar-flexion to dorsiflexion while the hip joint simultaneously moves from flexion into extension. The knee initially flexes but begins to extend before the lower limb and trunk reach vertical alignment (at which point it is still noticeably flexed), and the left leg at its mid-swing passes the right and continues to do so until the phase is completed. This phase occurs from about 10% to 45% of the gait cycle.

Heel-off to toe-off. During this phase (sometimes known as *push-off*), the right ankle plantar-flexes more rapidly while flexion of both the right hip and knee occurs, and the left leg achieves heel-strike. This phase occurs from about 45% to 60% of the gait cycle.

Swing phase. This phase commences as the right toe leaves the ground. The thigh accelerates from extension into flexion, imparting forward motion to the limb. Initially, the knee continues to maximum flexion while the ankle dorsiflexes from plantar-flexion to neutral to ensure ground clearance as the left leg reaches mid-stance with the right leg passing it halfway through swing phase. As flexion at the hip develops, the thigh decelerates, and the knee moves into extension in preparation for heel-strike, which completes the cycle. This phase of gait occurs from approximately 60% to 100% of the cycle.

There are also some subtle relationships occurring in the coronal plane. The trunk moves slightly toward the support side during the early stages of the stance phase and reverses this during the later stages, while the pelvis rotates downward slightly around the stance hip in mid-stance. Hardly any deviation occurs in hip or knee joints in the coronal plane, although supination and pronation of the foot respond to unevenness of the ground.

Vertical movements of the trunk inevitably occur as lower limbs flex and extend around the hip joint. These vertical deviations are attenuated, however, by knee flexion and slight hip adduction in mid-stance to reduce the peak rise, and foot plantar-flexion at the end of stance phase lessens the drop of the trunk. These subtle movements minimize the excursion of body center of gravity (Fig. 10–2) and thereby lessen the dynamic forces required to raise the mass of the body, reducing the energy cost of ambulation.

Any form of walking requires that the body has internal stabilization to prevent it from collapsing under its own weight, external stabilization so that it does not topple over, propulsive forces, and control of the stabilization and propulsive forces to ensure organized progression. The subtle interplay of the different phases and events in the normal gait cycle demands an excellent control system that organizes the muscles to provide internal stabilization (by balancing moments generated around the joints of the lower limbs), the posture so that body center of gravity is always within an effective (usually very small) support area, and the injection of propulsive forces to provide forward progression. Absence of effective control or muscle power inhibits walking ability and requires compromises to be made (involuntary or conscious), with the inevitable consequence that efficiency is diminished. Proper analysis of handicapped gait is essential if the most effective

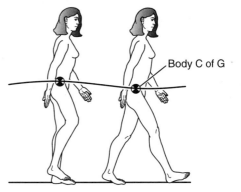

FIGURE 10–2 Vertical excursion of the body's center of gravity (C of G). (From ORLAU [Orthotic Research and Locomotor Assessment Unit], The Robert Jones and Agnes Hunt Orthopaedic and District Hospital, Oswestry, Shropshire, England SY10 7AG.)

compromise is to be achieved for each patient. This requires not only a good understanding of normal gait but also the means of establishing the temporal, force, and phasic relationships occurring in handicapped ambulation through appropriate methods of evaluation.

METHODS OF EVALUATION

One of the problems of judging the effectiveness of orthotic treatment has been the lack of evaluation techniques or instrumentation that can readily be applied in routine clinical situations. These are becoming available, and it seems likely that it will be increasingly possible to make valid scientific observations of the effect of applying an orthosis to ameliorate the problems created by biomechanical abnormalities. Three methods serve as an example of the means of monitoring patients to establish outcomes of orthotic treatment:

- Measuring ground reaction forces to permit qualitative and quantitative assessment of biomechanical alignment relative to the joints of the lower limbs
- Evaluating relative energy expenditure by measuring speed of walking and heart rate to produce a physiologic cost index (PCI)
- Classification of handicapped gait through allocation of appropriate categories that have specific determinants

MONITORING GROUND REACTION FORCES

Ground reaction forces are monitored by force platforms. These are devices placed within a walkway that follow the rapidly changing forces occurring between the foot and the ground during the stance phase of gait. The output from the force platform is given as force in three mutually perpendicular directions, referred to as F_x, F_y, F_z (Fig. 10–3A):

- The vertical (F_z)
- The horizontal in the line of walking (F_y)
- The horizontal at right angles to the line of walking (F_x)

These three planar outputs for a healthy subject walking at his or her usual pace are shown in Figure 10–3B, as a percentage of body weight. Although used widely in biomechanics, they are difficult to interpret for pathologic conditions because they give little indication of the effects that abnormalities have on the alignment of forces relative to the joints of the lower limb and the turning effects they therefore generate around

those joints. To permit a more immediately observable indication of the aberrant moments (turning effects) that may be present in a patient, the Video Vector Generator (VVG)[5] has been developed; it converts the force platform signals into a line on a video screen, accurately aligned to the image of the subject as he or she walks over the platform. This constitutes a vector of ground reaction force, the length of which is proportional to the magnitude and direction to the alignment. The video image, therefore, gives an immediate indication of the effect of ground reaction forces on the lower limb. In normal walking (Fig. 10–4), the ground reaction force in the sagittal plane remains close to the hip and knee joints throughout the stance phase of gait. The system shows any deviations from this due to pathologic conditions and allows an evaluation of their effects on an individual patient.

MONITORING RELATIVE ENERGY EXPENDITURE

Many orthotic treatments are intended to ease the burden of walking for severely handicapped patients. It is not always easy to determine subjectively whether that objective has been realized. Patients, for a variety of reasons, are not necessarily reliable reporters in this respect. It is a valuable adjunct to the rehabilitation process to have a quantitative analysis of relative effort for an individual patient walking before and after treatment. The scientifically preferred method of measuring oxygen uptake is not practical for many handicapped patients because the apparatus required (which incorporates tight-fitting face masks and cumbersome instrumentation) affects performance to an unacceptable degree. A simpler method for the patient is to monitor speed and heart rate. This can be done by picking up the electrocardiogram signal through two electrodes on the chest and transmitting it to instrumentation that processes it to give a frequently updated reading of heart rate. Speed can be calculated over an appropriate number of timed circuits of a suitable course depending on the level of handicap (e.g., a figure-of-eight 25-meter circuit) to establish a comparative standard. The raw data can be converted into a single figure of PCI by dividing the increase in heart rate from the resting rate by the speed of walking,[6–8] which gives a reading in beats per meter walked.

This method is comparatively simple to apply, does not create unacceptable difficulties for the patient, and, provided that the selected test is used rigorously before and after treatment, gives an outcome that is easy to interpret. Although there

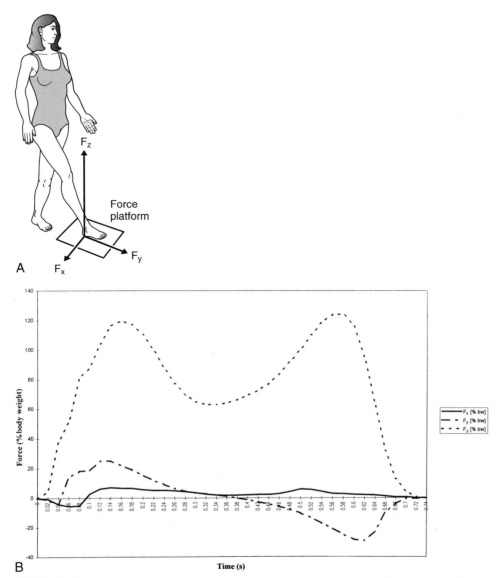

FIGURE 10–3 Ground reaction forces. *A*, The three force components of gait. *B*, Ground reaction forces in normal walking. (*A*, from ORLAU [Orthotic Research and Locomotor Assessment Unit], The Robert Jones and Agnes Hunt Orthopaedic and District Hospital, Oswestry, Shropshire, England SY10 7AG.)

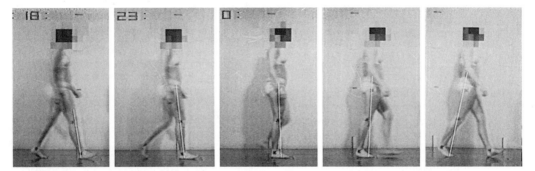

FIGURE 10–4 Video vector display of ground reaction force in a healthy subject during stance phase range.

is a wide spectrum of PCIs for healthy subjects (ranging from 0.2 to 0.6 beats/min[7]), patients have repeatable results. The test is not a good way of comparing different patients but is a valid method of monitoring change within a single subject as a result of rehabilitation treatment.

CLASSIFICATION OF HANDICAPPED GAIT

A simple but effective way of monitoring change in handicapped patients is to classify their walking ability according to well-defined categories. Hoffer and colleagues[9] defined four categories for a series of myelomeningocele patients for whom they were providing treatment. These categories, which have subsequently been widely used and slightly adapted, are now generally accepted as follows:

Chairbound patients: patients who never walk and use a wheelchair as their main means of locomotion

Therapeutic walkers: patients who use apparatus to walk primarily for therapeutic purposes and do so generally under supervision

Household walkers: patients who use apparatus to walk independently for functional purposes within the protected environment of home or special school

Community walkers: patients who use apparatus to walk independently within the community

None of these categories imply that patients have given up the use of a wheelchair, which remains the most efficient form of moving around on a flat surface for most severely handicapped patients.

Hoffer's classification[9] is a simple means of providing broad categories of ambulation for monitoring long-term change within an individual patient or for making general comparisons of outcome for different treatments. More refined systems of comparison have grown out of this simple (but effective) approach, and Garret and Meehan,[10] among others, have extended the concept for more sophisticated evaluation.

SUMMARY

These are but three examples of the means of making clinical comparisons to assess the effectiveness of rehabilitation treatments in which orthotics may play a part. Others exist to suit different situations, and an appropriate literature search could reveal more appropriate methods for particular situations. Alternatively, tests can be designed to cover comparisons for which suitable approaches have not be identified. In doing so, it is essential to ensure that the test has good repeatability and measures effectively the parameter of interest without interference from other factors. It is therefore best, if possible, to use a previously validated test procedure.

ENGINEERING CONSIDERATIONS

BIOMECHANICS

The most common objective of most orthotic devices is to resist moments generated around unstable joints. Each unstable joint requires a minimum of three forces to generate an equal and opposite moment to that which is causing the instability. For example, in Figure 10–5, body weight acting vertically produces a moment around the knee joint of 700 N times 0.15 m (i.e., 105 N m). This is resisted in the flail limb by the so-called three-point fixation of the caliper, which produces a balancing moment through the action of the three forces, F_1, F_2, and F_3, acting through their respective moment arms. The magnitude of the forces can be minimized by increasing the moment arms to the maximal practical distance available on the caliper.

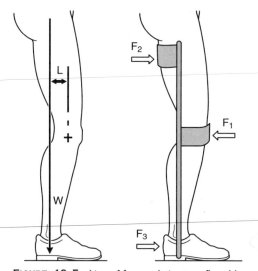

FIGURE 10–5 Line of force relative to a flexed knee and the equal and opposite moment generated by three-point fixation applied by a knee-ankle-foot orthosis *(dotted area)*. Knee moment = W × L (W = body weight; L = moment arm). $F_1 = F_2 + F_3$; together they produce the equal and opposite moment to W × L (F_1, F_2, and F_3 are the forces applied by the orthosis). (From ORLAU [Orthotic Research and Locomotor Assessment Unit], The Robert Jones and Agnes Hunt Orthopaedic and District Hospital, Oswestry, Shropshire, England SY10 7AG.)

Minimizing the forces is advantageous in that it reduces the loads applied directly to the patient through the orthosis. High interface pressures between the orthosis and the patient can lead to discomfort or, more seriously, particularly in anesthetic skin, to pressure sores. To reduce the risk, it is necessary not only to minimize the forces by creating the longest possible moment arms but also to spread the load over as large an area as possible.

Little research has been done to establish the loads applied to orthoses during patient activities. It is clear that the highest loads are likely to occur in lower limb orthoses as patients ambulate. In the absence of real research data, there is a temptation to imagine these as being related merely to patient body weight. This is to ignore the potential of dynamic loading during vigorous activity. Whenever a body changes speed or direction, forces over and above those required to maintain the status quo are required to produce those changes. These are known as *dynamic forces* and can be very significant.

During normal walking, the vertical ground reaction force rises to a maximum of 20% to 30% above body weight (see Fig. 10–3*B*). More vigorous activity causes the dynamic forces to rise dramatically. Running, for example, creates vertical ground reaction forces of about three times body weight. Unexpected incidents can lead to even higher forces, which are likely to lead to accidental overloads on orthotic structures. It is well within the bounds of possibility that loads 10 times body weight could occur, either from unexpected patient activity (e.g., jumping from a moving bus or abseiling for a hobby) or from unforeseeable accidents, and it is wise to bear these possibilities in mind when assessing the orthotic needs of a patient. Highly active patients

are more likely to produce overloads than those who are more sedentary, even if the latter are heavier.

MATERIALS

An objective of prescribing orthoses is usually to improve the function of the patient. Success inevitably leads to the generation of higher dynamic forces from increased activity, and it would be counterproductive to attempt to limit the function of the patient to protect the orthosis. It must be recognized that there is the possibility for overloads to occur on orthotic structures, and this must greatly influence the choice of material. One of the most important properties of a material is the way in which it fails, and there are essentially two modes of failure: brittle and ductile.

The characteristics of these two types of material failure are discernible from stress–strain diagrams (Fig. 10–6*A*, brittle, and Fig. 10–6*B*, ductile). A straight-line relationship between stress and strain implies an elastic material that stores strain energy. As stress increases (i.e., load is applied), equal increments of stress produce equal increments of strain (i.e., deformation). When the load is removed, both stress and strain return to zero (back down the straight line), and there is no net deformation.

Brittle materials are essentially purely elastic. They follow the straight-line relationship as load is increased until fracture occurs, which happens suddenly and with no warning. The area under a load deformation graph (i.e., stress–strain) represents the energy required to cause failure. With brittle materials (which are purely elastic), this energy is released at fracture, and fragments are imparted with kinetic energy, which, in orthotic

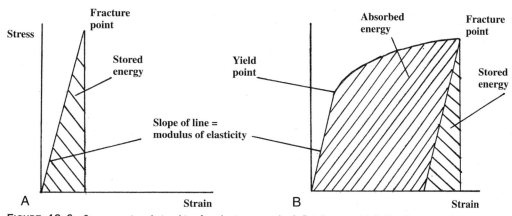

FIGURE 10–6   Stress–strain relationships for elastic materials. *A*, Brittle material. *B*, Ductile material.

devices that are overloaded, creates the potential for patient injury.

With ductile materials, the straight-line portion of the curve is followed by a change in characteristic. These materials reach a point at which they are no longer able to sustain elastic behavior, but they do not fracture when this occurs. Equal increments in stress produce greater increments of strain. The point at which this happens is known as the *yield point,* and the slope of the graph reduces dramatically. After yield has occurred, the deformation becomes permanent and is known as *plastic deformation.* In this phase, energy is absorbed within the material (mostly converted to heat).

The stress point at which a material fractures is known as the *ultimate strength* of the material. For ductile materials, the stress point at which yield occurs is the yield strength, and this is the point at which failure begins to occur.

A further important characteristic of materials is stiffness. The slope of the straight-line portion of the graph for elastic materials is known as the *modulus of elasticity.* It is a direct measure of the amount of deformation that occurs under applied stress and therefore defines the stiffness of the material. When deformation must be resisted, a high modulus of elasticity is necessary (i.e., a steep slope on the graph). For flexibility, a lower modulus of elasticity (less vertical slope) is required. Achieving an appropriate compromise for structural stiffness in an orthosis is often a challenge faced by designers. Material stiffness (as well as section modulus in the structure) plays an important role in ensuring the required characteristics in the device.

Figure 10–6*A* and *B* shows that for materials with the same ultimate strength and stiffness, a ductile material demands much greater energy to cause fracture than does a brittle material (although permanent deformation occurs earlier in the ductile material than does fracture in the brittle material). However, only the same amount of elastic strain energy is released when fracture finally does occur—the remainder having been safely absorbed by plastic deformation.

Typical examples of brittle materials are chalk and glass. Such materials require comparatively small amounts of energy to cause fracture and typically have jagged, sharp edges at the point of fracture. A good example of the properties of a ductile material is shown in a paper clip. It is comparatively easy to cause deformation and effective failure of the device but much more difficult to cause the material to fracture.

It is important to ensure maximum patient safety when providing orthoses for functional purposes. Brittle materials have low tolerance of overload and are therefore inherently unsafe. Ductile materials, on the other hand, can ensure that patients receive maximum protection from the potentially catastrophic consequences of a fracture in a material that may be very close to vulnerable areas of the body.

When materials are cyclically loaded, as many orthotic devices are (particularly those applied to the lower limb), fatigue failure becomes a possibility. This means that the material fails at load levels below those it can safely accommodate when it is new or when the load is not cyclically applied. The higher the loads relative to the strength of the device, the lower the number of load cycles to cause fatigue failure. This is an important failure mechanism throughout the field of orthopedic engineering but has particular relevance to lower limb orthoses. Failure commences at a point of high stress concentration, which is caused by sharp changes of section or holes within the device, scratches on the surface, or damage from general wear or manufacturing processes. The localized failure due to fatigue causes a crack in the material that does not lead to immediate fracture of the device. Propagation of the crack occurs as the cyclic load is continued, and this accelerates as the general strength of the device diminishes in response to the growth of the fatigue-induced flaw, eventually leading to catastrophic failure. Functional orthotic devices should be inspected regularly to ensure that they remain safe for the patient to use, and an examination for signs of fatigue should be a routine part of such a process.

STRUCTURAL PROPERTIES

As already indicated, the most common loads applied to orthotic structures are those that occur in bending. This is because an orthosis is usually expected to resist the moments generated around joints that do not have the muscle strength and power to do this.

The ability of a structural section to resist bending is related to the distribution of material around the bending axis. This principle is illustrated by bending a ruler around its long axis (Fig. 10–7). With the ruler flat (see Fig. 10–7*A*) it is easy to bend, whereas in the upright position (see Fig. 10–7*B*) it is difficult. The same amount of material is involved in both cases, but in the upright position, the distribution of material is more effectively spaced from the bending axis.

A useful fact that helps to reinforce the importance of this principle is that doubling the thickness of a section increases bending resistance by

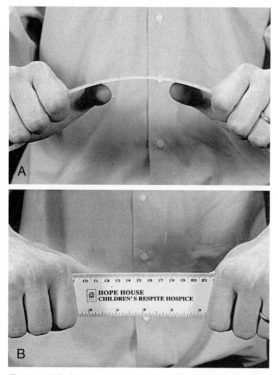

FIGURE 10-7 Bending a ruler in the flat *(A)* and upright *(B)* planes to indicate the difference in bending resistance made by distribution of material around the bending axis.

a factor of eight if the width remains the same. By the same token, halving the thickness reduces the bending resistance by a factor of eight. Figure 10-8, in which there are two beams of the same material, width and length, with one being twice the thickness, shows how the thinner beam deflects eight times as much under the same loading conditions.

LOWER LIMB ORTHOSES

Lower limb orthoses are subdivided into groups that cover the ankle-foot complex (AFO), the knee (KO), the knee-ankle-foot complex (KAFO), and the hip-knee-ankle-foot complex (HKAFO). Note that foot orthoses are treated as a separate entity and are not dealt with in this chapter. It is theoretically possible to have a hip orthosis, but these are rarely used and tend to be accepted as a special category.

To achieve the required control of each joint in the lower limb, a three-point force system is necessary to provide the equal and opposite moment to that being applied to the joint, which cannot be resisted by the patient's compromised control system. In general, an orthosis needs to be as long as possible so that the moment arms through which the orthosis applies its forces are at a maximum, reducing the magnitude of those forces.

ANKLE-FOOT ORTHOSES

AFO devices are the most commonly prescribed orthoses. They are intended to control the ankle and subtalar joints as well as the biomechanics of the knee or hip joint by ensuring appropriate alignment of ground reaction forces relative to those joints. A wide range of functions can be performed by AFO devices. Among the most common are the following:

- Resisting ankle plantar-flexion–dorsiflexion
- Controlling a drop-foot condition
- Controlling the range of ankle plantar-flexion–dorsiflexion
- Resisting valgus and varus at the ankle

Resisting Plantar-Flexion–Dorsiflexion

The most structurally demanding function for an AFO is to resist plantar-flexion–dorsiflexion moments around the ankle joint. During single stance, gait forces in excess of body weight are routinely generated. In conditions in which vaulting using the stance leg occurs, such forces can be considerable and may cause large moments around the

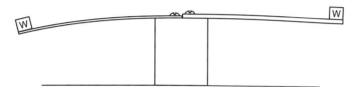

FIGURE 10-8 Deflexion of two beams under the same load (the beams are identical other than one being twice as thick as the other). The deflexion of the thinner beam is eight times greater. W, weight. (From ORLAU [Orthotic Research and Locomotor Assessment Unit], The Robert Jones and Agnes Hunt Orthopaedic and District Hospital, Oswestry, Shropshire, England SY10 7AG.)

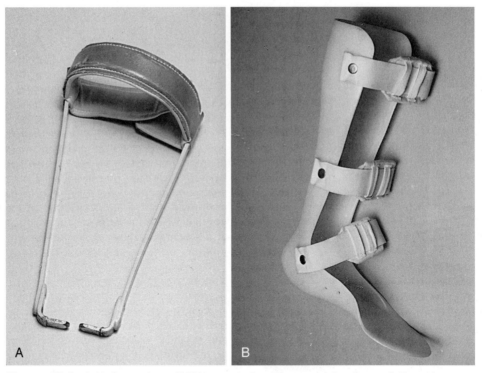

FIGURE 10–9 Ankle-foot orthoses (AFO) to resist plantar-flexion and dorsiflexion. *A*, Twin side-member AFO (note flat spurs to resist moments around the ankle joint). *B*, Molded plastic AFO (note depth of section at the ankle to resist moments around that joint).

ankle joint. Resisting those large moments may require a metal structure (Fig. 10–9A) to achieve sufficient stiffness to apply an effective three-point fixation system. Many patients are reluctant to wear such a device because of the inevitably poor cosmesis that results from this type of structure. An alternative plastic structure (Fig. 10–9B) can be used in the less structurally demanding situations involving pediatric, light-weight, or dynamically nonchallenging patients. Note that a very deep section around the ankle joint is required to produce sufficient bending resistance, even with the lower demands of these patients.

Controlling ankle plantar-flexion–dorsiflexion inevitably influences alignment of ground reaction forces relative to the knee and hip joints. Some patients may be able to compensate their gait to ensure that potentially adverse effects are limited when the objective is primarily to control an unstable ankle. However, the potential of fixed ankle orthoses to influence alignment of ground reaction forces can, in patients with lower limb control problems, either create unmanageable moments for the joints above the ankle or be put to good effect in achieving the desired alignment through careful tuning of the AFO shoe complex.

A good example of the use of an AFO to control knee mechanics is in cerebral palsy patients with a dynamic equinus condition. Although on examination the ankle may be correctable to neutral (or dorsiflexion), during walking, aberrant control leads to an equinus during stance phase and a consequent ground reaction force considerably ahead of the knee. Figure 10–10 shows the use of a VVG[5] to provide a video vector display of this condition (the on-screen line represents a vector of ground reaction force). This gives an indication of the excessive knee extending moment that results. The subject is a boy about 400 N in weight. In this figure, the moment on the knee can be calculated as follows:

Ground reaction force × moment arm
    (knee center to ground reaction force)

By inspection, the ground reaction force is about one third of the subject's body weight at maximum moment arm position (as illustrated in Fig. 10–10), and the moment arm is about 500 mm. On that basis, the moment is calculated as follows:

$$(400 \text{ N} \div 3) \times 500 \text{ mm} = 133 \text{ N}$$
$$\times 0.5 \text{ m} = 67 \text{ N m}$$

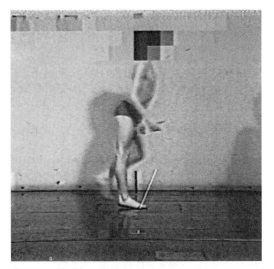

FIGURE 10–10   Dynamic equinus: typical ground reaction force alignment at mid-stance.

Abnormal stresses on the knee of the magnitude implied by this load are likely to lead to the development of a recurvatum unless the condition is alleviated. The use of a fixed-ankle AFO to prevent the equinus from developing might be expected to control the alignment problem. Experience shows, however, that achieving this objective requires careful tuning of the ankle–shoe complex by adjusting alignment with heel or sole raises on the shoe. Figure 10–11A shows the use of an AFO before tuning. It can be seen that surprisingly little effect has been achieved simply by preventing the equinus. After tuning with an appropriate heel raise (Fig. 10–11B), however, the alignment of the vector is much closer to the knee, and the excessive knee extending moment has been eliminated.

Long-term follow-up has been studied in a series of six cerebral palsy patients with a dynamic equinus while walking.[11] Each of eleven limbs with the condition showed a similar pattern of forward-facing vector relative to the knee joint when the subject walked without an AFO. In none of the cases was corrected alignment achieved with an AFO before tuning of the system. By monitoring the patients using a VVG, appropriate alignment was achieved for each of the limbs by tuning the AFO–shoe complex with heel or sole raises. Long-term follow-up showed that correcting the alignment had an effect on the patients' control systems. Over a period of 6 months or more, consistent use of the system led to an ability to maintain appropriate alignment when not using the orthosis. Some patients have been followed for more than 3 years after abandoning the orthosis

Without an AFO, this moment is resisted only by the skeletal structures around the knee, where the maximum moment arm would be about 50 mm. Thus, 67 N m equals the force in the knee structures times 0.05 meters (i.e., 50 mm). The potential force in the knee, therefore, is

$$67 \text{ N m}/0.05 \text{ m} = 1333 \text{ N}$$

Bearing in mind that 1 kg is almost 10 N, it can be seen that this force (equivalent to 133 bags of sugar at 1 kg each) has great destructive potential.

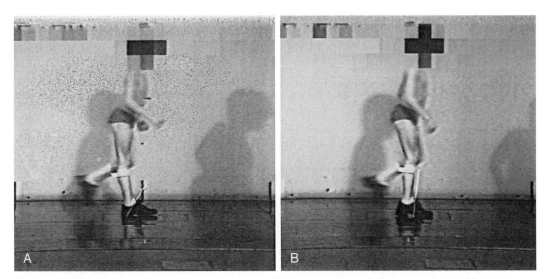

FIGURE 10–11   Provision of an orthosis to compensate for dynamic equinus. A, Before tuning the ankle-foot orthosis. B, After tuning the ankle-foot orthosis (using a video vector generator).

following achievement of corrected control, and they have maintained their improvement. This strongly suggests that mechanical orthoses can interact with a patient's control system and underlines the need to understand the mechanics of orthotic control of joints in individual cases.

The dynamic equinus condition is perhaps the most dramatic example of the potential to control the joints above the ankle with an AFO. Crouch gait can also be influenced beneficially by adjusting alignment, so that the ground reaction force passes closer to the knee and hip joints, reducing the flexing moments that the patient must resist with knee and hip extensors. Whenever a fixed-ankle AFO is used, it influences alignment; it is therefore appropriate to monitor the effects of this to ensure that optimal mechanics are achieved.

Controlling a Drop-Foot Condition

Some pathologic conditions, most notably stroke, can lead to a condition in which the patient has no effective dorsiflexors. The weight of the foot during the swing phase of gait creates a plantar-flexing moment around the ankle. Because of the loss of dorsiflexors, the patient is unable to generate the necessary balancing moment, and the foot drops into an equinus position. The consequence is that during swing phase, the patient needs to flex the knee to a greater extent than normal to create sufficient clearance for the foot to avoid contact with the ground. This not only leads to an abnormal gait pattern but also increases the energy cost of walking.

A drop-foot orthosis (Fig. 10–12) is intended to

cope with that condition. The moment generated around the ankle joint by the weight of the foot during swing phase is resisted by the structural section of the orthosis at the back of the ankle in the vicinity of the Achilles tendon. Because there is also a need to permit some dorsiflexion of the ankle during stance phase, this section requires a subtle compromise. Ideally, it should be stiff enough to prevent significant deformation from the moment caused by the weight of the foot in swing phase, but flexible enough to permit an appropriate range of dorsiflexion from the greater moments around the ankle joint under the influence of body weight during stance phase. If the orthosis is too stiff to permit an adequate dorsiflexion range, it can be adjusted by trimming the section of the orthosis in the area adjacent to the Achilles tendon. When this is done, the sensitivity of a bending section to a reduction in thickness is of great importance, and the general rule that, for a rectangular section, halving the thickness reduces resistance by a factor of eight should caution against overambitious trimming.

Controlling the Range of Ankle Plantar-Flexion–Dorsiflexion

Limiting the range of flexion and extension of the ankle joint is a function that can be performed by an AFO. To achieve this ideally requires an orthotic hinge in line with the ankle and stops attached to the structure to prevent the ankle joint from flexing or extending beyond the clinically specified range.

Because of the high dorsiflexing moment applied to the ankle joint during the stance phase of gait, the structural demands on an orthosis designed to achieve limitation of range can be considerable. Metal structures, with their greater strength and stiffness, are therefore frequently required for this function when patients are unable to provide balancing moments from their own musculoskeletal system.

In patients who are of light weight, have low levels of dynamic function, or can provide some of the biomechanical function themselves, the use of a plastic orthosis with flexion and extension stops becomes a much more practical option.

Resisting Valgus and Varus at the Ankle

To influence valgus or varus, an AFO must apply three-point fixation around the os calcis. A plastic fixed-ankle AFO can be molded to apply three-point fixation forces in both sagittal (to control plantar-flexion–dorsiflexion) and coronal planes to control ankle valgus or varus. This total blocking

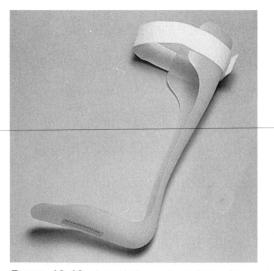

FIGURE 10–12 An ankle-foot orthosis designed to control a drop-foot condition.

of the ankle–subtalar complex is frequently considered unacceptable, and alternative orthoses that permit ankle plantar-flexion–dorsiflexion range are therefore necessary.

The weight of the patient, degree of dynamic activity, and extent of valgus and varus deformity determine the appropriate design of the orthotic structure to achieve the required control. When any of these is excessive, it may be necessary to resort to a metal structure to achieve sufficient structural stiffness to permit the required degree of control. Typically, such a device (Fig. 10–13A) has a metal side-member with a spur that fits into a socket insert in the heel of the patient's shoe. A T strap or Y strap applies the center control force at the level of the malleoli, with the counterforces applied by the shoe through the spur and socket and by the calf band of the orthosis. Not surprisingly, this device is not considered cosmetically acceptable by most patients and is increasingly used only in the most extreme biomechanical circumstances.

The use of plastic molded orthoses to control valgus and varus is now common. Although they may be biomechanically more compromised than the alternative metal structures, their greater acceptability to patients ensures that they are more likely to be regularly used. To achieve maximum effectiveness requires careful molding and cast rectification to ensure appropriate application of three-point fixation to the os calcis, and such devices therefore demand a high level of professionalism in casting, manufacture, and fitting.

A common requirement of an orthosis is to control valgus or varus at the ankle, so that a range of ankle flexion and extension is maintained. This makes it necessary either to have a hinge in line with the ankle joint (Fig. 10–13B) or to have sufficient structural flexibility in the sagittal plane to permit flexion and extension.

DYNAMIC ANKLE-FOOT ORTHOSES

A new category of orthosis that seeks to control the behavior of the ankle joint (and by reference the other joints of the lower limb) by influencing neurologic behavior is an interesting development.[12] These AFOs seek to achieve this through rectification of the positive mold to produce stimulating impressions on the orthosis relative to key neurologic receptor sites on the plantar surface of the foot. Some versions of these orthoses extend into and above the ankle joint region, whereas others remain below it. This suggests that those that do extend into the ankle region are intended to produce a combination of mechanical and neurologic effect, whereas those that remain below the ankle rely only on neurologic stimulation.

The diminished nature of the orthotic structure that the design allows provides major cosmetic benefits that could be an important encouragement for patients to persevere with the treatment. However, there is little published on the principles by which these devices achieve their intended aims and a dearth of clinical research to support the concept. In some clinical centers, the devices are used enthusiastically, suggesting that the evidence will accumulate and be published in the future. If

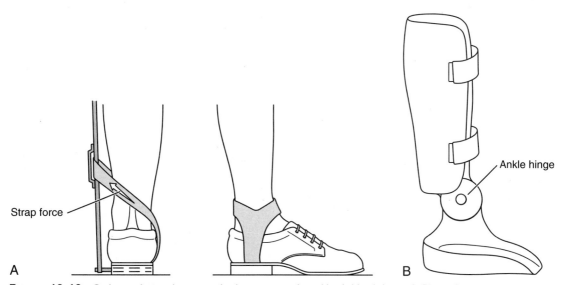

Strap force

Ankle hinge

FIGURE 10–13   Orthoses designed to control valgus-varus at the ankle. A, Metal design. B, Plastic design. (From ORLAU [Orthotic Research and Locomotor Assessment Unit], The Robert Jones and Agnes Hunt Orthopaedic and District Hospital, Oswestry, Shropshire, England SY10 7AG.)

the principles are elucidated clearly and supported by clinical evidence of success, these devices could revolutionize clinical practice.

Plastic molded AFO devices are now the most common type of orthosis for most forms of ankle control. Their attraction to patients in comparison with metal structures is obvious. They do, however, have some features that require careful consideration. Direct contact of nonpermeable materials with the patient can lead to overheating and perspiration. The molding process does not always give good control of material thickness in areas of high stress, and the overall strength of the structure can be compromised by this and possible adverse affects from overheating or underheating during the molding process. Not all plastic materials have good fatigue resistance, and inappropriate selection from ostensibly similar materials can cause premature failure.

Provided that these matters are effectively accommodated in the design of AFO devices, plastic materials have the potential to achieve most of their objectives. It is likely that technologic developments will result in new, more effective moldable materials that improve the position further, and to this extent, the future looks promising.

KNEE ORTHOSES

Knee orthoses are devices that span the knee joint only and do not seek to control other joints. They generally fall into one of two categories in terms of the type of patient they are intended to address: (1) vigorous patients who have suffered knee trauma and (2) more frail patients who are suffering a degenerative condition of the knee. Although the category of patient may influence the choice of orthosis, the principles through which such devices achieve their objectives remain the same. The following forms of control can be applied by knee orthoses:

- Resisting valgus and varus moments
- Limiting flexion and extension range
- Resisting anteroposterior relative movement between femur and tibia
- Limiting rotation of the femur on the tibia

The direct loads applied to the knee by the more frail patients are comparatively low. It is known that patients with severe osteoarthritis, for example, generate vertical ground reaction forces barely above body weight. Degenerative disease, however, usually leads to deformity of the joint, which in turn can mean that ground reaction force falls outside normal alignment, thereby producing excessively high moments around the joint. Figure 10–14A shows alignment of ground reaction force

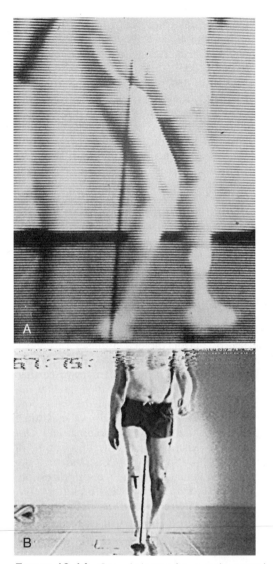

FIGURE 10–14 Ground reaction forces in the coronal plane (as indicated by the video vector generator). A, Patient with osteoarthritis of the knee. B, Healthy subject.

in the coronal plane (from a VVG analysis) on an osteoarthritic patient who has a severe valgus deformity of the knee. As a result of the degenerative process, the patient has a large valgus-deforming moment (calculated as being about 10 N m about the medial condyle) in comparison with a healthy subject (Fig. 10–14B), in whom it is effectively zero. Pathologic conditions of this kind present a severe challenge to knee orthoses.

The example of a frail patient with an osteoarthritic deformity demonstrates the potential for high moments to be generated around the knee joint even with comparatively low ground reaction forces inherent in such conditions. There is clearly a strong possibility for vigorous patients to generate large dynamic loads, and these might also be combined with abnormal alignment to produce even higher moments. Thus, the potential exists for very large moments around the knee joint to be generated in a variety of situations. Knee orthoses have short moment arms through which to produce resisting moments. It is therefore unrealistic to expect that excessive moments can be accommodated by an orthosis of this type because the large forces that would be required through the short moment arms would be intolerable for most patients.

Nevertheless, knee orthoses can deliver valuable functions, provided that their prescription is limited to objectives and applications that are realistic.

Resisting Valgus and Varus Moments

The line of force in the coronal plane during normal walking passes through the medial condyle of the knee (see Fig. 10–14B). Any deviation from this produces an abnormal moment. When a patient has a correctable deformity, an orthosis can be used to realign the knee joint. If this is achieved, the moment can be reduced to near-normal levels, and the orthosis will not have to bear excessive moments, except when aberrant alignments of force occur as a result of an accident or unusual activity.

Noncorrectable severe deformity produces unacceptable stresses on the knee joint. Some relief of those stresses can be provided through the use of an orthosis to transfer some of the loads to other parts of the affected limb. It is not realistic, however, to expect a complete relief of the applied moment because no acceptable orthotic structure could achieve this. The interface pressure created at the reaction points is also a cause of great concern, particularly in patients whose pathology compromises their skin condition.

Sports activity can produce large valgus and varus moments around the knee joint in the lateral plane (of the order 30 N m), particularly when side thrusts on the leg are necessary, such as occur when tennis or football players change direction suddenly. Patients with sports injuries are more able to tolerate interface pressures and accommodate the type of structure that would be necessary to produce large moments than are those with degenerative disease. Even in this situation, however, it is not realistic to expect complete relief of stress on the knee joint in the coronal plane.

When the only objective of the treatment is to resist valgus and varus moments, it is necessary for the structure to incorporate freely hinged knee joints. For the orthosis to be effective, these joints must bear the lateral moments required to achieve the required function. They must therefore have low friction under load and have strength and rigidity commensurate with the rest of the structure.

In regard to the magnitude of valgus and varus moments around the knee, informal measurements using a VVG have registered 10 N m at the lateral condyle for a frail, light-weight patient with a severe valgus deformity and 15 to 20 N m for an average adult male subject indulging in fairly light badminton activity while thrusting off sideways to make a shot. Such moments are not inconsiderable and indicate that the structural demands on a knee orthosis for a valgus and varus condition that is expected to do anything other than realign the joint during walking are high and therefore require sound engineering design.

Limiting Flexion and Extension Range

In normal walking, the ground reaction force passes close to the knee joint throughout the stance phase of gait, thereby producing very low flexing or extending moments. Pathologic conditions that result in a flexion (or less commonly, an extension) deformity can result in malalignment of ground reaction forces and lead to large moments around the knee in the sagittal plane. Sports frequently require vigorous use of the quadriceps to resist knee flexing moments generated in response to the athletic demands of the recreational activity. A knee orthosis can be used to resist any flexion and extension of the knee (usually in a pathologic condition) or to limit the range of flexion and extension to that which is clinically acceptable.

The biomechanical demand on such an orthosis depends on the type of patient and the required function. Holding the knee in a fixed position by resisting any flexion or extension requires that the orthosis be capable of sustaining the full flexion or extension moment around the joint in the position determined by deformity or clinical need. The greater the angle of the knee from neutral (in the sagittal plane), the larger the potential moment that will have to be resisted. Knee orthoses with short moment arms are unsuitable for applications in which there is excessive knee flexion because the high moment demands large orthotic forces. The knee should be kept as straight as possible for bracing within the clinical requirements of the treatment regimen being followed, to minimize the orthotic forces.

For sports or other trauma applications, it is likely that the objective is to limit the range of movement to that considered clinically necessary or desirable. In general use, the function of the orthosis is to act as a reminder to the patient not to exceed the prescribed limit. In those circumstances, used properly, loads are applied by the orthosis only when the patient inadvertently attempts to exceed the limit. There is the potential, however, for very high shock loads if the patient loses control over the knee range, and an orthosis needs to reflect the requirement to accommodate that situation. Knee-flexing moments of the order 160 N m have been monitored by a VVG for a healthy male subject during single-leg landing after playing a badminton shot. The impact this could create on the flexion end stop of a range-limiting orthosis is potentially high, and it is likely that the prescribed range would be exceeded in those circumstances.

Resisting Anteroposterior Relative Movement

When knee laxity is present, undesirable relative movement of the femur on the tibia may occur (this is frequently referred to as *drawer*). During any form of gait, horizontal components of force are applied to the lower limb. Depending on the direction of these, the femur will have a tendency to slide forward or backward on the tibia.

Some orthoses attempt to deal with this problem by providing general resistive support around the knee. Although this simple approach can be effective in coping with drawer, it can also have a resistive effect on other functions, such as permitting free flexion of the knee. An alternative approach is also adopted in which counter moments are applied by the orthosis to the leg above and below the knee joint. This is achieved by so-called four-point fixation of the knee (Fig. 10–15).

Depending on which way the forces are applied, posterior or anterior drawer can be resisted, so that the required alignment of femur and tibia can be achieved. Such an approach does not inhibit other functions, provided that the system is properly applied. This is important because the feature is often incorporated in an orthosis intended to achieve other objectives at the same time.

During normal walking, horizontal ground reaction forces of the order of 160 N have been registered by VVG monitoring, and it is these that have to be resisted to counteract drawer. Clearly, more vigorous activity would bring commensurate increases in the magnitude of this force.

Resisting Rotation of the Femur on the Tibia

Most activities that engage the lower limb involve the application of torque around the long axis of the bones. In gait, there are both internal and external moments around the axis of the lower limb during each full cycle. Joint laxity can lead to unacceptable rotations in response to these axial torques, and a function required of a knee orthosis can be to resist the turning moment along the axis of the limb. This is perhaps the most difficult of all the functions expected of a knee orthosis. There are no obvious solid reaction points around which to produce equal and opposite torque, and systems intended for this purpose have to rely on friction between the orthosis and the patient together with resilient strapping across the knee. Although this approach can provide some resistance, because these systems have to operate on a short moment arm (i.e., the width of the knee), the force to achieve a full compensatory torque is

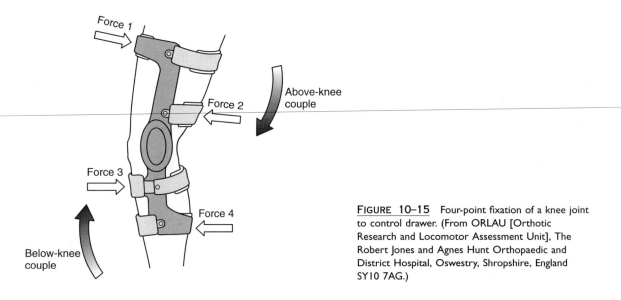

FIGURE 10–15 Four-point fixation of a knee joint to control drawer. (From ORLAU [Orthotic Research and Locomotor Assessment Unit], The Robert Jones and Agnes Hunt Orthopaedic and District Hospital, Oswestry, Shropshire, England SY10 7AG.)

inevitably very high. Because the reaction point is resilient, it must deform to a large degree to generate that force and thus allow a degree of rotation of the knee. That is not to say that support of this kind is worthless, but a cautionary note should be sounded about expecting too much of this orthotic function.

During normal walking, the torque around the long axis of the lower limb is about 10 N m. Fairly gentle badminton playing increases this to about 30 N m. A professional tennis player, cricketer, football or soccer player, or baseball pitcher could well exceed 100 N m during peak performance. This gives an indication of the task when an orthosis is to be used in sporting applications.

KNEE-ANKLE-FOOT ORTHOSES

KAFO devices encompass control of both the knee and the ankle and therefore have the potential to incorporate all of the elements of AFOs and KOs. Because of their much more comprehensive nature, KAFOs are intended to deal with greater levels of handicap and are inevitably more obtrusive, which makes them cosmetically less acceptable to patients. That these devices extend the whole length of the lower limb gives them the advantage of long moment arms through which to provide the controlling forces, and this enables them to cope with situations for which KOs would be impractical.

The primary functions of KAFO devices are to provide control of knee flexing and extending moments, knee valgus and varus moments, and any combination of these, along with weight relief of the lower limb. Any of the functions of AFO devices can also be incorporated, if necessary, by attaching to the lower end of the structure the appropriate orthotic components. Additional knee controls can be applied as described in the section on KOs, but the greater level of pathologic insult implied by the use of a KAFO makes this a less frequently applied option.

The primary indications for the prescription of KAFO devices are loss of control of the knee joint (as in paraplegia), severe weakness of the knee joint muscles, gross instability of the knee joint combined with excessive deformity, and structural weakness requiring weight relief.

In most applications, KAFOs resist knee flexion and extension. To be practical, these devices need to incorporate releasable knee joints so that patients can sit with their knees in a flexed position. Selection of these requires careful consideration of several important points, including joint specification, method of release, and location of the joint center.

Control of Knee Flexion and Extension

In normal walking, the line of force passes through or very close to the center of the knee joint for most of the stance phase of gait. This ensures minimal demands on the muscles around the knee to balance the small moments, which nevertheless inevitably develop. When there is no control of the quadriceps, it is essential to ensure that at no time is there a flexing moment because it is impossible for the patient to generate the equal and opposite moment. In those circumstances, it is necessary to use a KAFO to provide the requisite control at the knee (and also at the ankle) through three-point fixation to prevent collapse of the patient. The three points of force application (see Fig. 10–5) are at the back of the thigh through a thigh band, over the knee through a knee band (which usually incorporates a releasable fastening), and at the bottom of the shank, most commonly through the shoe (with spur and socket or in-shoe AFO section).

Control of Knee Valgus and Varus Moments

Excessive valgus or varus moments around the knee require resistance by three-point fixation in the lateral plane. These are applied laterally through the orthosis at the thigh and lower shank levels, with the opposing force applied through the knee strap at the side of the knee joint (medial for valgus, lateral for varus). Depending on the degree of deformity and the weight of the patient, valgus and varus stabilizing forces can be considerable, and the orthotic structure must have adequate strength and stiffness in the lateral plane to cope with these.

Combination of Orthotic Function

Patients usually need control of both flexion and extension and valgus and varus of the knee (together with controls of the ankle joint). When a KAFO has an adequate structure, these functions can be readily combined into one orthosis. In this situation, attention must be paid to the patient support strap arrangements to ensure that all the necessary forces are applied in the appropriate directions.

Weight-Relieving Orthoses

A function that is occasionally required of KAFO devices is the relief loading on the lower limb. This requires that the thigh section of the device extend to the level at which loads can be transmitted through the patient's ischial tuberosities, and the shank section should incorporate a ground reaction support plate under the patient's shoe. To ensure that no ground reaction forces are transmitted through the leg, there must be clearance between the shoe and the support plate. Such an arrangement demands a raise on the opposite side to compensate.

Transmitting loads through the ischial tuberosities causes discomfort to the patient, and the additional raise is also an unwelcome inconvenience. Because the orthosis, in these circumstances, is required to carry all the dynamic ground reaction forces in the stance phase of gait, the structure must be robust and therefore comparatively heavy. The musculoskeletal system of the lower limb (if intact) can also continue to function and generate loads internally, minimizing the relief of skeletal stress. It is for these reasons that this orthotic function is only occasionally invoked.

Structural Design Considerations

The magnitude of the stabilizing forces that the orthosis is required to generate (and therefore the design that needs to be adopted) depends on the weight of the patient, the degree of knee flexion deformity, the level of dynamic activity undertaken by the patient, and the spacing of the stabilizing forces (the farther apart they are, the lower they will be). In stabilizing orthoses (i.e., those seeking only to resist moments generated around the knee), the patient's skeletal structure is intended to carry the ground reaction forces. Inevitably, because of friction at the orthosis location points, an indeterminable proportion of the loads along the long axis of the lower limb are carried by the KAFO. This makes it necessary to have a generous safety margin in the design of these devices (particularly because there are also significant fatigue implications), which is in conflict with the patient requirements of light weight and inobtrusiveness. A careful compromise, therefore, has to be struck to achieve the solution most acceptable to the patient in line with adequate function and safety within the structure of the orthosis. Fig. 10–16A shows a typical metal KAFO.

For light-weight patients with no significant knee flexion contracture, it is possible to use a plastic molded structure incorporating a thigh cuff and in-shoe AFO connected by metal knee joints riveted to the above-knee and below-knee components (Fig. 10–16B). This is widely known as a *cosmetic caliper*[13] and has obvious attractions to many patients. When used appropriately, this device is an eminently satisfactory solution to the design dilemma. The temptation to use it in situations in which it is too close to the limit of its

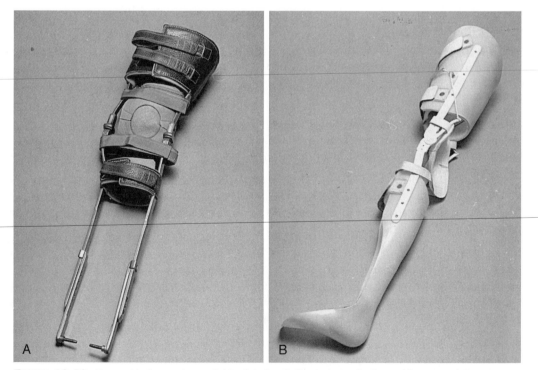

FIGURE 10–16 Knee-ankle-foot orthoses. *A,* Metal design. *B,* Plastic design (with metal knee joints) for improved cosmesis.

capabilities is great, however, and can lead to its being prescribed unwisely. Before a decision is taken to opt for this type of design, an investigation of the activities of the patient should be undertaken to ensure they are compatible with the structural specification of the orthosis. Cases have occurred in which ostensibly ideal patients experienced frequent structural failure of the orthosis. Subsequent discussion with the patients usually identified a hobby, such as abseiling, to be the likely cause. Although not always feasible, gait analysis can also confirm that the line of ground reaction force is not producing excessive knee-flexing moments.

When a patient is heavy or indulges in vigorous dynamic activity, it is essential to use substantial orthotic structures to produce a viable device capable of safely sustaining the very high bending loads that will be applied to control knee flexion and extension. This approach usually requires the use of standard metal sections to form the side-members of the orthotic structure. The choice of material is typically stiff, inexpensive steel or light-weight, lower-ductility aluminum alloy. In selecting the material, a major influencing factor is the likelihood of the patient's overloading the orthosis. A frail elderly woman with a low level of activity, for example, would need the advantage of the light-weight structure made possible by aluminum alloy. An active, young, heavy man could be expected to have a propensity to overload the orthotic structure in some unexpected manner. The high level of ductility possessed by steel and the consequently high level of energy it absorbs before fracturing (after the yield point has been exceeded) makes it the ideal choice for this situation, even though the greater weight of the material is a necessary penalty. For patients between those two extremes, the choice becomes increasingly difficult as they approach the midpoint of the compromise range. Fatigue performance of the two materials is fairly similar, although steel would be expected to be less likely to suffer this mode of failure, all other things being equal.

Joint Specification

Patient safety is of paramount importance, and the design of an orthotic knee joint used in KAFO devices must reflect that requirement. Bending is clearly the most demanding mode of loading that will be applied, and the joint strength must obviously be sufficient to withstand that which can reasonably be anticipated during any function the patient might be expected to undertake. Because overload is an ever-present possibility, the failure mode of the joint (when locked) in all planes

should ideally be ductile in nature, so that energy can be absorbed before fracture occurs. When a joint does have a brittle failure mode, the orthotic structure should incorporate a "mechanical fuse" that will fail in a safe manner before the joint is overloaded.

Method of Release

To enable patients to achieve full independence, it is essential to provide a practical means of releasing the lock on an orthotic knee joint. Two commonly used solutions to this problem are the ring lock and the bale lock.

With the ring lock (Fig. 10–17A), a sliding ring on the upper section of the side-member of the KAFO overlaps a tongue on the lower section of the side-member above the hinge, thus preventing the hinge from rotating until the ring is raised above the tongue. Simple methods of retaining the ring in the lower (locked) or upper (unlocked) position on the KAFO side-member are usually employed. This system demands conscious operation by the patient for both locking and unlocking (although simple "automatic" gravity locking can be used if means of retaining the ring in the upper position are not employed).

In bale lock arrangements (Fig. 10–17B), the stop is operated using a lever extending upward from the rear of the joint hinge. The lever is usually spring biased to the locked position, so that as the joint is straightened, the lock closes automatically. Unlocking can then be effected manually by the patient or automatically as the lever comes into contact with a seat edge when the patient descends into the seated position.

To operate either of these two types of orthotic knee joint, it is necessary for the patient to relieve the knee-flexing moment on the joint when he or she releases the lock. An inability to do this will compromise the independence of the patient.

Location of Orthotic Joint Center

Orthotic joints are normally aligned as closely as possible to the appropriate anatomic joint of the patient. This ensures that there is minimal relative movement between the patient and the orthosis as the two joints move through their permitted range. Severe malalignment can lead to interface problems from rubbing of the orthosis on skin (particularly when there is insensitivity) or excess interface pressure due to migration of the orthosis from its optimal position. Orthoses that cross more than one joint are particularly prone to raising interface pressures when malalignment leads to effective

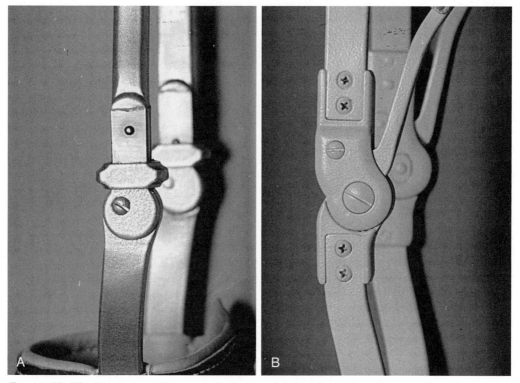

FIGURE 10–17 Commonly used knee joint designs. A, Ring lock joint. B, Bale lock joint.

shortening of the distance between the orthotic joints relative to anatomic joints.

HIP-KNEE-ANKLE-FOOT ORTHOSES

Orthoses of this generic type can achieve all of the functions available in AFO and KAFO devices together with required controls of the hip joint. Three-point fixation of the hip is achieved by providing forces at the thoracic and sacral levels and on the thigh in the relevant directions for the selected control. The main purpose of HKAFO devices is to facilitate ambulation for severely handicapped patients who have inadequate or aberrant control of the hip joint. Typically, patients have complete spinal lesions at L1 or above, which implies that there is no motor control of the hip joint at all. It is not a realistic expectation that these patients will achieve as efficient locomotion on a flat surface as they can anticipate in a wheelchair, and it is therefore necessary to identify the justification for prescription of such devices. Those who advocate walking for the severely handicapped have two main objectives:

1. To provide therapeutic benefit
2. To increase independence and allow patients to undertake activities not possible in a wheelchair

Menelaus,[1] Rose,[14] Carroll,[15] and others have all cited clinical experience suggesting that ambulation can achieve these objectives. More recently, Mazur and colleagues[16] showed in a study of matched groups that nonwalkers have five times the number of pressure sores and twice the number of bone fractures. Additionally, walkers were able to perform a series of activities of daily living in significantly greater numbers than the nonwalkers and were three times more likely to be independently mobile within the community. The case for providing orthoses to enable such patients to walk is therefore strong, provided that a practical, financially viable system that is acceptable to patients is available. What is practical and acceptable varies among patients and generally is judged against the following factors:

Walking style
Energy cost of walking
Ease of applying and removing the system
Overall cost of all elements of treatment, including ongoing service

As indicated earlier, any form of walking requires control of both internal and external stabilization forces. Severe handicap inhibits the necessary control, and an HKAFO is therefore required to compensate. In particular, an orthosis provides appropriate control at the hip joint for the style of ambulation in question, which (together with the support for other lower limb joints) provides internal stabilization and a larger area of support (sometimes in combination with other walking aids) than is necessary for a healthy subject to ensure good external stabilization. Propulsive forces are injected by the upper limbs (by an additional walking aid) or through inertial forces generated by truncal movement.

Many different walking systems have evolved, and the means of hip control (and control of other distal joints) is a fundamental determining factor in the style of walking they provide and their consequent ability to satisfy the needs of patients. The other factors are dependent on detail design of individual orthotic systems. Overall effectiveness of service delivery (e.g., patient assessment, production of orthosis, fitting and training the patient, ongoing regular review) are of primary importance in ensuring a practical outcome for any form of walking system for severely handicapped patients.

Walking Style

Several different walking styles are employed by patients with complete absence of control in the lower limbs. Those most commonly adopted include the following:

Swing-through gait
Swivel walking
Reciprocal walking

The choice of style depends on patient and clinician preference, the physical characteristics and functional capabilities of the patient, and the physical therapy, orthotic, and financial resources available. Apart from swivel walking, an additional walking aid such as walking frame or crutches is also necessary.

Swing-Through Gait

For swing-through gait, the patient's hips and knees are held in a fixed position by the HKAFO (the ankles may be either fixed or allowed to flex and extend, depending on the pathology of the ankle). This enables a walking frame or crutches to be used to raise the whole weight of the body (and orthosis) from the ground using the upper limbs. The legs are then swung forward in space to land a complete stride forward. The performance of the patient depends on his or her strength and control and is further influenced by the weight of the orthosis and its ability to provide the required stability, particularly in the lateral plane, during the stance phase.

In most applications, unlockable joints at the hips and knees are required to permit the patient to sit while wearing the orthosis. The structural demands on these (and other elements of the orthosis) are dictated by the deformities of the patient. When there are large contractures at the anatomic joints, the moments that the orthosis must resist are correspondingly great, and the structure needs to reflect the increased stresses that result.

Although swing-through gait is probably the simplest means of providing walking for severely handicapped patients, it is physically demanding and is the least efficient of the available options. The conventional orthotic structures generally used for swing-through gait (Fig. 10–18A) are difficult to put on and take off, and this inhibits independence. Although more modern designs of orthosis address some of the difficulties[17] (Fig. 10–18B), many patients find the challenges of adopting this type of ambulation too great. A review of the literature[18–20] reveals that the average energy cost for swing-through gait in patients with thoracic lesions is about 30 J/kg/m, which is almost 10 times that for normal walking.

Swivel Walking

Swivel walking requires an orthosis that provides internal stabilization of the patient by resisting moments around all the joints of the lower limbs (i.e., at hips, knees, and ankles) to avoid collapse of the skeletal structure. Swivel walking also incorporates footplates to give an adequate support area for external stabilization, to prevent the patient from falling over.

The footplates also need a mechanism that permits them to swivel forward alternately on the grounded footplate as the patient rocks from side to side. Ambulation is achieved by the patient's injecting an inertial force into the orthosis by thrusting the trunk sideways (Fig. 10–19A). This leads to several interactive mechanical reactions, as indicated in Fig. 10–19B. Being slightly angled (dihedral angle), the footplates rest on their inner border, and the orthosis rocks onto the footplate coincident with the direction of inertial thrust (I). The bearing center of the footplates are arranged to be behind the patient's center of gravity, so that the sideways inertial thrust, I_f, normally produces a forward rotating moment around the grounded footplate to advance the swivel walker in the generally preferred direction. To ambulate backward, the inertial thrust, I_r, must be arranged to lie behind the footplate bearing center. This is more difficult (but not impossible) for the patient to achieve.

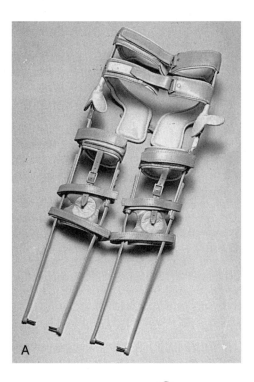

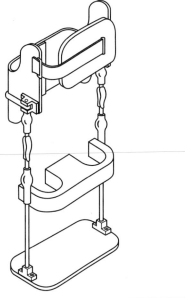

FIGURE 10–18 Hip-knee-ankle orthoses for swing-through gait. A, Conventional orthosis. B, Parapodium. (B, From ORLAU [Orthotic Research and Locomotor Assessment Unit], The Robert Jones and Agnes Hunt Orthopaedic and District Hospital, Oswestry, Shropshire, England SY10 7AG.)

In addition to the inertial forces, there is a small component of gravitational force (K) because of the angle of the body relative to the ground when the swivel walker is on one footplate. This can be useful when setting up a swivel walker because it

leads to forward rotation of the swivel walker if the footplate is held on the ground (e.g., by stepping on it), provided that the center of gravity of the patient is forward of the footplate bearings.

A typical example of a swivel walker is shown in Figure 10–20, including the four primary fixation points necessary to achieve the required internal stabilization of the patient.

Swivel walking is performed without the use of additional walking aids such as crutches, but as a consequence, it is limited to flat, smooth surfaces, which are only common indoors. It is comparatively easy to perform, requiring coordination of upper body movements rather than strength, and is therefore suited to very young patients (it can be adopted from the age of 1 year) and to those with upper limb involvement that prevents the use of crutches.

The structural design that can be adopted for this type of orthosis permits a more ready accommodation of the increased moments generated by stabilizing joints with contractures. This enables ambulation to be provided for much greater levels of physical handicap than any other form of walking. In addition, it is possible to build in a high degree of structural rigidity, and this influences the ease of walking by increasing the efficiency of transferring the inertial forces required to produce ambulation.

Several manifestations of this type of orthosis exist, and they generally fall into one of two categories:

1. Those providing hip joints (and knee joints in some cases) to permit sitting[21, 22]
2. Those designed to ease putting on and taking off, so that the orthosis can be readily discarded for sitting[23, 24]

For patients who can transfer easily from a wheelchair while wearing a cumbersome orthosis, there are some potential advantages to the first category if ambulation is interspersed with periods of sitting. Most patients are likely to use a swivel walker for set periods of ambulation, and in this situation the second category offers more comfort and safety when sitting. Careful analysis of the most appropriate compromise is needed to ensure that patients are provided with the best solution for their individual needs.

Reciprocal Walking

Swing-through gait and swivel walking do have significant disadvantages. Both have a style that emphasizes disability; the former is difficult and has a high energy consumption, and the latter is slow and limited to flat surfaces. More recent

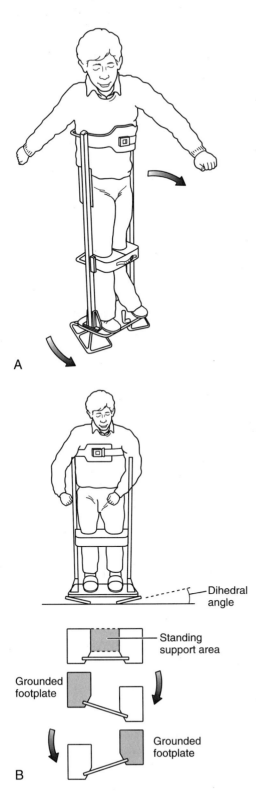

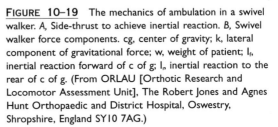

FIGURE 10–19 The mechanics of ambulation in a swivel walker. *A,* Side-thrust to achieve inertial reaction. *B,* Swivel walker force components. cg, center of gravity; k, lateral component of gravitational force; w, weight of patient; I_f, inertial reaction forward of c of g; I_n, inertial reaction to the rear of c of g. (From ORLAU [Orthotic Research and Locomotor Assessment Unit], The Robert Jones and Agnes Hunt Orthopaedic and District Hospital, Oswestry, Shropshire, England SY10 7AG.)

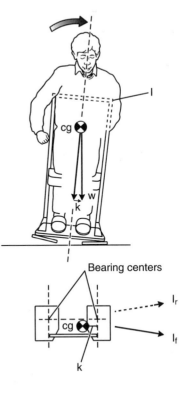

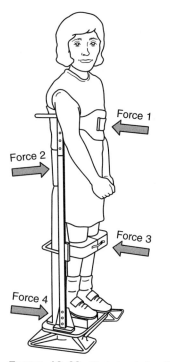

FIGURE 10–20 Typical swivel walker with four points of force required to provide internal stabilization for a paraplegic patient. (From ORLAU [Orthotic Research and Locomotor Assessment Unit], The Robert Jones and Agnes Hunt Orthopaedic and District Hospital, Oswestry, Shropshire, England SY10 7AG.)

orthotic developments have sought to overcome those difficulties by making reciprocal walking possible. This style mimics much more closely normal walking by allowing flexion and extension of the hip joint under orthotic control while maintaining stabilization of the other joints of the lower limbs. Because there is no active power in the paralyzed hip joint, propulsive forces have to be injected through walking frame or crutches, and these also serve to provide increased external stabilization by increasing the support area.

The essential features of reciprocal walking are that at least one leg is on the ground supporting the weight of the subject at any stage of the gait cycle and that the trunk advances over the stance leg while the swing leg moves from a relatively extended to a flexed position before landing to initiate a double support phase.

For healthy subjects, this means of progression is the most efficient form of ambulation, and its translation to handicapped patients held the hope of more practical solution to walking. This has proved to be the case for those with good upper limb function, limited deformities, lack of obesity, and good coordination. The main principles of orthotic reciprocal walking are as follows:

Swing-leg clearance is achieved by tilting or lifting the body through the walking frame (or crutches). Tilting is easier but requires a high degree of lateral rigidity in the HKAFO.

Swing-leg progression by hip flexion is initiated by gravity on a freely hinged orthotic hip joint, or through a cross-linkage from the opposite orthotic hip joint to allow progression on the stance side to drive this requirement.

Advancing the trunk over the stance leg is achieved through the use of latissimus dorsi to pull the trunk forward by the arms, via the crutches or walking frame reacting on the ground.

These principles are indicated diagrammatically in Fig. 10–21 for one practical manifestation of orthotic reciprocal walking.

A number of reciprocal walking systems are routinely available. These fall into two main categories:

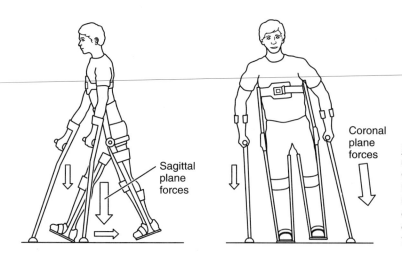

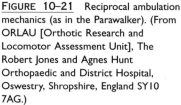

FIGURE 10–21 Reciprocal ambulation mechanics (as in the Parawalker). (From ORLAU [Orthotic Research and Locomotor Assessment Unit], The Robert Jones and Agnes Hunt Orthopaedic and District Hospital, Oswestry, Shropshire, England SY10 7AG.)

Those with linkages between the two orthotic hip joints, constraining them to move in unison, but with opposite rotation. Typical manifestations of this approach have been described by Douglas and associates,[25] Lissons[26] and Motloch.[27]

Those with freely hinged hip joints with a controlled range of flexion and extension. This approach has been proposed by Rose,[28] and an orthosis that uses this mechanism is shown in Figure 10–22.

The linked hip joint mechanisms are intended to ensure that the anatomic hip joints remain under orthotic control at all times, whereas a limited free range of the orthotic hip joints provides gravitational drive of the swing phase and greater flexibility of use of the anatomic hip joints. Little published evidence is available to support the competing claims of the benefits of the two approaches to the hip joint mechanisms.

Other aspects of overall design have been examined in some detail. The theoretical case for lateral rigidity of the orthotic structure has been proposed by Stallard and Major.[29] The ORLAU Parawalker[30] is widely acknowledged as the reciprocal walking orthosis with the greatest lateral rigidity, and a modification of this device, which brought about an increase in stiffness of 10%, has lent further support to the importance of that property by

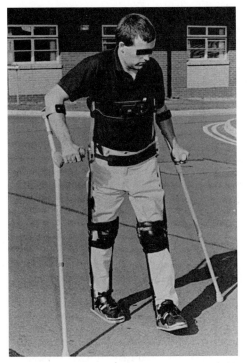

FIGURE 10–22 A reciprocal walking orthosis (Parawalker).

showing a measurable increase in efficiency of ambulation. Each of three patients with long experience in the use of the system significantly reduced the energy cost of walking[31] in the stiffer orthosis. Although this is the only direct evidence of the theoretical benefit of lateral rigidity, there is much other evidence that the orthosis with the greatest stiffness provides the most efficient walking. It cannot be ruled out that other features of this orthosis (which has freely hinged hip joints with limited flexion range) also contribute to ease of walking for the patient.

Energy Cost of Walking

In a review of six patients using two types of orthoses, Bowker and colleagues[32] showed that the energy cost in the orthosis with the lower lateral rigidity was on average significantly greater. Banta and colleagues,[33] using a different methodology on four other patients, reported almost identical quantitative findings.

An important factor in the practical value of a walking orthosis is the additional walking aids required to make the system viable. Crutches are considerably less cumbersome than a walking frame and much more convenient to transport; they are more difficult to use, however, and rely more heavily on the orthotic structure to supplement the patient input. In a study of several types of reciprocal walking orthoses, Bernardi and coworkers[34] found that for the orthosis with the greatest lateral rigidity, all patients used crutches, whereas for those with less stiffness, many patients used walking frames.

Although rigidity does confer higher levels of efficiency in walking, the structural design necessary to achieve this is judged by some observers to carry a penalty in terms of cosmesis. Others consider that overall functional performance (including an ability to put on and take off the orthosis as well as efficiency of walking) determines the degree to which walking orthoses can provide therapeutic and independence benefits. In the final analysis, it is the regular, ongoing use of the walking system that holds the key to success. Three studies of the Parawalker on different groups of patients[35–37] showed that 60% of subjects or more continued to use the system for 3 years or considerably longer. It was concluded that an important factor in the superiority of these results to those reported in similar studies of equivalent patients using conventional orthoses was the routine regular review of patients using the Parawalker. Nevertheless, the level of compliance reported in different groups gives encouragement to the concept that reciprocal walking is a viable option for severely handicapped patients.

As with other types of lower limb orthoses, contractures of hips, knees, or ankles increase the moments that the orthosis must resist to ensure internal stabilization for the patient. They may also inhibit the available range of hip flexion and extension and thereby limit the capacity for effective reciprocal walking. Ease of ambulation and strength of the orthotic structure have an important bearing on the practicality of a system for these patients, and extra caution should be exercised when assessing patients who fall into this category.

REALISM OF TREATMENT OBJECTIVES

Important advances have been made in the field of orthotics in the whole range of devices, from AFOs to HKAFOs. When they are used in the context of a multidisciplinary team assessing the most appropriate treatment options for an individual patient, they do have the potential to provide effective and long-term benefit. The limitations of orthoses must always be borne in mind when they are a treatment option being considered against other systems that may also be appropriate. To be effective, an orthosis must always interface with the patient, and the loads that have to be applied to achieve the treatment objectives must be practical for both the patients and the orthosis.

Orthoses that can achieve subtle effects by influencing neurologic plastic change are being developed, but this demands accurate alignment of forces relative to specific joints. In those circumstances, it is essential to have instrumentation available to permit tuning of the orthosis–patient relationship. The increasing availability of clinical gait laboratories makes it more practical to consider this option. Without that facility, it is not possible to be certain that the required effects are being achieved, and inappropriate outcomes would be likely to occur.

New materials are being developed that hold much promise for important advances in the field of orthotics. Greater strength and stiffness can lead to less obtrusive devices with yet further improvements in patient performance. In considering these new opportunities, designers must not lose sight of the potential for accidental overload with handicapped patients who have compromised control and should consider carefully the failure mode of the materials they specify.

References

1. Menelaus MBD: Progress in the management of the paralytic hip in myelomeningocele. Orthop Clin North Am 11:17, 1987.
2. Rose GK: Surgical/orthotic management of spina bifida. *In* Murdoch G (ed): The Advance of Orthotics. London, Edward Arnold, 1976, pp 403–413.
3. ISO 15032: Structural testing of hip joints, 1996.
4. Major RE, Butler PB: Discussion of segmental stability with implications for motor leaning. Clin Rehabil 9:167, 1995.
5. Tait JH, Rose GK: The real time video vector display of ground reaction forces during ambulation. J Med Eng Technol 3:252, 1979.
6. MacGregor J: The evaluation of patient performance using long term ambulatory monitoring technique in the domiciliary environment. Physiotherapy 67:30, 1981.
7. Butler PB, Englebrecht M, Major RE, et al: Physiological cost index of walking for normal children and its use as an indicator of physical handicap. Dev Med Child Neurol 26:607, 1984.
8. Nene AV, Jennings SJ: Physiological cost index of paraplegic locomotion using the ORLAU Parawalker. Paraplegia 30:246, 1992.
9. Hoffer M, Feiwell E, Perry R, et al: Functional ambulation of patients with myelomeningocele. J Bone Joint Surg 55A:137, 1973.
10. Garrett M, Meehan C: Classification of walking handicap in the spinal cord injured population: A pilot study. *In* Pedotti A, Ferrarin M (eds): Restoration of Walking for Paraplegics: Recent Advances and Trends. Oxford, UK, IOS Press, 1992, pp 343–349.
11. Butler PB, Thompson N, Major RE: Improvements in walking performance of children with cerebral palsy: Preliminary results. Dev Med Child Neurol 34:567, 1992.
12. Hylton N: The use of dynamic ankle foot orthoses and their impact on balance and upper body function. Neurol Rep 13:15, 1989.
13. Tuck W: The Stanmore cosmetic caliper. J Bone Joint Surg 56B:115, 1974.
14. Rose GK: Orthoses for the severely handicapped: Rational or empirical choice? Physiotherapy 66:76, 1980.
15. Carroll N: The orthotic management of the spina bifida child. Clin Orthop 102:108, 1974.
16. Mazur JM, Shurtleff D, Menelaus M, Colliver J: Orthopaedic management of high-level spina bifida. J Bone Joint Surg 71A:56, 1989.
17. Motloch W: The Parapodium: An orthotic device for neuromuscular disorders. Artif Limbs 15:36, 1971.
18. Clinkingbeard JR, Gesten JW, Hoehn D: Energy cost of ambulation in traumatic paraplegia. Am J Phys Med 43:157, 1964.
19. Huang CT, Kuhlemeier KV, Moore MB, Fine PR: Energy cost of ambulation in paraplegic patients using Craig Scott braces. Arch Phys Med Rehabil 60:595, 1979.
20. Merkel KD, Miller NE, Westbrooke PR, Merritt JL: Energy expenditure of paraplegic patients standing and walking with two knee ankle foot orthoses. Arch Phys Med Rehabil 65:121, 1984.
21. Griffiths JC, Henshaw JT, Heywood OB, et al:

Clinical applications of the paraplegic swivel walker. Biomed Eng 2:250, 1980.

22. Motloch WM, Elliott J: Fitting and training children with swivel walkers. Artif Limbs Autumn:27, 1966.

23. Edbrooke H: Clicking splint. Physiotherapy 56:148, 1970.

24. Butler PB, Farmer IR, Poiner R, Patrick JH: Use of the ORLAU Swivel Walker for the severely handicapped patient. Physiotherapy 68:324, 1982.

25. Douglas R, Larson P, D'Ambrosia R, McCall RE: The LSU Reciprocating Gait Orthosis. Orthopedics 6:834, 1983.

26. Lissons MA: Advanced Reciprocating Gait Orthosis in paraplegic patients. ISPO World Congress, Chicago, June 28 to July 3, 1992.

27. Motloch W: Principles of orthotic management for child and adult paraplegia and clinical experience with the Isocentric RGO. *In* Zupko P (ed): Proceedings of the 7th World Congress of the ISPO, Chicago, June 28 to July 3, 1992, p 28.

28. Rose GK: The principles and practice of hip guidance articulations. Prosthet Orthot Int 3:37, 1979.

29. Stallard J, Major RE: The case for lateral stiffness in walking orthoses for paraplegic patients. Part H. J Eng Med 207:1, 1993.

30. Butler PB, Major RE: The Parawalker: A rational approach to the provision of reciprocal ambulation for paraplegic patients. Physiotherapy 73:393, 1987.

31. Stallard J, Major RE: The influence of orthosis stiffness on paraplegic ambulation and its implications for functional electrical stimulation (FES) walking systems. Prosthet Orthet Int 19:108, 1995.

32. Bowker P, Messenger N, Ogilvie C, Rowley D: The energetics of paraplegic walking. J Biomed Eng 14:344, 1992.

33. Banta JV, Bell KJ, Muik EA, Fezio J: Parawalker: Energy cost of walking. Eur J Pediatr Surg 1(Suppl I):7, 1991.

34. Bernardi M, Canale I, Castellano V, et al: The efficiency of walking of paraplegic patients using a reciprocating gait orthosis. Paraplegia 33:409, 1995.

35. Moore P, Stallard J: A clinical review of adult paraplegic patients with complete lesions using the ORLAU Parawalker. Paraplegia 29:191–196, 1991.

36. Major RE, Patrick JH, Stallard J: A review of adult paraplegic patients using the ORLAU Parawalker. Proceedings of ISPO World Congress, Melbourne, April 2–7, 1995.

37. Stallard J, Major RE, Patrick JH: The use of the ORLAU Parawalker by adult myelomeningocele patients: A seven year retrospective study—preliminary results. Eur J Pediatr Surg 5(Suppl I):24, 1995.

INDEX

Note: Page numbers in *italics* refer to illustrations; page numbers followed by t refer to tables.